Novel Therapeutics for Rare Lymphomas

Christopher Dittus
Editor

Novel Therapeutics for Rare Lymphomas

Springer

Editor
Christopher Dittus
Department of Medicine, Division of Hematology and Oncology
University of North Carolina at Chapel Hill
Chapel Hill, NC
USA

ISBN 978-3-030-25612-8 ISBN 978-3-030-25610-4 (eBook)
https://doi.org/10.1007/978-3-030-25610-4

This Springer imprint is published by the registered company Springer Nature Switzerland AG
The registered company address is: Gewerbestrasse 11, 6330 Cham, Switzerland

Preface

Common diseases have many advantages: a large pool of people to contribute donations, research interest, and significant clinical experience among providers. Conversely, rare diseases have few treatment options, and those they do have are based on limited scientific evidence. Arriving at a diagnosis is often difficult, and many patients are misdiagnosed initially. Only certain academic centers have capabilities to adequately treat rare diseases limiting access to care for the majority of patients with these disorders. Many people are impacted by this because rare diseases, as a whole, affect a large number of individuals. In order to level the playing field, rare diseases need disproportionate attention.

Cancer, taken together, is not rare. In fact, it is the second leading cause of death in the United States (after cardiovascular causes) [1]. This is misleading, though, because cancer is comprised of hundreds of distinct diseases. Few types of cancer exemplify this better than lymphoma, which is broadly divided into Hodgkin and non-Hodgkin lymphoma (NHL), but, in fact, consists of more than 60 unique diseases [2]. Including chronic lymphocytic leukemia (CLL), there are approximately 100,000 cases of lymphoma in the United States each year [3]. Of these, only two groups have over 20,000 cases per year: CLL (20,980 cases in 2016) and diffuse large B-cell lymphoma (DLBCL; 25,380 cases in 2016). None of the remaining subtypes have more than 15,000 cases per year, and most have fewer than 10,000.

In this context, we turn to the focus of this book: novel therapeutics for rare lymphomas. As therapeutic advances race forward for many types of cancer, rare cancers are often lagging behind. New medications are often tested on common cancers to ensure there is ample financial support for the drug. Eventually, a small clinical trial, or often retrospective review, may evaluate the new drug in a rare cancer. Often, one study will make up the entire evidence base for many years. The aim of this book is to highlight research advances in a group of diseases that are often overlooked. This book serves as a single repository of information on the most recent advances in targeted small molecule inhibitors, monoclonal antibodies, and immunotherapy, as they pertain to rare types of lymphoma.

Experts and leaders in the field of lymphoma have been selected for each chapter, and the book will serve as a guide for community oncologists as well as academic oncologists. Each chapter begins with background information on the specific type of lymphoma and then describes standard treatment approaches; the remainder of each chapter focuses on novel treatment approaches.

The reader will find a book that is highly readable, clinically relevant, and easily accessible. The first chapter in the book focuses on hematopathology, which is where all of oncology begins – obtaining an accurate diagnosis. This is particularly important for lymphoma, which needs a subtype diagnosis. This can be difficult, even for common types. For rare lymphomas, hematopathology is particularly crucial, as an inexperienced hematopathologist may mistake the diagnosis for a more common lymphoma subtype.

Moving through the book chapters, we focus on both indolent and aggressive B-cell lymphomas, including lymphoplasmacytic lymphoma, plasmablastic lymphoma, mantle cell lymphoma, and primary CNS lymphoma. Certain chapters focus on rare variants of more common types of lymphoma, such as primary mediastinal B-cell lymphoma and TP53-altered chronic lymphocytic leukemia. Additionally, we devote a chapter to an important new treatment approach as it pertains to Hodgkin lymphoma: chimeric antigen receptor (CAR) T-cell therapy.

The latter portion of the book focuses on very rare variants of T-cell lymphomas, including the viral-associated subtypes, adult T-cell leukemia/lymphoma, and extranodal NK/T-cell lymphoma. Other chapters include anaplastic large cell lymphoma, enteropathy-associated T-cell lymphoma, and hepatosplenic T-cell lymphoma. The book concludes with a thorough review of cutaneous T-cell lymphoma.

I hope this book will serve as a reference for practicing oncologists, as well as other interested physicians, residents, and students. It was a great experience bringing together experts and leaders in the field from around the country, and it is my hope that readers will appreciate the depth of knowledge these specialists bring to this volume.

Chapel Hill, NC, USA — Christopher Dittus

References

1. Heron M. Deaths: leading causes for 2016. In: National vital statistics reports, vol 67, no 6. Hyattsville: National Center for Health Statistics; 2018.
2. Swerdlow SH, Campo E, Harris NL, Jaffe ES, Pileri SA, Stein H, Thiele J, editors. WHO classification of tumours of haematopoietic and lymphoid tissues. Revised 4th ed. Lyon: IARC; 2017.
3. Teras LR, DeSantis CE, Cerhan JR, Morton LM, Jemal A, Flowers CR. 2016 US lymphoid malignancy statistics by World Health Organization subtypes. CA Cancer J Clin. 2016;66(6);443–59.

Contents

Contributors

Anne W. Beaven, MD Division of Hematology and Oncology, Lineberger Comprehensive Cancer Center, The University of North Carolina at Chapel Hill, Chapel Hill, NC, USA

Renee Betancourt, MD Department of Pathology and Laboratory Medicine, University of North Carolina at Chapel Hill, Chapel Hill, NC, USA

Edith V. Bowers, MD, PhD Department of Dermatology, The University of North Carolina at Chapel Hill, Chapel Hill, NC, USA

Jorge J. Castillo, MD Bing Center for Waldenström Macroglobulinemia, Dana-Farber Cancer Institute, Harvard Medical School, Boston, MA, USA

Luis Malpica Castillo, MD Division of Hematology and Oncology, University of North Carolina at Chapel Hill, Chapel Hill, NC, USA

Catherine C. Coombs, MD Department of Medicine, Division of Hematology and Oncology, University of North Carolina at Chapel Hill, Chapel Hill, NC, USA

Christin B. DeStefano, MD Uniformed Services University, Bethesda, MD, USA

Christopher Dittus, DO, MPH Department of Medicine, Division of Hematology and Oncology, University of North Carolina at Chapel Hill, Chapel Hill, NC, USA

Kieron Dunleavy, MD George Washington University Hospital, Washington, DC, USA

Yuri Fedoriw, MD Department of Pathology and Laboratory Medicine, University of North Carolina at Chapel Hill, Chapel Hill, NC, USA

Natalie Sophia Grover, MD Department of Medicine, Division of Hematology and Oncology, University of North Carolina at Chapel Hill, Chapel Hill, NC, USA

Thomas A. Guerrero-Garcia, MD Division of Hematologic Malignancies, Dana-Farber Cancer Institute, Harvard Medical School, Boston, MA, USA

Eric Jacobsen, MD Harvard Medical School, Dana-Farber Cancer Institute, Boston, MA, USA

Shekeab Jauhari, MD Medical Oncology and Cellular Therapy, Duke University Medical Center, Durham, NC, USA

Christopher R. Kelsey, MD Department of Radiation Oncology, Duke University Medical Center, Durham, NC, USA

Austin Kim, MD Harvard Medical School, Dana-Farber Cancer Institute, Boston, MA, USA

Catherine Lai, MD, MPH MedStar Georgetown University Hospital, Washington, DC, USA

Zanetta S. Lamar, MD Wake Forest Baptist Medical Center, Winston Salem, NC, USA

Matt McKinney, MD Division of Hematologic Malignancies, Department of Medicine, Duke University School of Medicine, Durham, NC, USA

Neha Mehta-Shah, MD Division of Oncology, Washington University Medical School, St. Louis, MO, USA

Yara Park, MD Department of Pathology and Laboratory Medicine, The University of North Carolina at Chapel Hill, Chapel Hill, NC, USA

Craig A. Portell, MD Division of Hematology/Oncology, University of Virginia, Charlottesville, VA, USA

Raghuveer Ranganathan, MD Department of Medicine, Division of Hematology and Oncology, University of North Carolina at Chapel Hill, Chapel Hill, NC, USA

Daniel R. Reed, MD Division of Hematology/Oncology, University of Virginia, Charlottesville, VA, USA

Shayna Sarosiek, MD Section of Hematology and Medical Oncology, Boston University Medical Center, Boston, MA, USA

Mary Beth Seegars, MD Wake Forest Baptist Medical Center, Winston Salem, NC, USA

Thomas C. Shea, MD Department of Medicine, Division of Hematology and Oncology, University of North Carolina at Chapel Hill, Chapel Hill, NC, USA

Stephanie Teja, MD Washington University School of Medicine in St. Louis, St. Louis, MO, USA

Timothy J. Voorhees, MD Department of Medicine, Division of Hematology and Oncology, The University of North Carolina at Chapel Hill, Chapel Hill, NC, USA

Chapter 1
The Hematopathology and Diagnostic Challenges of Rare Lymphomas

Renee Betancourt and Yuri Fedoriw

Introduction

Modern tumor classification systems aim to provide a framework to distinguish biologically and/or clinically unique tumors into reproducible diagnoses. As the understanding of disease mechanism and biology evolves, so too does the capacity to more granularly refine categories. This evolution is reflected in the growing number of unique diagnoses, and accurate classification requires access to an ever-growing panel of ancillary studies and capacity to summarize the data from this testing [1]. For common lymphoma subtypes that have been extensively investigated, such as diffuse large B-cell lymphoma (DLBCL), diagnostic markers of disease, ranging from conventional histology to genomic alterations, are more readily appreciated [1]. While a comprehensive understanding of these diseases is far from complete, assigning diagnoses and enrolling patients into clinical trials is possible and, in many instances, expected [2]. However, patients with rare lymphoma subtypes are further challenged by inconsistencies in diagnosis and treatment, in part reflecting under-appreciation of distinguishing diagnostic or predictive features. The clinical teams managing these patients rely heavily on small, retrospective case series and expert opinion. Even among expert pathologists, for example, interobserver variability is high for less common lymphoma subtypes [3].

R. Betancourt · Y. Fedoriw (✉)
Department of Pathology and Laboratory Medicine, University of North Carolina at Chapel Hill, Chapel Hill, NC, USA
e-mail: renee.betancourt@unchealth.unc.edu; yuri.fedoriw@unchealth.unc.edu

C. Dittus (ed.), *Novel Therapeutics for Rare Lymphomas*,
https://doi.org/10.1007/978-3-030-25610-4_1

B-Lineage Neoplasms

Whether rare variants of common lymphomas are more frequently encountered than common variants of rare lymphomas is difficult to address. B-lineage neoplasms account for the majority of lymphoid tumors, but rarer B-cell lymphomas and lymphoma subtypes are nonetheless challenging to classify and treat.

Classic Hodgkin Lymphoma

Typical cases of classic Hodgkin lymphoma (CHL) have such specific morphologic and immunophenotypic features that accurate classification is straightforward. The archetypal Hodgkin and Reed-Sternberg (H/R-S) cells can be readily identified, highlighted by expression of CD30, CD15, and dim PAX5, and lacking appreciable CD20 staining by immunohistochemistry (IHC) (Fig. 1.1). These cells are

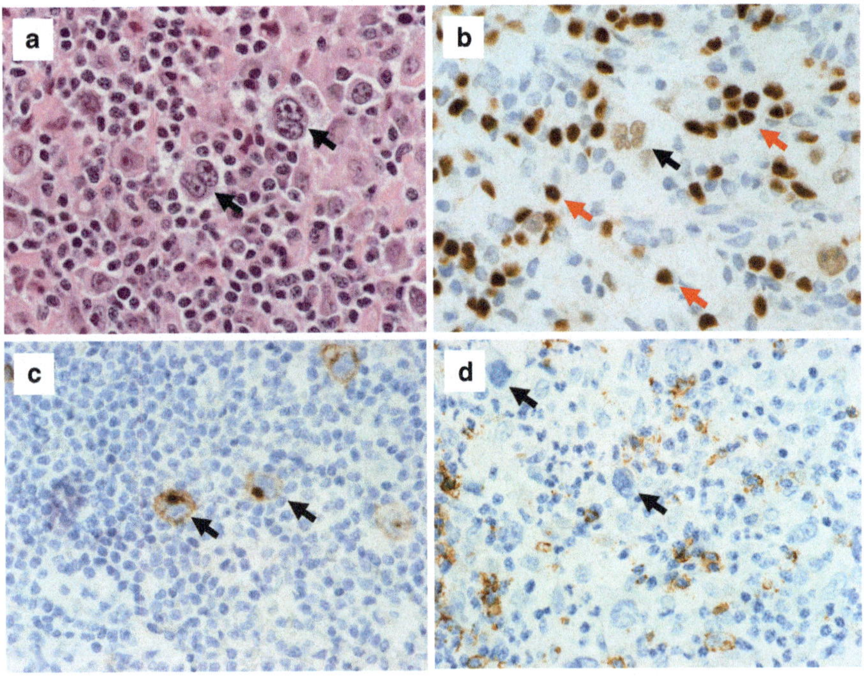

Fig. 1.1 Classic Hodgkin lymphoma. The hematoxylin and eosin (H&E) stained section (**a**) demonstrates the characteristic cytologic features of classic H/R-S cells: large, sometimes binucleate (arrows) or multinucleate, with inclusion-like dark red nucleoli, and abundant eosinophilic cytoplasm. The neoplastic cells show faint PAX5 staining (**b**: black arrow), while the background reactive B-lymphocytes show intense staining (**b**: red arrow). CD30 (**c**) shows membranous and Golgi staining within the H/R-S cells. CD20 (**d**) is negative in the H/R-S cells (black arrow) and highlights the background reactive B-lymphocytes. (Original objective magnification ×20)

frequently found in a polymorphous background of small lymphocytes, plasma cells, and eosinophils [1]. However, diagnostic pitfalls reflecting limitations of morphology and our evolving appreciation of distinct lymphoma subtypes make classification challenging. Cells practically indistinguishable from classic H/R-S cells can be seen in other lymphoma subtypes (Table 1.1; Fig. 1.2) [4]. In the case of angioimmunoblastic T-cell lymphoma (AITL), these H/R-S-like cells represent Epstein-Barr virus (EBV) proliferations in part driven by the neoplastic cells of T-follicular helper cell origin. While AITL is a well-described peripheral T-cell lymphoma, CHL is far more frequent, and the identification of H/R-S-like cells may distract from appropriate classification and diagnostic work-up. Rarely, cases of T-cell lymphomas, such as ALK-negative anaplastic large cell lymphoma (ALCL), can resemble CHL not only in the overlapping morphology of the malignant cells but also in background cellular milieu. In this setting, the immunophenotype can be sufficiently distinct to avoid misdiagnosis, but T-cell markers are frequently identified in CHL by IHC, while commonly being absent in ALCL [1, 5, 6].

Table 1.1 Hodgkin/Reed-Sternberg cells and mimics

	Cell of origin	Histologic features	Tumor immunophenotype
Classic Hodgkin lymphoma (CHL)	Germinal center B-cell	Scattered rare neoplastic cells with large nucleoli in an inflammatory background comprised of eosinophils, histiocytes, and/or neutrophils	CD30+, CD15+, CD20 variable, PAX-5 dim, CD45− (T-cell antigens can be aberrantly expressed by H/RS cells in up to 15% of cases)
Angioimmunoblastic T-cell lymphoma (AITL)	Alpha/beta T-cell	Clusters of neoplastic T-immunoblasts (often perivascular) Proliferation of high endothelial venules	Pan T-cell marker+ (CD2, CD3, CD5, CD7)
		Polymorphic reactive background Contains EBV+ B-cell immunoblasts	T-follicular helper cell marker+ (CD4, CD10, PD1, BCL6)
Anaplastic large cell lymphoma (ALCL)	T-cell	Neoplastic cells are large, atypical, and bizarre – often with polylobated nuclei (but vary from small to large, which helps to distinguish from CHL)	CD30+, CD15−, CD20−, PAX-5−, ALK+/−
Gray zone lymphoma (intermediate between CHL and DLBCL)	B-cell (thymic or nodal)	Intratumoral heterogeneity with large, atypical H/RS-like cells and centroblasts in a sparsely inflammatory background in some areas, whereas other areas more closely resemble DLBCL or PMBL	CD30+/−, CD15+/−, CD20+ (often bright), CD45+ (staining characteristics overlap between CHL and DLBCL)

EBV Epstein-Barr virus, *DLBCL* diffuse large B-cell lymphoma, *PMBL* primary mediastinal B-cell lymphoma

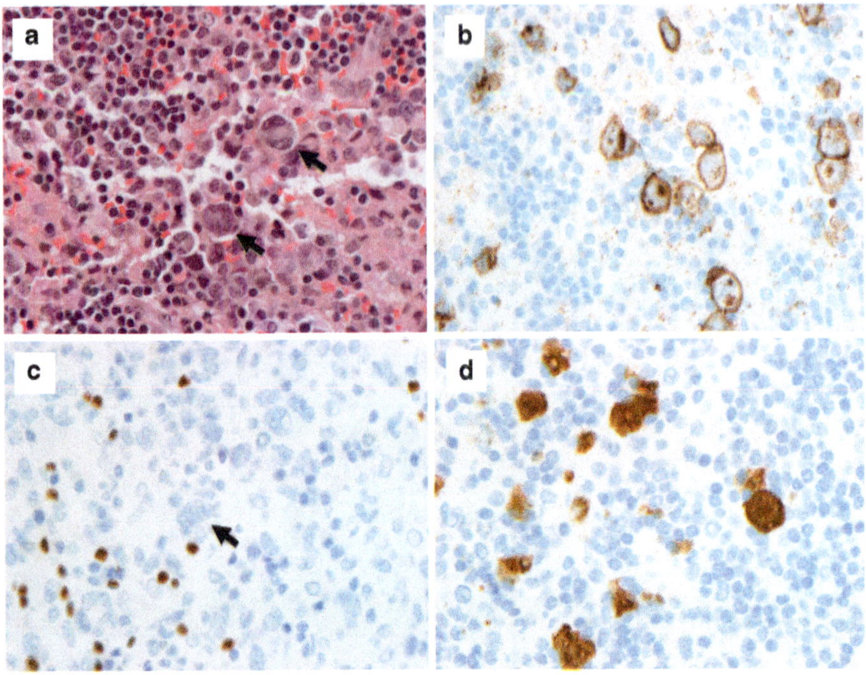

Fig. 1.2 Anaplastic large cell lymphoma, ALK-positive. H&E stained sections reveal large, abnormal neoplastic cells showing morphologic overlap with CHL (**a**). The neoplastic cells are strongly CD30 positive (**b**), negative for PAX5 (**c**: black arrow), and show intense nuclear and cytoplasmic staining with ALK (**d**). (Original objective magnification ×20)

Interpretation of IHC and other immunophenotyping is far from binary, and subtle expression differences can reflect distinct biology associated with markedly different prognoses. Otherwise typical cases of CHL with strong, diffuse CD20 expression may more accurately represent B-cell lymphoma unclassifiable with features intermediate between DLBCL and CHL (Fig. 1.3) [1, 7, 8]. These so-called "gray zone" lymphomas have a markedly worse prognosis compared to CHL and require a different approach to management [9]. While in many cases the morphology and immunophenotype are overlapping, the diagnosis may rely heavily on overexpression of CD20 by IHC [1]. While the distinction between these neoplasms is clinically relevant, strict or uniform criteria for assessing degree of CD20 expression are lacking, and thus, the assessment is qualitative and subjective.

Plasmablastic and Primary Effusion Lymphomas

Current classification is similarly challenging for the uncommonly encountered and virally associated non-Hodgkin lymphoid neoplasms including

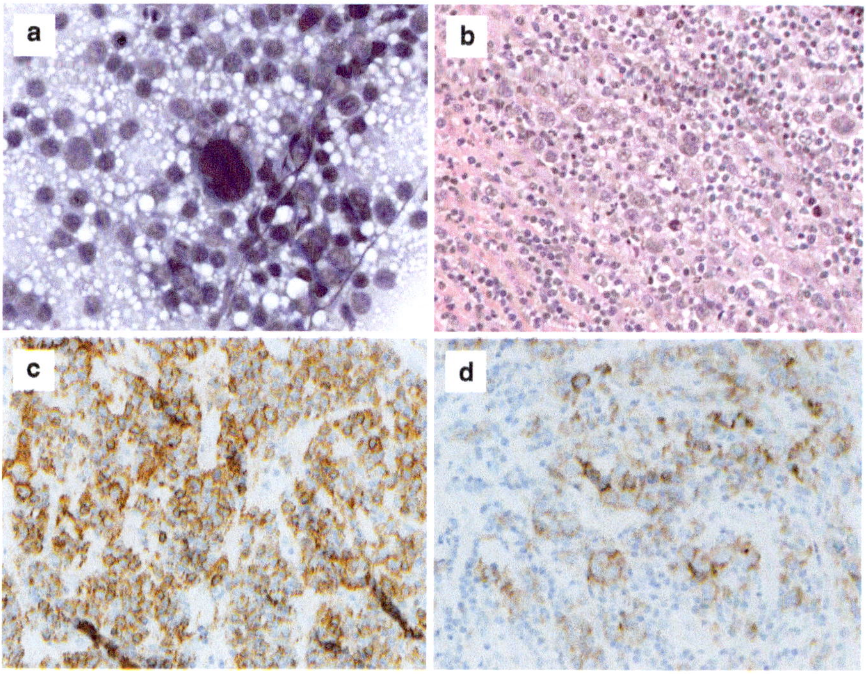

Fig. 1.3 Gray zone lymphoma (between diffuse large B-cell lymphoma and classic Hodgkin lymphoma). Wright-Giemsa stained touch preparation reveals readily identifiable neoplastic cells closely resembling H/R-S cells (**a**) (Original objective magnification ×60). H&E sections (**b**) show an abnormal infiltrate of neoplastic cells ranging from large, pleomorphic R-S forms to intermediate-to-large mononuclear cells. All neoplastic cells are CD20 positive (**c**) and a subset show expression of CD30 (**d**). (Original objective magnification ×20)

plasmablastic lymphoma (PL) and primary effusion lymphoma (PEL). While the clinical presentation including HIV status and biopsy site are telling clues to these diagnoses, the broad spectrum of morphologic, immunophenotypic, and clinical variants is significant [1, 10]. Both PL and PEL are classically associated with HIV infection and, like the majority of lymphomas arising in this population, morphologically and immunophenotypically resemble more mature and near terminally differentiated B-cells [10, 11]. As such, these tumors express the plasma cell markers CD38, CD138, and MUM1 and are negative for CD19, CD20, and PAX5 [10, 12]. Both are typically EBV-positive, and PEL additionally shows co-expression of the human herpes virus 8 (HHV-8) and latency-associated nuclear antigen-1 (LANA-1). In the most classic HIV-associated cases, PL presents as an oral cavity lesion, while PEL is identified in pulmonary and peritoneal effusions (Fig. 1.4) [13, 14].

However unique these tumors may appear, the relatively low frequency with which classic forms of these diseases are identified in the United States and their morphologic overlap with other malignant neoplasms significantly complicates the

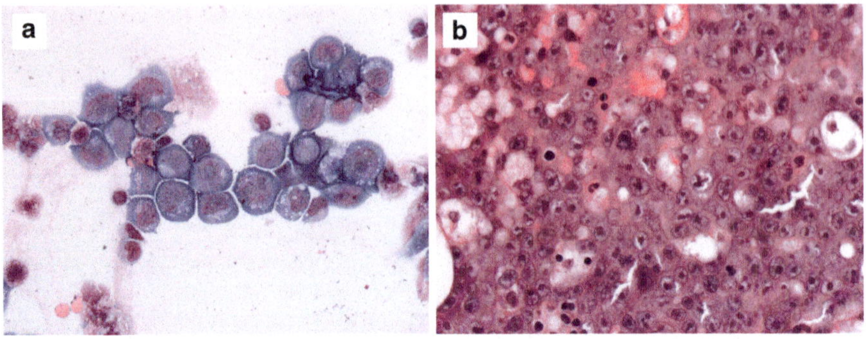

Fig. 1.4 Primary effusion lymphoma and plasmablastic lymphoma. The left panel (**a**) shows large abnormal lymphoid cells with characteristic morphology of primary effusion lymphoma in a Wright-Giemsa stained pleural effusion specimen. The H&E stained section on the right (**b**) shows a dense, monotonous infiltrate of large plasmacytoid-appearing cells typical of plasmablastic lymphoma. (Original objective magnification ×60)

diagnostic work-up. PEL and PL arise in the HIV-uninfected patients, particularly in immunocompromised hosts after organ transplantation or advanced age [15]. Solid variants of PEL have more recently been appreciated that can morphologically resemble PL, DLBCL, and anaplastic myelomas [1, 14, 16, 17]. Thorough IHC assessment, including evaluation of LANA-1 expression, is paramount to accurate diagnosis and treatment [18].

T-Cell Lymphomas

T-cell lymphoproliferations, as a whole, are not only difficult to classify but often difficult to establish as *neoplastic* in the first place. Unlike in other hematolymphoid neoplasms, defining cytogenetic aberrations are relatively uncommon in T-cell lymphomas. With the exception of systemic ALCL harboring rearrangements of ALK, recurrent karyotypic changes are far less frequent. Furthermore, while establishing "clonality" of a T-cell proliferation is reasonably straightforward with conventional T-cell receptor (TCR) rearrangement analyses, clonal but nonneoplastic T-cell populations are frequent in the setting of reactive dermatoses and autoimmune disease [19]. Moreover, TCR subtypes cannot generally be used as an independent surrogate for clonality. In contrast to the generally consistent systemic ratio of kappa/lambda light chain expressing B-cells, the overwhelming population of T-cells express the alpha/beta receptor, while peripheral gamma/delta proliferations can be identified in reactive settings. As such, qualifying the TCR subtype is often useful once the neoplastic nature of the T-cell proliferation has been established, and immunophenotyping can impact diagnostic category.

Mycosis Fungoides

Mycosis fungoides (MF), the most common T-cell neoplasm, represents more than half of all cutaneous lymphomas. Accurate and timely diagnosis remains challenging due to its overlapping characteristics with some benign dermatoses. Reactive, inflammatory, and autoimmune dermatologic entities can closely mimic MF by exhibiting similar histomorphologic, immunophenotypic, and molecular features. To date, clinicopathologic correlation remains the gold standard for reliably distinguishing early MF from other benign dermatoses, as there is currently no single confirmatory test. With low concordance rates among pathologists for the histologic interpretation of MF, especially at primary presentation, serial biopsies obtained from various sites at different time points are often required.

MF has the propensity to present at various stages and also exists as different variants including folliculotropic MF, pagetoid reticulosis, and granulomatous slack skin, further confounding the diagnostic picture. Classic MF tends to follow a relatively indolent course, evolving as the disease progresses over several years to decades. The earliest stages are often represented clinically by pruritic erythematous patches or plaques, with the histologic appearance of a mild lichenoid infiltrate with single-cell epidermotropism. Later stages present with biopsy findings of a dense band-like infiltrate of atypical lymphocytes with convoluted, "cerebriform" nuclei and microabscesses adjacent to the epithelium (Fig. 1.5).

As the disease continues to evolve, the neoplastic lymphocytes form a nodular dermal infiltrate and often lose the characteristic epidermotropism that is useful for histologic diagnosis. In the nodular/tumor stage, the lymphocytes are large and atypical, often with expression of CD30. Large cell transformation can occur following this stage and is characterized by the presence of >25% large T-cells, portending a poorer overall prognosis.

Immunophenotypically, MF classically shows CD3+ T-cells with expression of CD4 and a CD4/CD8 ratio often >6 (Fig. 1.5). However, this T helper phenotype is not always present, and rare CD8+ positive cases of MF have been reported. It has been proposed that a more sensitive and specific IHC finding is loss of CD7 expression by the clonal T-cell population, but even this feature has been proven to have limited utility, as it can be seen in some reactive dermatoses as well and other reactive T-cell proliferations [20]. T-cell clonality can be confirmed by the detection of TCR alpha/beta or gamma/delta gene rearrangement by polymerase chain reaction (PCR) amplification followed by capillary electrophoresis. Reports of sensitivity range from 40% to 90% and appear to be stage-dependent, with more advanced disease having a higher likelihood of harboring a dominant clone [20, 21].

An algorithm published by the International Society for Cutaneous Lymphomas (ISCL) in 2005 provides standardized guidelines for pathologists and clinicians, incorporating both clinical and pathologic parameters in a point-based scoring system [21, 22]. Subsequent attempts at validating this algorithm demonstrate a need for further diagnostic refinement, with one study documenting a sensitivity of 87.5% and specificity of 60% [21, 23].

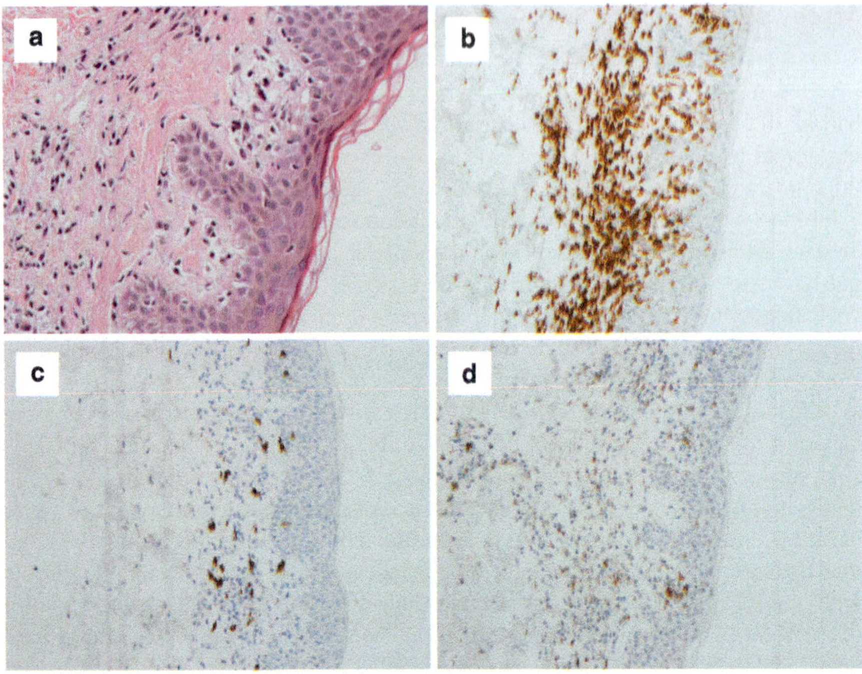

Fig. 1.5 Mycosis fungoides. H&E stained skin biopsy (**a**) reveals a subtle infiltrate of small-to-intermediate-sized lymphoid forms within clusters in the superficial dermis and small lymphocytes extending into the epidermis (epidermotropism). The infiltrate is predominantly composed of CD4-staining T-cells (**b**), with only rare CD8-positive cells identified (**c**). There is aberrantly decreased expression of CD7 (**d**). (Original objective magnification ×20)

While immunophenotypic aberrancy and the presence of a T-cell clone by TCR studies are useful adjuncts in identifying and confirming clonal populations, these findings do not elucidate whether the clone is reactive or neoplastic. However, in cases where a common clone is identified in multiple biopsies separated spatially and temporally, these findings would support the diagnosis of MF in the appropriate clinical context.

As the pathogenesis and molecular biology of MF become more clear, additional analytical techniques will be increasingly utilized for early diagnosis. Next-generation sequencing assays promise to substantially increase sensitivity of clonal detection, while distinct microRNA signatures have recently been identified in MF cases and may help to provide the specificity our current diagnostic methodologies lack [21, 24].

Anaplastic Large Cell Lymphomas

Anaplastic large cell lymphoma (ALCL) was initially described in 1985 as a hematologic malignancy characterized by large, anaplastic lymphoid cells expressing the lymphocyte activation marker CD30 [25]. The histologic appearance was highly variable but often showed a cohesive growth pattern within lymph node sinuses and in a perivascular distribution. Invariably present were pleomorphic neoplastic cells with abundant eosinophilic cytoplasm and kidney-shaped eccentric nuclei (so-called "hallmark" cells). Binucleated and multinucleated cells were also identified in some cases, at times raising Hodgkin lymphoma as a diagnostic consideration in the context of a neoplasm with large cells and CD30 positivity (Fig. 1.2). Recognition of T-cell lineage in ALCL was elucidated soon thereafter, as were its distinct features setting it apart from other peripheral and cutaneous T-cell lymphomas.

Less than a decade later, the discovery of a novel chromosomal translocation in approximately half of ALCL cases demonstrated surprising biologic heterogeneity in what was previously defined as a single entity. This finding was among the first chromosomal rearrangements identified in lymphoma and resulted in broad segregation of ALCL into two separate subgroups defined by the presence or absence of a t(2;5) translocation [26, 27]. Rearrangement and fusion of the anaplastic lymphoma kinase (*ALK*) gene on chromosome 2 to a partner (most often the nucleophosmin (*NPM*) gene on chromosome 5) were shown to result in constitutive tyrosine kinase activity, ALK protein expression, and subsequent lymphomagenesis. Notably, ALK protein expression is essentially absent from normal postnatal human tissues, with the exception of rare neural cells and a handful of non-hematologic neoplasms (e.g. lung, soft tissue). This confers increased utility and practicality to ALK IHC and fluorescent in situ hybridization for the identification of *ALK* rearranged (ALK+) and *ALK* rearrangement-negative (ALK−) ALCL cases [1].

The 2008 World Health Organization classification recognized ALK− ALCL as a provisional entity which was somewhat poorly understood. At that time, it was defined as a lymphoma within the morphologic spectrum of ALK+ ALCL, with strong and uniform CD30 staining but lacking expression of the oncogenic ALK protein. It was becoming increasingly evident that although ALK+ and ALK− ALCL share some common phenotypic features, they also display marked clinical heterogeneity in addition to the established biologic differences. Studies have shown that ALK expression is more often observed in younger populations and importantly identifies a group of patients with a superior prognosis [25]. When treated with standard chemotherapy, 5-year overall survival (OS) of patients with ALK+ disease is 80–85%, in contrast to ALK− disease, for which the 5-year OS is <50% [1, 28]. However, recent genetic substratification of ALK− cases has identified widely disparate clinical outcomes even within this category.

As our understanding of cancer genetics continues to evolve, many previously homogeneous entities are being further subdivided into more distinct diagnoses with specific genetic profiles. ALK− ALCL is an illustrative example of this phenomenon, demonstrating how advances in molecular technology and increased access to genetic data lend essential prognostic information and guide therapeutic decisions. Recent identification of mutually exclusive rearrangements of *ALK*, *DUSP22*, and *TP63* has elucidated genetic heterogeneity with critical differences in outcome among the subtypes. Approximately 30% of ALK− ALCLs harbor *DUSP22* rearrangements, 8% have *TP63* rearrangements, and 42% lacked all three.

Correlation with clinical outcomes showed that DUSP22-rearranged cases identify a particular subset of ALK− ALCL with an excellent prognosis comparable to ALK+ patients receiving similar treatment. In addition to a unifying chromosomal translocation, this subgroup was also found to be characterized by a unique gene expression profile and a more classic ALCL histologic appearance with sheets of "hallmark cells" [29]. *TP63* rearrangements were associated with refractoriness or failure to standard chemotherapy and therefore have a more aggressive course and dismal prognosis [28, 30]. Cases without identification of *ALK*, *DUSP22*, or *TP63* rearrangements had intermediate outcomes and may represent a currently undefined homogeneous entity or, more likely, one with genetic and clinical heterogeneity that is yet to be delineated.

Biomarkers

Treatment of rare cancer subtypes is not standardized, as data from large clinical trials of afflicted patients are lacking. However, ongoing drug development and comprehensive molecular characterization of uncommon lymphoma subtypes have provided rationale for therapeutic selection. The role of pathology is concomitantly expanding to provide and effectively document prognostic and predictive markers of disease. While large-scale sequencing technologies that aim to identify targetable genetic mutations and cellular pathways are growing increasingly available, conventional histopathology and cytogenetic studies are currently the cornerstone of disease assessment. Assessment of prognostic and predictive biomarkers in DLBCL, for example, is now the standard of care and includes IHC evaluation of CD20 and CD30 expression, cell-of-origin classification, and cytogenetic analysis of *MYC*, *BCL2*, and *BCL6* rearrangement status, among others [1]. In rare lymphoma subtypes, the breadth of available markers to guide therapy is less developed but expanding as new therapies are introduced and drugs originally approved for other indications are shown to be effective.

Effective biomarker testing and reporting also continues to evolve as the oncology community gains experience with their use and applicability. For example, after the development of the anti-CD30 antibody-drug conjugate, brentuximab vedotin (BV), evaluation of tumoral CD30 expression rapidly grew beyond its conventional use as a *diagnostic* marker [31–38]. Within a few years after BV's original approval for a subset of patients with CHL, the *prognostic* and *predictive* implications of CD30 expression were reported across a broad range of lymphoma subtypes and for which BV has now gained additional FDA approvals [32, 39–41]. However, pathologists and clinicians should be aware that the degree of CD30 expression by IHC does not linearly correlate with response to therapy [42, 43]. In tumors for which CD30 is not a sine qua non for classification, multiple studies have shown that staining in even a small subset of malignant cells associates with response to therapy [41, 44]. This phenomenon highlights both our incomplete understanding of disease biology and the imperfect test characteristics of currently available phenotypic assays.

Conclusions

Lymphomas represent a heterogenous group of tumors that are often difficult to diagnose and accurately classify. This challenge is exaggerated when approaching rare lymphoma subtypes that share many diagnostic features with common neoplasms but carry distinctly different prognoses and expected responses to therapy. Appreciation for the spectrum of lymphoma subtypes, complexity in their underlying biology, diagnostic work-up, and evolving therapeutics can assist in improved comprehensive care for patients.

References

1. Swerdlow S, Campo E, Harris N, Jaffe E, Pileri S, Stein H, et al. WHO classification of tumors of Haematopoietic and lymphoid tissues. Lyon: International Agency for Research on Cancer (IARC); 2017.
2. Rimsza L, Fedoriw Y, Staudt LM, Melnick A, Gascoyne R, Crump M, et al. General biomarker recommendations for lymphoma. J Natl Cancer Inst. 2016;108(12):pii: djw250.
3. Pongpruttipan T, Sukpanichnant S, Assanasen T, Bhoopat L, Kayasut K, Kanoksil W, et al. Interobserver variation in classifying lymphomas among hematopathologists. Diagn Pathol. 2014;9:162.
4. Gomez-Gelvez JC, Smith LB. Reed-Sternberg-like cells in non-Hodgkin lymphomas. Arch Pathol Lab Med. 2015;139(10):1205–10.
5. Venkataraman G, Song JY, Tzankov A, Dirnhofer S, Heinze G, Kohl M, et al. Aberrant T-cell antigen expression in classical Hodgkin lymphoma is associated with decreased event-free survival and overall survival. Blood. 2013;121(10):1795–804.
6. Tzankov A, Bourgau C, Kaiser A, Zimpfer A, Maurer R, Pileri SA, et al. Rare expression of T-cell markers in classical Hodgkin's lymphoma. Mod Pathol. 2005;18(12):1542–9.
7. Garcia JF, Mollejo M, Fraga M, Forteza J, Muniesa JA, Perez-Guillermo M, et al. Large B-cell lymphoma with Hodgkin's features. Histopathology. 2005;47(1):101–10.
8. Traverse-Glehen A, Pittaluga S, Gaulard P, Sorbara L, Alonso MA, Raffeld M, et al. Mediastinal gray zone lymphoma: the missing link between classic Hodgkin's lymphoma and mediastinal large B-cell lymphoma. Am J Surg Pathol. 2005;29(11):1411–21.
9. Dunleavy K, Wilson WH. Primary mediastinal B-cell lymphoma and mediastinal gray zone lymphoma: do they require a unique therapeutic approach? Blood. 2015;125(1):33–9.
10. Chadburn A. Immunodeficiency-associated lymphoid proliferations (ALPS, HIV, and KSHV/HHV8). Semin Diagn Pathol. 2013;30(2):113–29.
11. Delecluse HJ, Anagnostopoulos I, Dallenbach F, Hummel M, Marafioti T, Schneider U, et al. Plasmablastic lymphomas of the oral cavity: a new entity associated with the human immunodeficiency virus infection. Blood. 1997;89(4):1413–20.
12. Castillo JJ, Bibas M, Miranda RN. The biology and treatment of plasmablastic lymphoma. Blood. 2015;125(15):2323–30.
13. Alexanian S, Said J, Lones M, Pullarkat ST. KSHV/HHV8-negative effusion-based lymphoma, a distinct entity associated with fluid overload states. Am J Surg Pathol. 2013;37(2):241–9.
14. Harmon CM, Smith LB. Plasmablastic lymphoma: a review of clinicopathologic features and differential diagnosis. Arch Pathol Lab Med. 2016;140(10):1074–8.
15. Morscio J, Dierickx D, Nijs J, Verhoef G, Bittoun E, Vanoeteren X, et al. Clinicopathologic comparison of plasmablastic lymphoma in HIV-positive, immunocompetent, and posttransplant patients: single-center series of 25 cases and meta-analysis of 277 reported cases. Am J Surg Pathol. 2014;38(7):875–86.

16. Ahn JS, Okal R, Vos JA, Smolkin M, Kanate AS, Rosado FG. Plasmablastic lymphoma versus plasmablastic myeloma: an ongoing diagnostic dilemma. J Clin Pathol. 2017;70(9):775–80.
17. Kim Y, Leventaki V, Bhaijee F, Jackson CC, Medeiros LJ, Vega F. Extracavitary/solid variant of primary effusion lymphoma. Ann Diagn Pathol. 2012;16(6):441–6.
18. Shimada K, Hayakawa F, Kiyoi H. Biology and management of primary effusion lymphoma. Blood. 2018;132(18):1879–88.
19. Ritz N, Sahar D, Bergman R. T-cell receptor gene rearrangement studies using the GeneScan technique as an adjunct to the histopathological diagnosis of mycosis fungoides. Am J Dermatopathol. 2015;37(3):210–3.
20. Jawed SI, Myskowski PL, Horwitz S, Moskowitz A, Querfeld C. Primary cutaneous T-cell lymphoma (mycosis fungoides and Sezary syndrome): part I. diagnosis: clinical and histopathologic features and new molecular and biologic markers. J Am Acad Dermatol. 2014;70(2):205.e1–16; quiz 21–2.
21. Vandergriff T, Nezafati KA, Susa J, Karai L, Sanguinetti A, Hynan LS, et al. Defining early mycosis fungoides: validation of a diagnostic algorithm proposed by the International Society for Cutaneous Lymphomas. J Cutan Pathol. 2015;42(5):318–28.
22. Pimpinelli N, Olsen EA, Santucci M, Vonderheid E, Haeffner AC, Stevens S, et al. Defining early mycosis fungoides. J Am Acad Dermatol. 2005;53(6):1053–63.
23. Ferrara G, Di Blasi A, Zalaudek I, Argenziano G, Cerroni L. Regarding the algorithm for the diagnosis of early mycosis fungoides proposed by the International Society for Cutaneous Lymphomas: suggestions from routine histopathology practice. J Cutan Pathol. 2008;35(6):549–53.
24. Sufficool KE, Lockwood CM, Abel HJ, Hagemann IS, Schumacher JA, Kelley TW, et al. T-cell clonality assessment by next-generation sequencing improves detection sensitivity in mycosis fungoides. J Am Acad Dermatol. 2015;73(2):228–36.e2.
25. Savage KJ, Harris NL, Vose JM, Ullrich F, Jaffe ES, Connors JM, et al. ALK- anaplastic large-cell lymphoma is clinically and immunophenotypically different from both ALK+ ALCL and peripheral T-cell lymphoma, not otherwise specified: report from the International Peripheral T-Cell Lymphoma Project. Blood. 2008;111(12):5496–504.
26. Taylor J, Xiao W, Abdel-Wahab O. Diagnosis and classification of hematologic malignancies on the basis of genetics. Blood. 2017;130(4):410–23.
27. Morris SW, Kirstein MN, Valentine MB, Dittmer KG, Shapiro DN, Saltman DL, et al. Fusion of a kinase gene, ALK, to a nucleolar protein gene, NPM, in non-Hodgkin's lymphoma. Science. 1994;263(5151):1281–4.
28. Parrilla Castellar ER, Jaffe ES, Said JW, Swerdlow SH, Ketterling RP, Knudson RA, et al. ALK-negative anaplastic large cell lymphoma is a genetically heterogeneous disease with widely disparate clinical outcomes. Blood. 2014;124(9):1473–80.
29. Luchtel RA, Dasari S, Oishi N, Pedersen MB, Hu G, Rech KL, et al. Molecular profiling reveals immunogenic cues in anaplastic large cell lymphomas with DUSP22 rearrangements. Blood. 2018;132(13):1386–98.
30. Pedersen MB, Hamilton-Dutoit SJ, Bendix K, Ketterling RP, Bedroske PP, Luoma IM, et al. DUSP22 and TP63 rearrangements predict outcome of ALK-negative anaplastic large cell lymphoma: a Danish cohort study. Blood. 2017;130(4):554–7.
31. Wasik MA, Jimenez GS, Weisenburger DD. Targeting CD30 in malignant tissues: challenges in detection and clinical applications. Pathobiology. 2013;80(5):252–8.
32. Senter PD, Sievers EL. The discovery and development of brentuximab vedotin for use in relapsed Hodgkin lymphoma and systemic anaplastic large cell lymphoma. Nat Biotechnol. 2012;30(7):631–7.
33. Barberio E, Thomas L, Skowron F, Balme B, Dalle S. Transformed mycosis fungoides: clinicopathological features and outcome. Br J Dermatol. 2007;157(2):284–9.

34. Delabie J, Holte H, Vose JM, Ullrich F, Jaffe ES, Savage KJ, et al. Enteropathy-associated T-cell lymphoma: clinical and histological findings from the international peripheral T-cell lymphoma project. Blood. 2011;118(1):148–55.
35. Edinger JT, Clark BZ, Pucevich BE, Geskin LJ, Swerdlow SH. CD30 expression and proliferative fraction in nontransformed mycosis fungoides. Am J Surg Pathol. 2009;33(12):1860–8.
36. Hu S, Xu-Monette ZY, Balasubramanyam A, Manyam GC, Visco C, Tzankov A, et al. CD30 expression defines a novel subgroup of diffuse large B-cell lymphoma with favorable prognosis and distinct gene expression signature: a report from the International DLBCL Rituximab-CHOP Consortium Program Study. Blood. 2013;121(14):2715–24.
37. Ohtsuka E, Kikuchi H, Nasu M, Takita-Sonoda Y, Fujii H, Yokoyama S. Clinicopathological features of adult T-cell leukemia with CD30 antigen expression. Leuk Lymphoma. 1994;15(3–4):303–10.
38. Slack GW, Steidl C, Sehn LH, Gascoyne RD. CD30 expression in de novo diffuse large B-cell lymphoma: a population-based study from British Columbia. Br J Haematol. 2014;167(5):608–17.
39. Younes A, Gopal AK, Smith SE, Ansell SM, Rosenblatt JD, Savage KJ, et al. Results of a pivotal phase II study of brentuximab vedotin for patients with relapsed or refractory Hodgkin's lymphoma. J Clin Oncol. 2012;30(18):2183–9.
40. Horwitz S, O'Connor OA, Pro B, Illidge T, Fanale M, Advani R, et al. Brentuximab vedotin with chemotherapy for CD30-positive peripheral T-cell lymphoma (ECHELON-2): a global, double-blind, randomised, phase 3 trial. Lancet. 2019;393(10168):229–40.
41. Prince HM, Kim YH, Horwitz SM, Dummer R, Scarisbrick J, Quaglino P, et al. Brentuximab vedotin or physician's choice in CD30-positive cutaneous T-cell lymphoma (ALCANZA): an international, open-label, randomised, phase 3, multicentre trial. Lancet. 2017;390(10094):555–66.
42. Blum KA. CD30: seeing is not always believing. Blood. 2015;125(9):1358–9.
43. Jacobsen ED, Sharman JP, Oki Y, Advani RH, Winter JN, Bello CM, et al. Brentuximab vedotin demonstrates objective responses in a phase 2 study of relapsed/refractory DLBCL with variable CD30 expression. Blood. 2015;125(9):1394–402.
44. Fanale MA, Horwitz SM, Forero-Torres A, Bartlett NL, Advani RH, Pro B, et al. Brentuximab vedotin in the front-line treatment of patients with CD30+ peripheral T-cell lymphomas: results of a phase I study. J Clin Oncol. 2014;32(28):3137–43.

Chapter 2
Novel Therapeutics in the Management of Waldenström Macroglobulinemia

Shayna Sarosiek and Jorge J. Castillo

Introduction/Epidemiology

Waldenström macroglobulinemia (WM) is an indolent B-cell lymphoproliferative disorder that was first described by Jan Waldenström in 1944 [1]. The etiology of this rare, indolent lymphoma is a lymphoplasmacytic clone that produces a circulating IgM monoclonal protein. WM is seen most frequently in older, male patients and has an age-adjusted incidence of 3.8 per million persons per year. The age of onset differs between races, with a median age at diagnosis of 63 years for blacks and 73 years for whites [2]. In addition, there seems to be an overrepresentation of WM in individuals of Ashkenazi Jewish ancestry, and cases of familial WM have been described [3].

Clinical Presentation

Patients with WM are often diagnosed incidentally upon discovery of a circulating monoclonal IgM and may not have any clinical signs or symptoms of the disease at the time of diagnosis. Although many patients are asymptomatic at diagnosis, others may present with signs or symptoms of the disease related to the burden of clonal

S. Sarosiek (✉)
Section of Hematology and Medical Oncology, Boston University Medical Center, Boston, MA, USA
e-mail: Shayna.Sarosiek@bmc.org

J. J. Castillo
Bing Center for Waldenström Macroglobulinemia, Dana-Farber Cancer Institute, Harvard Medical School, Boston, MA, USA
e-mail: JorgeJ_Castillo@dfci.harvard.edu

C. Dittus (ed.), *Novel Therapeutics for Rare Lymphomas*,
https://doi.org/10.1007/978-3-030-25610-4_2

cells in the bone marrow; anemia is the most common criterion to treat patients with WM. Occasionally, patients may present more acutely with an elevated serum IgM level causing symptoms of hyperviscosity (e.g., nosebleeds, headaches, and blurred vision). Other presenting symptoms may also be attributed to disorders associated with WM, including mixed type II cryoglobulinemia, peripheral neuropathy, AL amyloidosis, or cold agglutinin hemolytic anemia [4, 5]. Rarely, WM can cause symptomatic extramedullary disease such as renal dysfunction and pleural effusions. Additionally, patients with relapsed disease, and occasionally those with a new diagnosis, can present with Bing-Neel syndrome which is characterized by the involvement of the cerebral spinal fluid, meninges, or cerebral parenchyma by the clonal WM cells. Bing-Neel syndrome can result in headaches, cognitive deficits, changes in gait, cranial nerve impairment, visual changes, or hearing impairment [6].

Diagnosis, Staging, and Workup

Diagnostic criteria for WM include the discovery of a lymphoplasmacytic infiltrate in the bone marrow and the presence of a circulating IgM monoclonal protein [7]. The typical immunoprofile of clonal lymphocytes in the marrow demonstrates expression of the B-cell markers CD19, CD20, CD22, and CD79a. In addition, there is often a population of clonal plasma cells that are CD38 and CD138 positive. Due to overlapping features with other hematologic disorders, WM should be distinguished from other similar diseases, such as light chain (AL) amyloidosis, IgM monoclonal gammopathy of undetermined significance (MGUS), marginal zone lymphoma (MZL), and IgM multiple myeloma. In cases in which IgM multiple myeloma is suspected, it is helpful to evaluate the bone marrow sample for t(11;14) and/or cyclin D1 expression, as these markers are distinctively common in this condition [8].

Diagnostic workup for WM typically includes baseline laboratory testing, such as complete blood count, comprehensive metabolic panel, serum immunofixation electrophoresis, serum protein electrophoresis, quantitative immunoglobulins, and serum viscosity. Additionally, viral serologies for HIV and hepatitis B should be sent, as well as a lactate dehydrogenase (LDH) and beta-2-microglobulin. For patients presenting with peripheral neuropathy, testing for both anti-myelin-associated glycoprotein (MAG) antibodies and antiganglioside antibodies (GM-1) is an important component of the initial workup. Baseline CT scans (with or without PET imaging) of the chest, abdomen, and pelvis are also recommended. Genetic testing to evaluate for mutations of myeloid differentiation factor 88 (MYD88) or CXCR4 is also recommended.

These mutational analyses can aid in diagnosis, as MYD88 mutations are present in >90% of patients with WM [9]. The presence of a leucine to proline substitution at amino acid position 265, called MYD88 L265P, is the most common mutation, although a few additional mutations have been identified using Sanger sequencing. MYD88 mutations are also detected in >50% of patients with IgM MGUS and 5% of patients with MZL. MYD88 mutations have not been detected in IgM myeloma

[8]. CXCR4 mutations, as seen congenitally in warts, hypogammaglobulinemia, infection, and myelokathexis (WHIM) syndrome, are found in 40% of patients with WM [10]. There are more than 30 known mutations involving this gene, including frameshift (FS) and nonsense (NS) mutations. The MYD88 and CXCR4 mutational status in WM is known to affect clinical presentation, with those patients with MYD88^{L265P} and CXCR4$^{WHIM/NS}$ having a higher level of bone marrow involvement, higher serum IgM levels, lower rates of lymphadenopathy, and increased risk of hyperviscosity, while those patients with MYD88^{WT} and CXCR4^{WT} have the lowest degree of bone marrow involvement [11]. CXCR4 mutations have also been associated with acquired von Willebrand disease in WM patients [12].

Prognosis

In recent years, the disease-specific survival of WM has increased and has now reached approximately 11 years [13, 14]. The International Prognostic Scoring System (IPSS) for WM can be used to assess prognosis in newly diagnosed individuals using the following criteria: age >65 years, hemoglobin ≤11.5 g/dL, platelet count ≤100,000/μL, β2 microglobulin >3 mg/L, and monoclonal IgM >7 g/dL. Based on these clinical criteria, a median survival can be approximated. Patients with low-, intermediate-, or high-risk disease have an estimated 5-year overall survival of 87%, 68%, and 36%, respectively [15].

This prognostic scoring system will likely be refined in the future using more recently discovered information about genetic alterations. New data demonstrate that MYD88 and CXCR4 status may affect not only disease presentation but also response to treatment and overall survival. MYD88 wild-type patients have a worse overall survival than patients with MYD88 mutations [11]. This was demonstrated in another study which showed an increased risk of death with wild-type MYD88 versus mutated MYD88, with 10-year overall survival of 73% and 90%, respectively [16]. In addition, patients with wild-type MYD88 have an increased risk of development of a diffuse large B-cell lymphoma (15% vs. 1%) [16]. CXCR4 mutations have not been shown to affect overall survival in WM patients, but have been associated with a slower time to treatment response, shorter duration of response, more superficial treatment response, and resistance to therapy with ibrutinib, ixazomib, and everolimus [17–20].

Conventional Treatment Approach

Despite the diagnosis of WM, not all patients require treatment at presentation. Initiation of therapy should be considered in those with constitutional symptoms affecting quality of life, symptomatic lymphadenopathy or splenomegaly, hemoglobin ≤10 g/dL or platelets <100 K/μL due to marrow infiltration, or development of specific complications related to the disease such as symptomatic extramedullary disease, amyloidosis, peripheral neuropathy, hyperviscosity, or symptomatic cryoglobulinemia [21]. Additionally, asymptomatic patients with an IgM level above 6 g/dL are at high risk of developing symptomatic hyperviscosity (370-fold odds), and therefore treatment in these patients is also recommended [22]. Owing to the rarity of WM, the majority of treatment recommendations are based on single-arm or Phase II studies rather than large randomized controlled trials, but many treatment options are available to control the underlying lymphoplasmacytic clone. Some patients presenting with symptomatic hyperviscosity may also require initial treatment with plasmapheresis as a bridge to more definitive therapy.

If treatment is indicated, there are multiple established regimens that may be utilized. Traditionally, treatment of WM has included rituximab, a CD20 monoclonal antibody, as the mainstay of treatment, given as a single agent or in combination with alkylating agents and/or proteasome inhibitors. Although rituximab is very effective in WM, this medication should be held during initiation of treatment (or plasmapheresis may be initially offered) to prevent complications of hyperviscosity associated with an IgM flare in patients with IgM levels >4000 mg/dL [23]. Bendamustine with rituximab (Benda-R) is a commonly used regimen in newly diagnosed and relapsed WM. This regimen is generally well tolerated and has an ORR of approximately 90–95% in newly diagnosed patients and 80% in those with relapsed disease [24–26]. The efficacy of rituximab in combination with bortezomib and dexamethasone (BDR) has also been demonstrated in several studies, with an ORR ranging from 90% to 95% and PFS of 40–60 months [27–29]. In part due to the increased risk of neuropathy with bortezomib, the CARD regimen (carfilzomib, rituximab, and dexamethasone) was tested in proteasome inhibitor- and rituximab-naïve patients with WM and was found to have an ORR of approximately 81% with a median PFS of 46 months (range, 2–63). The length of PFS with the CARD regimen was associated with the depth of response achieved [30, 31]. In place of a proteasome inhibitor, cyclophosphamide can also be combined with rituximab and dexamethasone (CDR). This regimen has a slightly lower ORR of 80–87% with a median PFS of about 32–36 months [32, 33]. Despite the availability of multiple combination therapies, rituximab administered as a single agent remains the most utilized treatment in older patients with WM, according to a recent population-based study from the SEER-Medicare database [34], although the response rate is only 30–55% and the time to response is prolonged [35, 36]. Maintenance rituximab therapy can also be considered in patients with WM after completing one of the above listed regimens, which has been associated with improved PFS and OS rates in retrospective studies [24, 37].

Although all the previously mentioned regimens have activity in WM, the appropriate regimen should be chosen based on specific patients' symptoms, comorbidities, preference, and genomic profile, with additional guidance on treatment from retrospective and prospective studies. A recent retrospective study comparing Benda-R, BDR, and CDR showed no difference in response rates, but time to best response and PFS rates were lower with CDR. Major response was more commonly achieved in patients on rituximab maintenance (97 vs. 68%) with an extension in

PFS from 2.8 to 6.8 years and an OS benefit for those patients who received maintenance rituximab. Five-year overall survival in this study was 95%, 96%, and 81% for Benda-R, BDR, and CDR, respectively [24].

After years of using the previously mentioned chemoimmunotherapy regimens, ibrutinib became the first Food and Drug Administration (FDA)-approved treatment for WM in January 2015 based on data showing a 91% overall response rate in patients with relapsed disease [18]. Ibrutinib is a small molecule, oral inhibitor of Bruton's tyrosine kinase (BTK) which is known to cause apoptosis in WM cells. Since the time of its initial approval, ibrutinib demonstrated efficacy in patients with rituximab-refractory disease [18, 38], as well as those who were newly diagnosed [39]. Individual patient responses can be affected by the CXCR4 status and MYD88 status, with a lower overall response rate and decreased major responses in those with a CXCR4 mutation [18] and shorter ibrutinib responses in patients with wild-type MYD88 [11, 18]. In a recent study, previously treated patients that subsequently received ibrutinib therapy had an ORR of approximately 90%, but the PFS varied based on mutational status of MYD88 and CXCR4. The longest PFS, which was not reached, was seen in those patients with mutated MYD88 and wild-type CXCR4. Patients with mutations in both of these genes had a PFS of about 45 months, and those with wild-type MYD88 and CXCR4 had a PFS of only about 21 months [17].

Despite multiple existing treatment options, many patients do not achieve a complete response, and countless others develop resistance to standard therapies. Additional treatment options, including everolimus, immunomodulatory therapies, and nucleoside analogs, are available, but the benefit-toxicity ratio with these regimens is less favorable [40–43]. In select refractory patients, autologous or allogeneic stem cell transplantation (SCT) may be considered, although the role of these therapies in WM is not clearly defined [44–46]. A recent position paper based on international consensus recommends consideration of autologous SCT in young patients with WM who have progressed after exposure to alkylators, proteasome inhibitors, anti-CD20 antibodies, and BTK inhibitors, while the value of allogeneic SCT should be properly evaluated in the context of clinical trials [47].

Novel Agents and Ongoing Clinical Trials

Additional treatment options are needed for patients with refractory disease, and many novel therapies, as well as innovative combinations of medications, are being developed.

Due to the success of bortezomib in the treatment of WM, ixazomib, a proteasome inhibitor with lower rates of neurotoxicity, has been tested in patients with WM. Recently reported data show an ORR of 96% and an 18-month PFS rate of 90% in a Phase II single-arm study evaluating the combination of ixazomib, rituximab, and dexamethasone (IDR) in newly diagnosed patients [19]. The response rates, as well as the benign toxicity profile, were comparable to Benda-R. Preclinical data have also demonstrated the antitumor effects of ixazomib as a single agent or in combination with ibrutinib, even in ibrutinib-resistant cell lines. These data provide the foundation for a potential treatment strategy in patients with disease progression on ibrutinib [48]. More recently, oprozomib, another proteasome inhibitor, has shown activity in WM cells, and a Phase Ib/II clinical trial has completed enrollment with early data demonstrating responses, even in disease that has been refractory to other proteasome inhibitors [49, 50].

Due to the effectiveness of rituximab in WM, additional anti-CD20 monoclonal antibodies are being studied. Ofatumumab, an anti-CD20 monoclonal antibody with more potent complement-dependent cytotoxicity when compared to rituximab, has demonstrated very rapid disease responses with an ORR of 51% after one cycle of treatment and an ORR of 77% after two cycles. The median time to response in this recently published trial was 78.5 days, and the median PFS was 536 days. This treatment appears promising, but will require additional investigation, potentially as part of combination therapy with other existing or novel therapies [51]. Currently NCCN and IWWM recommend considering ofatumumab in patients who are intolerant to rituximab, which can be seen in about 7% of WM patients [23, 52, 53].

Although ibrutinib is an effective therapy in many patients, there is a potential for improving ORR by evaluating ibrutinib in combination with other novel therapies. One such therapy is ulocuplumab, a monoclonal antibody against CXCR4, which is known to prevent cell survival when tested in chronic lymphocytic leukemia cells in vitro [54]. Due to the known presence of CXCR4 mutations in 40% of patients with WM, this therapy is being evaluated on a clinical trial in combination with ibrutinib for patients with a CXCR4 mutation (NCT03225716). Rituximab has also been used in combination with ibrutinib, and recently published data demonstrate an improvement in progression-free survival at 30 months (82% vs. 28%) and higher rates of major response (72% vs. 32%) with ibrutinib-rituximab compared with placebo-rituximab, although there were increased rates of atrial fibrillation and hypertension in patients on ibrutinib.

Additional BTK inhibitors are also being investigated for patients with relapsed or refractory disease. A Phase II trial with a second-generation irreversible BTK inhibitor, acalabrutinib, has recently completed enrollment (NCT02180724), and the preliminary data reveal overall response rates of 93% and 94% for treatment naïve and relapsed/refractory patients, respectively [55]. Early data from investigation of this agent also demonstrate a lower risk of bleeding and atrial fibrillation, both of which are side effects of ibrutinib, and therefore this drug may be a safer alternative [56]. Additionally, BGB-3111 (zanubrutinib), another potent and irreversible BTK inhibitor, has shown efficacy in Phase I trials [57, 58]. While these were small Phase I trials, the patients with WM who enrolled in the trial demonstrated objective responses, with increasing rates of very good partial responses (VGPR) with continued treatment with zanubrutinib [59]. A Phase III randomized trial investigating the efficacy and safety of this drug is now recruiting (NCT03053440).

Due to the nature of the underlying clonal lymphoplasmacytic population of cells in WM, some therapies with activity in multiple myeloma may also prove to be effective in WM. One such therapy, daratumumab, an anti-CD38 monoclonal antibody, has shown to be active in selected WM cell lines [60]. CD38, a plasma cell receptor, is known to be highly expressed on plasma cells in WM [61, 62]. This agent is currently being investigated as a single agent in a Phase II trial in patients with relapsed or refractory WM (NCT03187262). In the future, this well-tolerated monoclonal antibody may prove to be effective in combination with other treatments targeting B cells and potentially provide an opportunity for complete disease eradication.

Apoptotic proteins are known to play a role in the development of many hematologic disorders. In particular, venetoclax, an oral BCL2 inhibitor, has led to significant improvement in the care of patients with chronic lymphocytic leukemia and may also become a promising treatment for WM. Recent results from a Phase I trial in patients with relapsed or refractory non-Hodgkin lymphoma demonstrated a 100% ORR in the four patients with WM treated on the trial [63]. Further investigation into the use of this treatment in WM is now ongoing (NCT02677324), and interim results demonstrate an overall response rate of 80% with a major response rate of 53% and an acceptable toxicity profile in previously treated patients [64].

The phosphatidylinositol 3-kinase (PI3K)/AKT pathway is known to have an important role in the growth of WM cells. Everolimus is an inhibitor of mTOR, which is a serine-threonine kinase located downstream of the PI3K/AKT pathway, that has demonstrated activity in WM, but the toxicity profile was limiting. In addition, a Phase II study evaluating idelalisib, a first in class PIKδ inhibitor, in WM patients was stopped after enrolling 5 of 30 patients due to high rates of grade 3 and 4 hepatotoxicity [65]. Alternative manners of targeting the PI3K/ATK pathway are being pursued in hopes of finding an effective therapy with a tolerable safety profile. Umbralisib, a PI3Kδ and casein kinase-1ε inhibitor, which has been shown to have activity in relapsed and refractory lymphomas [66], is currently being offered as monotherapy in a Phase II clinical trial in patients with non-Hodgkin lymphoma, including WM.

Immunotherapies, such as pembrolizumab and nivolumab, have demonstrated efficacy in many solid malignancies, and the safety of immunotherapy is now actively being investigated in patients with B-cell lymphomas, including WM. Currently multiple Phase 1 and 2 clinical trials are enrolling. These trials include pembrolizumab or nivolumab alone or in addition to other therapies, such as lenalidomide, ibrutinib, idelalisib, and acalabrutinib (NCT03015896, NCT03498612, NCT02332980, NCT02950220, NCT02362035). As knowledge of the host immune system activation is gained, the role of chimeric antigen receptor T (CAR-T) cells will be defined. This recently approved treatment for diffuse large B-cell lymphoma is also being investigated in patients with relapsed and refractory WM (NCT01815749).

Promising Early Phase/Preclinical Agents

In addition to the ongoing clinical trials mentioned above, there have been many recently published reports regarding agents with promising preclinical results. Many of these in vitro studies are utilizing novel targeted therapies to address specific receptors, kinases, or regulatory pathways, such as FGFR-1 or SYK, that are activated in WM. One of the more recent publications of preclinical data has demonstrated enrichment of FGFR-1 and FGF-2,-12,-17, and -18 in WM cells. FGFR-1 is known to be one of the most upregulated genes in WM cells, and anti-WM activity has been demonstrated with blockade of FGF/FGFR axis, both in the IgM-secreting clonal cells and bone marrow-derived mesenchymal stromal cells. These results suggest that bone marrow angiogenesis may be an active target in this disease that should be further developed [67]. Another recently discovered mechanism of growth in WM cells is through the activation of SYK in MYD88 mutant WM cells. In vitro the SYK inhibitor R406 has demonstrated cytotoxic effects as a single agent and has shown synergistic activity when combined with ibrutinib. These findings confirm the role of SYK and warrant further investigation, as targeting BTK and SYK may lead to a meaningful clinical response [68]. These, and other, preclinical agents may prove to offer more effective treatment options for patients with WM.

Recommended Treatment Approach for Frontline and Relapsed Disease

Continued investigation is required to discern the most appropriate treatment regimens for patients with WM, including a distinction regarding the need for maintenance or fixed duration therapy. Current recommendations for treatment of newly diagnosed patients include a rituximab-based regimen, such as Benda-R, BDR, or CRD. Other options, such as single-agent rituximab or ibrutinib, can also be considered. In the setting of relapsed disease, a clinical trial is always the preferred manner of treatment, as this is the way in which future WM therapies will be developed. Many additional, targeted therapies are in development at this time. As research continues hopefully treatments will become more personalized, based on patient and disease-specific characteristics, such as MYD88 and CXCR4 status, with the ultimate goal of complete eradication of WM.

References

1. Waldenström J. Incipient myelomatosis of "essential" hyperglobulinemia with fibrinogenopenia – a new syndrome? Acta Med Scand. 1944;117(3–4):216–47.
2. Wang H, Chen Y, Li F, Delasalle K, Wang J, Alexanian R, et al. Temporal and geographic variations of Waldenstrom macroglobulinemia incidence: a large population-based study. Cancer. 2012;118(15):3793–800.
3. Treon SP, Hunter ZR, Aggarwal A, Ewen EP, Masota S, Lee C, et al. Characterization of familial Waldenström's macroglobulinemia. Ann Oncol. 2006;17(3):488–94.
4. Stone M, Merlini G, Pascual V. Autoantibody activity in Waldenstrom's macroglobulinemia. Clin Lymphoma. 2005;5(4):225–9.

5. Thakral B, Kanagal-Shamanna R. Systemic AL amyloidosis associated with Waldestrom macroglobulinemia: an unusual presenting complication. Blood. 2016;127(1):168.
6. Minnema MC, Kimby E, D'Sa S, Fornecker L-M, Poulain S, Snijders TJ, et al. Guideline for the diagnosis, treatment and response criteria for Bing-Neel syndrome. Haematologica. 2017;102(1):43–51.
7. Owen RG, Treon SP, Al-Katib A, Fonseca R, Greipp P, McMaster M, et al. Clinicopathological definition of Waldenstrom's macroglobulinemia: consensus panel recommendations from the Second International Workshop on Waldenstrom's macroglobulinemia. Semin Oncol. 2003;30(2):110–5.
8. Castillo JJ, Jurczyszyn A, Brozova L, Crusoe E, Czepiel J, Davila J, et al. IgM myeloma: a multicenter retrospective study of 134 patients. Am J Hematol. 2017;92(8):746–51.
9. Treon SP, Xu L, Yang G, Zhou Y, Liu X, Cao Y, et al. MYD88 L265P somatic mutation in Waldenström's macroglobulinemia. N Engl J Med. 2012;367(9):826–33.
10. Hunter ZR, Xu L, Yang G, Zhou Y, Liu X, Cao Y, et al. The genomic landscape of Waldenström macroglobulinemia is characterized by highly recurring MYD88 and WHIM-like CXCR4 mutations, and small somatic deletions associated with B-cell lymphomagenesis. Blood. 2014;123(11):1637–46.
11. Treon SP, Cao Y, Xu L, Yang G, Liu X, Hunter ZR. Somatic mutations in MYD88 and CXCR4 are determinants of clinical presentation and overall survival in Waldenstrom. Blood. 2014;123(18):2791–7.
12. Castillo JJ, Gustine J, Meid K, Dubeau T, Severns P, Xu L, et al. Low levels of von Willebrand markers associate with high serum IgM levels and improve with response to therapy, in patients with Waldenström macroglobulinaemia. Br J Haematol. 2019;184(6):1011–4.
13. Ghobrial IM, Fonseca R, Gertz MA, Plevak MF, Larson DR, Therneau TM, et al. Prognostic model for disease-specific and overall mortality in newly diagnosed symptomatic patients with Waldenstrom macroglobulinaemia. Br J Haematol. 2006;133(2):158–64.
14. Castillo JJ, Olszewski AJ, Kanan S, Meid K, Hunter ZR, Treon SP. Overall survival and competing risks of death in patients with Waldenström macroglobulinaemia: an analysis of the surveillance, epidemiology and end results database. Br J Haematol. 2015;169(1):81–9.
15. Morel P, Duhamel A, Gobbi P, Dimopoulos M, Dhodapkar M, McCoy J, et al. International prognostic scoring system (IPSS) for Waldenström's macroglobulinemia (WM). Blood. 2006;108:127.
16. Treon SP, Gustine J, Xu L, Manning RJ, Tsakmaklis N, Demos M, et al. MYD88 wild-type Waldenstrom macroglobulinaemia: differential diagnosis, risk of histological transformation, and overall survival. Br J Haematol. 2018;180(3):374–80.
17. Treon SP, Meid K, Gustine J, Bantilan KS, Dubeau T, Severns P, et al. Long-term follow-up of previously treated patients who received ibrutinib for symptomatic Waldenstrom's macroglobulinemia: update of pivotal clinical trial. Blood. 2017;130:2766.
18. Treon SP, Tripsas CK, Meid K, Warren D, Varma G, Green R, et al. Ibrutinib in previously treated Waldenström's macroglobulinemia. N Engl J Med. 2015;372(15):1430–40.
19. Castillo JJ, Meid K, Gustine JN, Dubeau T, Severns P, Hunter ZR, et al. Prospective clinical trial of ixazomib, dexamethasone and rituximab as primary therapy in Waldenström macroglobulinemia. Clin Cancer Res. 2018;24:3247–52.
20. Treon SP, Meid K, Tripsas C, Heffner LT, Eradat H, Badros AZ, et al. Prospective, multicenter clinical trial of everolimus as primary therapy in Waldenstrom macroglobulinemia (WMCTG 09-214). Clin Cancer Res. 2017;23(10):2400–4.
21. Kyle R, Treon S, Alexanian R, Barlogie B, Björkholm M, Dhodapkar M, et al. Prognostic markers and criteria to initiate therapy in Waldenstrom's macroglobulinemia: consensus panel recommendations from the Second International Workshop on Waldenstrom's macroglobulinemia. Semin Oncol. 2003;30(2):116–20.
22. Gustine JN, Meid K, Dubeau T, Hunter ZR, Xu L, Yang G, et al. Serum IgM level as predictor of symptomatic hyperviscosity in patients with Waldenström macroglobulinaemia. Br J Haematol. 2017;177(5):717–25.

23. Leblond V, Kastritis E, Advani R, Ansell S, Buske C, Castillo J, et al. Treatment recommendations from the Eighth International Workshop on Waldenstrom's macroglobulinemia. Blood. 2016;128(10):1321–9.
24. Castillo JJ, Gustine JN, Meid K, Dubeau TE, Severns P, Xu L, et al. Response and survival for primary therapy combination regimens and maintenance rituximab in Waldenström macroglobulinaemia. Br J Haematol. 2018;181(1):77–85.
25. Tedeschi A, Picardi P, Ferrero S, Benevolo G, Margiotta Casaluci G, Varettoni M, et al. Bendamustine and rituximab combination is safe and effective as salvage regimen in Waldenström macroglobulinemia. Leuk Lymphoma. 2015;56(9):2637–42.
26. Rummel MJ, Niederle N, Maschmeyer G, Banat GA, Von Grünhagen U, Losem C, et al. Bendamustine plus rituximab versus CHOP plus rituximab as first-line treatment for patients with indolent and mantle-cell lymphomas: an open-label, multicentre, randomised, phase 3 non-inferiority trial. Lancet. 2013;381(9873):1203–10.
27. Dimopoulos MA, Gavriatopoulou M, Morel P, Kyrtsonis M, Michalis E, Kartasis Z, et al. Primary therapy of Waldenstrom macroglobulinemia (WM) with weekly bortezomib, low-dose dexamethasone, and rituximab (BDR). Blood. 2013;122(19):3276–82.
28. Ghobrial IM, Xie W, Padmanabhan S, Badros A, Rourke M, Leduc R, et al. Phase II trial of weekly bortezomib in combination with rituximab in untreated patients with Waldenström macroglobulinemia. Am J Hematol. 2010;85(9):670–4.
29. Treon SP, Ioakimidis L, Soumerai JD, Patterson CJ, Sheehy P, Nelson M, et al. Primary therapy of Waldenström macroglobulinemia with bortezomib, dexamethasone, and rituximab: WMCTG clinical trial 05-180. J Clin Oncol. 2009;27(23):3830–5.
30. Treon SP, Tripsas CK, Meid K, Kanan S, Sheehy P, Chuma S, et al. Carfilzomib, rituximab, and dexamethasone (CaRD) treatment offers's a neuropathy-sparing approach for treating Waldenstrom macroglobulinemia. Blood. 2014;124(4):503–10.
31. Meid K, Dubeau T, Severns P, Gustine J, Ghobria IM, Castillo JJ, et al. Long-term follow-up of a prospective clinical trial of carfilzomib, rituximab and dexamethasone (CaRD) in Waldenstrom's macroglobulinemia. Blood. 2017;130:2772.
32. Kastritis E, Gavriatopoulou M, Kyrtsonis M, Roussou M, Hadjiharissi E, Symeonidis A, et al. Dexamethasone, rituximab, and cyclophosphamide as primary treatment of Waldenstrom macroglobulinemia: final analysis of a phase 2 study. Blood. 2015;126(11):1392–4.
33. Paludo J, Abeykoon JP, Kumar S, Shreders A, Ailawadhi S, Gertz MA, et al. Dexamethasone, rituximab and cyclophosphamide for relapsed and/or refractory and treatment-naïve patients with Waldenstrom macroglobulinemia. Br J Haematol. 2017;179(1):98–105.
34. Olszewski AJ, Treon SP, Castillo JJ. Evolution of management and outcomes in Waldenström macroglobulinemia: a population-based analysis. Oncologist. 2016;21(11):1377–86.
35. Dimopoulos M, Zervas C, Zomas A, Hamilos G, Gika D, Efstthiou E, et al. Extended rituximab therapy for previously untreated patients with Waldenström's macroglobulinemia. Clin Lymphoma Myeloma Leuk. 2002;3(3):163–6.
36. Gertz MA, Abonour R, Heffner LT, Greipp PR, Uno H, Rajkumar SV. Clinical value of minor responses after 4 doses of rituximab in Waldenström macroglobulinaemia: a follow-up of the eastern cooperative oncology group E3A98 trial. Br J Haematol. 2009;147(5):677–80.
37. Treon SP, Hanzis C, Manning RJ, Ioakimidis L, Patterson CJ, Hunter ZR, et al. Maintenance rituximab is associated with improved clinical outcome in rituximab naïve patients with Waldenstrom macroglobulinaemia who respond to a rituximab-containing regimen. Br J Haematol. 2011;154(3):357–62.
38. Dimopoulos MA, Trotman J, Tedeschi A, Matous JV, Macdonald D, Tam C, et al. Ibrutinib for patients with rituximab-refractory Waldenström's macroglobulinaemia (iNNOVATE): an open-label substudy of an international, multicentre, phase 3 trial. Lancet Oncol. 2017;18(2):241–50.
39. Treon SP, Gustine J, Meid K, Dubeau T, Severns P, Patterson C, et al. Ibrutinib is highly active as first line therapy in symptomatic Waldenstrom's macroglobulinemia. Blood. 2017;130:2767.
40. Leblond V, Johnson S, Chevret S, Copplestone A, Rule S, Tournilhac O, et al. Results of a randomized trial of chlorambucil versus fludarabine for patients with untreated Waldenström

macroglobulinemia, marginal zone lymphoma, or lymphoplasmacytic lymphoma. J Clin Oncol. 2013;31(3):301–7.
41. Roccaro AM, Sacco A, Jia X, Banwait R, Maiso P, Azab F, et al. Mechanisms of activity of the TORC1 inhibitor everolimus in Waldenstrom macroglobulinemia. Clin Cancer Res. 2012;18(24):6609–22.
42. Treon SP, Soumerai JD, Branagan AR, Hunter ZR, Patterson CJ, Ioakimidis L, et al. Thalidomide and rituximab in Waldenstrom macroglobulinemia. Blood. 2008;112(12):4452–7.
43. Dimopoulos M, Tsatalas C, Zomas A, Hamilos G, Panayiotidis P, Margaritis D, et al. Treatment of Waldenstrom's macroglobulinemia with single-agent thalidomide or with the combination of clarithromycin, thalidomide and dexamethasone. Semin Oncol. 2003;30(2):265–9.
44. Kyriakou C, Canals C, Cornelissen JJ, Socié G, Willemze R, Ifrah N, et al. Allogeneic stem-cell transplantation in patients with waldenström macroglobulinemia: report from the lymphoma working party of the european group for blood and marrow transplantation. J Clin Oncol. 2010;28(33):4926–34.
45. Kyriakou C, Canals C, Sibon D, Cahn JY, Kazmi M, Arcese W, et al. High-dose therapy and autologous stem-cell transplantation in Waldenström macroglobulinemia: the lymphoma working party of the European group for blood and marrow transplantation. J Clin Oncol. 2010;28(13):2227–32.
46. Cornell RF, Bachanova V, D'Souza A, Woo-Ahn K, Martens M, Huang J, et al. Allogeneic transplantation for relapsed Waldenström macroglobulinemia and lymphoplasmacytic lymphoma. Biol Blood Marrow Transplant. 2017;23(1):60–6.
47. Kyriakou C, Advani R, Ansell S, Buske C, Castillo J, Dreger P, et al. Indications for hematopoietic stem cell transplantation in patients with Waldenstrom's macroglobulinemia: a consensus project of the EBMT Lymphoma Working Party (LWP)/ European Consortium for Waldenstrom's Macroglobulinemia (ECWM)/International Waldenstrom. Blood. 2017;130:2026.
48. Paulus A, Manna A, Akhtar S, Singh N, Kumar A, Basu K, et al. The Oral proteasome inhibitor ixazomib, alone and in combination with ibrutinib, induces lethality in Waldenstrom macroglobulinemia cells that are resistant to ibrutinib. Blood. 2017;130:1260.
49. Chauhan D, Singh AV, Aujay M, Kirk CJ, Bandi M, Ciccarelli B, et al. A novel orally active proteasome inhibitor ONX 0912 trigger in vitro and in vivo cytotoxicity in multiple myeloma. Blood. 2010;116(23):4906–15.
50. Siegel D, Kaufman J, Raje N, Mikhael J, Kapoor P, Treon S, et al. Updated results from a multicenter, open-label, dose-escalation phase 1b/2 study of single-agent oprozomib in patients with Waldenström macroglobulinemia (WM). Blood. 2014;124:1715.
51. Furman R, Eradat H, DiRienzo C, Hofmeister C, Haymnan S, Leonard J, et al. A phase 2 study of ofatumumab in Waldenström's macroglobulinaemia. Lancet Haematol. 2017;4(1):e24–34.
52. Castillo J, Kanan S, Meid K, Manning R, Hunter Z, Treon S. Rituximab intolerance in patients with Waldenstrom macroglobulinaemia. Br J Haematol. 2016;174:631–57.
53. Waldenstrom's Macroglobulinemia/Lymphoplasmacytic Lymphoma. National Comprehensive Cancer Network. 2018. https://www.nccn.org/professionals/physician_gls/p.
54. Kashyap MK, Kumar D, Jones H, Amaya-Chanaga CI, Choi MY, Melo-Cardenas J, et al. Ulocuplumab (BMS-936564 / MDX1338): a fully human anti-CXCR4 antibody induces cell death in chronic lymphocytic leukemia mediated through a reactive oxygen species-dependent pathway. Oncotarget. 2016;7(3):2809–22.
55. Owen R, McCarthy H, Rule S, D'Sa S, Thomas S, Forconi F, et al. Acalabrutinib in patients with Waldenstrom macroglobulinemia. EHA Learn Cent. 2018:S853.
56. Byrd JC, Harrington B, O'Brien S, Jones JA, Schuh A, Devereux S, et al. Acalabrutinib (ACP-196) in relapsed chronic lymphocytic leukemia. N Engl J Med. 2016;374(4):323–32.
57. Tam C, Grigg A, Opat S, Ku M, Gilbertson M, Anderson M, et al. The BTK inhibitor, Bgb-3111, is safe, tolerable, and highly active in patients with relapsed/ refractory B-cell malignancies: initial report of a phase 1 first-in-human trial. Blood. 2015;126:832.

58. Zhu J, Li J, Zhou J, Song Y, Qi J, Xu W, et al. BGB-3111, a highly specific BTK inhibitor, is well tolerated and highly active in Chinese patients with relapsed/refractory B-cell malignancies: initial report of a phase 1 trial in China. Blood. 2017;130:5347.
59. Trotman J, Tam C, Marlton P, Gottlieb D, Simpson D, Cull G, et al. Improved depth of response with increased follow-up for patients with Waldenstrom macroglobulinemia treated with Bruton's tyrosine kinase inhibitor zanubrutinib. EHA Learn Cent. 2018:PS1186.
60. Paulus A, Akhtar S, Bashir Y, Paulus S, Yousaf H, Roy V, et al. Drug resistance alters CD38 expression and in vitro response to daratumumab in Waldenstrom macroglobulinemia cells. Blood. 2016;128:3018.
61. Paulus A, Chitta KS, Wallace PK, Advani PP, Akhtar S, Kuranz-Blake M, et al. Immunophenotyping of Waldenströms macroglobulinemia cell lines reveals distinct patterns of surface antigen expression: potential biological and therapeutic implications. PLoS One. 2015;10(4):1–17.
62. Barakat FH, Medeiros LJ, Wei EX, Konoplev S, Lin P, Jorgensen JL. Residual monotypic plasma cells in patients with waldenstrom macroglobulinemia after therapy. Am J Clin Pathol. 2011;135(3):365–73.
63. Davids MS, Roberts AW, Seymour JF, Pagel JM, Kahl BS, Wierda WG, et al. Phase I first-in-human study of venetoclax in patients with relapsed or refractory non-Hodgkin lymphoma patient demographic and clinical characteristics. J Clin Oncol. 2017;35(8):826–33.
64. Castillo J, Gustine J, Meid K, Dubeau T, Allan J, Furman R, et al. Prospective phase II study of venetoclax in patients with previously treated Waldenstrom macroglobulinemia. EHA Learn Cent. 2018:S85.
65. Castillo J, Gustine J, Meid K, Dubeau T, Yang G, Xu L, et al. Idelalisib in Waldenström macroglobulinemia: high incidence of hepatotoxicity. Leuk Lymphoma. 2017;58(4):1002–4.
66. Burris HA, Flinn IW, Patel MR, Fenske TS, Deng C, Brander DM, et al. Umbralisib, a novel PI3Kδ and casein kinase-1ε inhibitor, in relapsed or refractory chronic lymphocytic leukaemia and lymphoma: an open-label, phase 1, dose-escalation, first-in-human study. Lancet Oncol. 2018;19(4):486–96.
67. Sacco A, Affo L, Ghedini G, Lanzi G, Giacomini A, Motta M, et al. Targeting lymphoplasmacytic lymphoma through a novel anti-FGF-based therapeutical strategy. Blood. 2017;130:2818.
68. Munshi M, Liu X, Chen J, Xu L, Tsakmaklis N, Demos M, et al. Mutated MYD88 activates the BCR component SYK and provides a rationale therapeutic target in Waldenstrom's macroglobulinemia. Blood. 2017;130:2539.

Chapter 3
Immunotherapy in Hodgkin Lymphoma and Other CD30+ Lymphomas

Raghuveer Ranganathan and Thomas C. Shea

Hodgkin Lymphoma

Background/Epidemiology

Hodgkin lymphoma (HL) is an uncommon, B-lymphocyte-derived malignancy, comprising about 11% of all lymphomas seen in the United States and 0.5% of all new cancer cases in the United States. It has an approximate annual incidence of 2.6 new cases per 100,000 men and women per year, with an estimated 8260 new cases occurring in 2017 across the United States [3]. HL is traditionally associated with a bimodal distribution of occurrence, with a median age at diagnosis of 39 years [3]. Siblings of HL patients seem to have an increased risk of developing the disease. Interestingly, siblings of the same gender have been shown to be at twice the risk of siblings of the opposite gender [4]. Studies suggest a possible predilection between ethnicity, socioeconomic status, and HL incidence. Certain HL histologic subtypes like mixed cellularity and lymphocyte-depleted occur more in patients of Hispanic origin with lower socioeconomic status, while another subtype, nodular sclerosis HL, happens more frequently in patients with higher socioeconomic standard of living [5].

Histopathology/Pathogenesis

Based on differences in the histology and phenotype of the tumor cells, HL is divided into two discrete disease entities: classical HL and nodular lymphocyte-predominant

---

R. Ranganathan (✉) · T. C. Shea
Department of Medicine, Division of Hematology and Oncology,
University of North Carolina at Chapel Hill, Chapel Hill, NC, USA
e-mail: rrangana@email.unc.edu; tom_shea@med.unc.edu

C. Dittus (ed.), *Novel Therapeutics for Rare Lymphomas*,
https://doi.org/10.1007/978-3-030-25610-4_3

HL [6]. Classical HL (cHL) is further split into four subsets: nodular sclerosis, mixed cellularity, lymphocyte-rich, and lymphocyte-depleted. While there are minor variations between the cHL subtypes in clinical presentation, the overall prognosis and treatment for these subtypes are similar. On the other hand, nodular lymphocyte-predominant HL (NLPHL) is distinct in immunophenotypic and genomic features, presentation, prognosis, and treatment. Importantly, it is usually negative for CD30, but positive for CD20 and is treated in a fashion analogous to indolent non-Hodgkin lymphomas. Since it lacks the CD30 antigen, NLPHL will not be included in this discussion.

The characteristic pathologic feature of cHL is the presence of Reed-Sternberg (RS) cells, which are large, multinucleated cells present within a dense, reactive cellular environment made of granulocytes, lymphocytes, dendritic cells, and monocytes. The actual occurrence of RS cells within the cellular background is quite rare, another hallmark of cHL, generally comprising just 1–2% of the cell population [7]. Although RS cells definitively express CD30, they possess an atypical immunophenotype capable of mixed co-expression of myeloid, granulocytic, T cell, and B cell markers [8]. As is the case with most hematologic malignancies, the disease cause is likely multifactorial. RS cells originate from mature germinal center B cells, based on studies showing these cells carrying clonal and somatically mutated immunoglobulin heavy- and light-chain gene rearrangements [9]. However, they have a universal paucity of B cell gene expression, by specifically downregulating expression of B cell transcription factors which causes loss of B cell receptor (BCR) expression on the surface [10]. Normally, the loss of BCR surface expression would shunt a B cell to rapid apoptosis, which indicates that RS cell precursors acquire additional pathogenetic steps that allow for escape from this fate.

Interestingly, in 40–50% of cHL, the RS cells are latently infected with Epstein-Barr virus (EBV) [11]. Since the RS cells are clonally infected, it raises the possibility that EBV infection can be an early and critical step for cHL formation [12]. The RS cells express the EBV-encoded antigens EBNA1, LMP1, and LMP2a, which are weakly immunogenic but may confer a survival benefit on RS cells by mimicking the CD40 receptor and BCR stimulatory signaling [13, 14]. RS cells also show genomic gains of genes that specifically result in dysregulated and constitutive activity of the transcription factor NF-κB and JAK/STAT pathways [15–18]. Genes for TNFAIP3 and SOCS1 that negatively regulate these same pathways are often found to be mutated or inactivated which further promote proliferation and survival of malignant cells [19, 20].

cHL also dictates the composition of its tumor microenvironment by selectively recruiting cells that support cHL survival through either cell-cell interactions or by inhibiting immune antitumor activity, the latter of which is a mechanism also employed by many solid tumor malignancies [21, 22]. RS cells produce chemokines such as MDC/CCL122, IL-10, and TARC/CCL17, which attract regulatory T cells (Tregs) and helper T cells (Th2); these cells then suppress and impair the activity of the few cytotoxic T lymphocytes that gain access to the tumor site [23, 24]. RS cells also overexpress PD-L1 due to gains in chromosomal region 9p24, which further suppresses antitumor activity [25]. This aspect of cHL biology will be addressed further in the section on therapies for this disease since it results in susceptibility of the tumor cells to checkpoint inhibitors such as nivolumab and pembrolizumab [26–30].

Clinical Presentation

The majority of cHL patients present with palpable but painless supradiaphragmatic lymphadenopathy, commonly in the cervical, axillary, supraclavicular, and mediastinal regions. Subdiaphragmatic lymphadenopathy, bone marrow involvement with resultant cytopenias, splenic involvement, and extra-nodal disease are less frequent presentations. About 35% of cases present with constitutional "B" symptoms, which include fevers/chills, drenching night sweats, and unintentional weight loss of greater than 10% in the preceding 6 months. Other possible systemic symptoms include early satiety, fatigue, shortness of breath, persistent cough, generalized pruritus (often severe and precedes lymphadenopathy), and pain upon alcohol ingestion [31]. These symptoms tend to more commonly occur in patients with bulky or extra-nodal involvement in the spleen, liver, bone marrow, lungs, or a combination of these regions.

Staging/Workup and Diagnosis

Initial workup consists of a comprehensive physical exam and detailed history of symptoms. The physical exam should focus on identifying palpable lymphadenopathy in the cervical, supraclavicular, axillary, inguinal, and popliteal areas. Examination for the presence of hepatomegaly or splenomegaly should also be a focus of the exam. Typical laboratory workup includes a complete blood count with differential, basic metabolic panel, liver function tests, erythrocyte sedimentation rate (ESR), lactate dehydrogenase, and viral studies checking for HIV and hepatitis B. Glucose-6-phosphate dehydrogenase and tumor lysis syndrome (TLS) tests can also be done, but generally cHL does not present with TLS. PET-CT is the standard for imaging cHL due to its improved accuracy compared to CT scans for staging nodal and extra-nodal sites and has replaced the need for bone marrow biopsy to evaluate for marrow involvement [32, 33]. Patients are staged using the modified Ann Arbor staging system [34].

A definitive diagnosis relies upon procuring a full excisional lymph node biopsy for pathology review, since fine needle aspirates and core needle biopsies often do not provide enough tissue sample for an accurate diagnosis. The predominant immunophenotype of cHL RS cells is CD15+, CD30+, MUM1+, CD19−, and CD45−. CD20 can be weakly positive in some RS cells but is generally considered to be negative in cHL.

Additional treatment-related workup includes an echocardiogram to assess a patient's cardiac ejection fraction prior to anthracycline therapy. Pulmonary function testing with a measurement of the diffusion capacity of the lung for carbon monoxide (DLCO) is required prior to bleomycin treatment. Fertility preservation is typically discussed with patients, although most patients treated with standard frontline therapy regain fertility.

Prognosis

cHL patients are generally sorted into three primary prognostic risk groups: early favorable risk (stages I–II with no unfavorable factors), early unfavorable risk (stages I–II having any one of the unfavorable factors), and advanced stage [35]. The determining prognostic risk factors for early-stage disease are elevated ESR, involvement of >3 lymph node regions, B symptoms; and extra-nodal presentation [36]. The NCCN further delineates the early unfavorable risk group into those with and without bulky disease [37]. The International Prognostic Score identifies several predictive disease factors that project freedom from progression (FFP) and overall survival (OS) in patients with advanced disease. These features include age >45 years, albumin <4 g/dL, hemoglobin <10.5, male gender, stage IV disease, white blood cell count >15,000/μL, and lymphocyte count <600/μL [38]. The more cumulative features a cHL patient has, the worse the prognostic outcome overall for the patient [35–38].

Interim PET-CT (iPET-CT) represents a critical element for prognosticating a patient's overall course and progression-free survival (PFS), with studies showing that it supersedes a patient's IPS score [39]. A negative iPET after two cycles of chemotherapy with ABVD portends a significantly greater PFS than a positive iPET regardless of the disease stage, IPS score, or risk group stratification [39, 40].

Treatment

Standard of care for early-stage HL differs from advanced stage HL. Combination chemotherapy has not changed greatly since the early 1970s in the United States, with ABVD (doxorubicin, bleomycin, vinblastine, and dacarbazine) being the most commonly used regimen [41]. The German Hodgkin Lymphoma Study Group devised a different, more intensive approach consisting of bleomycin, etoposide, doxorubicin, cyclophosphamide, vincristine, procarbazine, and prednisone, or BEACOPP, with standard and escalated variants [42]. BEACOPP is more toxic than ABVD and is not given to patients older than 65 years of age [43]. It also has an increased risk for MDS/AML, treatment-related deaths, and a much higher infertility rate [44, 45].

Treatment for HL can result in secondary malignancies in the breast, lung, and GI tract primarily from the use of radiation therapy [46]. Cardiovascular risk with diastolic dysfunction, myocardial infarction, and cerebrovascular risk can also occur after receiving XRT to the mediastinum or neck [46]. However, there has been incremental improvement in long-term survival among HL patients due to ongoing modifying of treatment regimens to limit long-term toxicities, especially in early stage HL [47]. The NCCN favors a risk-based approach for early-stage HL divided into three categories: early favorable, early unfavorable non-bulky disease, and early unfavorable bulky disease. The standard approach for early favorable risk is ABVD × 2 cycles followed by 20 Gy of involved site radiotherapy (ISRT) or ABVD alone × 4 cycles to minimize XRT exposure if mediastinal disease is present [48, 49]. Early unfavorable non-bulky disease can be treated with ABVD × 4 cycles plus 30 Gy of ISRT or ABVD alone × 6 cycles especially if mediastinal disease is present [49, 50]. Early unfavorable bulky disease has a similar approach, although these patients are often treated as advanced stage disease.

For advanced stage cHL (stages III–IV), treatment is primarily with ABVD, with an iPET after cycle 2 determining modulation or intensification of further therapy. Studies have investigated treatment with ABVD versus BEACOPP in advanced stage HL. BEACOPP tended to show improved FFP over ABVD, but at the expense of increased hematologic and non-hematologic toxicities along with the aforementioned higher rates of MDS/AML, infertility, and intolerability in patients above age 65 [51]. Importantly, there was no difference in OS between the two groups. There was a slightly higher proportion of patients with relapsed/refractory disease treated with frontline ABVD compared to BEACOPP, but salvage therapy nullified possible FFP and OS differences between the two treatment groups [51]. In subset analyses of high-risk advanced stage cHL patients, defined as having an IPS score of 3 or greater, there was equivalent EFS and OS between ABVD- and BEACOPP-treated patients [52]. As such, the standard treatment for advanced stage HL in the United States has remained ABVD × 6 cycles. The role of PET-CT-adapted therapy has recently redefined treatment methodologies in advanced stage cHL. If the iPET is negative (defined as Deauville 1–3) after two cycles of ABVD, then bleomycin can be stopped, and the remaining four cycles can be completed with just AVD [53]. This treatment approach is now supported by the NCCN guidelines and would reduce potential pulmonary toxicity from bleomycin. Escalating therapy in patients with a positive iPET from ABVD to eBEACOPP is an option, but has not been evaluated in a randomized fashion [40].

About 15% of patients have primary refractory disease, and additional 15–25% have relapse after an initial complete response. In these patients, the standard treatment is high-dose salvage chemotherapy with subsequent autologous stem cell transplant (auto-SCT). Common salvage regimens include ifosfamide with etoposide and carboplatin (ICE), dexamethasone with cytarabine and cisplatin (DHAP), or gemcitabine-containing regimens (GDP, GVD, BeGEV) [54–58]. Trials comparing salvage chemotherapy with and without auto-SCT showed better disease-free survival with patients receiving auto-SCT [59, 60]. Pre-transplant PET-CT is highly predictive of the outcome with auto-SCT, as patients with a negative pre-transplant PET-CT had a vastly superior EFS compared to patients who had a positive PET prior to auto-SCT [61]. Allogeneic stem cell transplant can be offered as a third-line option if a patient fails auto-SCT.

Anaplastic Large Cell Lymphoma and Other CD30-Expressing Lymphomas

Anaplastic large cell lymphoma (ALCL) is a rare form of NHL, accounting for 3% of all NHLs, and is a subtype of peripheral T cell lymphoma. There are four variants: primary systemic ALCL which is positive for anaplastic lymphoma kinase (ALK) gene rearrangement, ALK-negative primary systemic ALCL, primary cutaneous, and breast-implant-associated. Systemic ALCL has a worse prognosis than the cutaneous or breast-implant-associated subtypes [62]. It has a similar bimodal age of incidence as cHL, but is a disease that occurs more often in the preteen or adolescent age groups [63]. The systemic variants generally have an aggressive presentation with rapidly progressive lymphadenopathy and systemic B symptoms. ALCL has strong CD30 expression, no expression of B cell antigens, and the majority expressing one or more T cell-associated antigens (CD3, CD43, CD45RO). In contrast to HL, they are predominantly negative for CD15 expression. Staging and workup of systemic ALCL is similar to the workup for other aggressive lymphomas with blood work, PET-CT, and excisional biopsy required for definitive diagnosis of systemic disease. Primary systemic ALK-positive ALCL patients have a better prognosis than ALK-negative ALCL patients [64, 65]. Additional prognostic indications include the patient's age at diagnosis, beta-2 microglobulin, and the IPI score [66]. Treatment is usually six cycles of an anthracycline-based regimen such as CHOP, CHOEP, or ACBVP, with patients above age 60 primarily receiving CHOP while those below age 60 receiving the more aggressive treatment regimens [66–68].

In addition to HL and ALCL, various other lymphomas have variable positive expression of CD30. DLBCL can have CD30 expression in approximately 20–25% of cases, while T cell and NK/T cell lymphomas can express CD30 close to 60% of the time [69, 70].

Brentuximab Vedotin

Brentuximab vedotin is a CD30-targeting antibody-drug conjugate linking an anti-CD30 monoclonal antibody with the anti-microtubule agent monomethyl auristatin E (MMAE). Initial studies with the naked CD30 antibody only yielded mediocre results, which led to the conjugation of the antibody to MMAE [71]. In the first phase I trial with brentuximab vedotin (BV), 45 patients with relapsed/refractory CD30+ lymphoma were administered varying doses of the drug to find the maximum tolerated dose (MTD), which was eventually determined to be 1.8 mg/kg intravenously (IV). Out of 12 patients who received the 1.8 mg/kg dose, 6 (50%) achieved an objective response with 4 complete responses (CRs) and 2 partial responses (PRs) [72]. Thirty-six out of forty-two evaluable patients (86%) had discernible tumor regression. The most common adverse events seen were fatigue, pyrexia, diarrhea, nausea, and neutropenia. These results led to a pivotal phase II trial, which had 102 patients with relapsed or refractory HL unresponsive to auto-SCT receiving BV 1.8 mg/kg IV every 3 weeks for up to 16 cycles [73]. The overall response rate (ORR) was 75%, with 34% of all patients achieving CR. In those patients with an objective response, the median duration of response was 6.7 months; it was 20.5 months in patients reaching CR. Median PFS and OS were 9.3 and 40.5 months in all patients, respectively, and 21.7 months and not reached, respectively, in the CR patients. In long-term follow-up, 13 out of the 34 patients who originally achieved CR (38%) remained in CR [74]. The phase III AETHERA trial looked at 329 relapsed/refractory HL patients with high risk features (defined as refractory to frontline therapy, relapse < 12 months after frontline therapy, or relapse greater than or equal to 12 months with extranodal disease) being apportioned to receive, after auto-SCT, either placebo or up to 16 cycles of BV to assess whether BV could improve PFS when given as consolidative therapy. The median PFS in the BV arm was 42.9 months compared to 24.1 in the placebo arm, leading to BV being approved for treatment of HL patients who had failed at least two prior chemotherapy regimens or auto-SCT, and for use as consolidative therapy in HL patients with high risk features [75, 76].

A multicenter, single-arm, phase I–II trial looked at combining BV with bendamustine, with the hopes of establishing the combination as a possible alternative salvage regimen before proceeding to auto-SCT in relapsed/refractory HL and ALCL patients [77]. Overall, 32% of the patients across both phase I and II achieved a CR. The most serious adverse effects were grade 3 lung infection in 14% of patients in the phase II, and 25% of patients across phases I and II had grade 3–4 neutropenia, with no treatment-related deaths in the study. A second phase I–II study also similarly looked at salvage BV-bendamustine treatment prior to auto-SCT and demonstrated ORR of 92.5% and CR of 73.6% out of 55 evaluable patients [78]. Based on these two clinical trials, the combination of bendamustine with BV appears to be an effective alternative to standard salvage chemotherapy regimens.

BV as first-line treatment in Hodgkin lymphoma has been evaluated. In an early phase I study comparing BV in combination with standard ABVD or combined with a modified standard AVD, a very high rate of pulmonary toxicity was detected in the BV plus ABVD arm [79]. This was not seen in the BV plus AVD arm, so subsequent studies focused on this particular combination. A randomized phase III trial, ECHELON-1, compared first-line BV in combination with AVD against ABVD in patients with stage III or IV cHL [80]. The BV plus AVD arm showed similar efficacy to ABVD and was deemed to demonstrate superior risk reduction in progression, death, and need for additional anticancer therapy compared to the ABVD arm. However, there was a substantial proportion of patients in the BV plus AVD arm who developed peripheral neuropathy (67%), with 31% of patients having grade 2 or higher neuropathy. While the neuropathy was reported to be largely reversible, longer follow-up data is needed to fully study the issue. There were also discrepancies with the mortality and hospitalization rates of patients in the ABVD arm, as they were higher than historical rates with ABVD treatment. Due to these issues, we feel that BV + AVD should not replace ABVD for frontline treatment of Hodgkin lymphoma. However, this remains an excellent option for patients who cannot receive bleomycin due to pre-existing pulmonary disease or abnormal pulmonary function tests.

A recent phase I study investigated the frontline use of BV in combination with cyclophosphamide, doxorubicin, and prednisone (BV-CHP), followed by up to ten cycles of consolidative BV monotherapy in patients with CD30+ peripheral T cell lymphomas (PTCL). Twenty-six patients were evaluated overall, with 19 having systemic ALCL. One hundred percent of the patients demonstrated an objective response, with a CR of 92% and no patient receiving consolidative stem cell transplant [81]. After 60 months, median PFS and OS were not reached, with estimated 5-year PFS and OS being 52% and 80%, respectively. The primary adverse effect observed was peripheral neuropathy, which resolved or improved in 95% of patients. Based on these results, BV-CHP was evaluated in a phase III trial in CD30-positive PTCL, with CHOP as the comparator arm [82]. This study randomized 226 patients to each regimen, and the results favored BV-CHP in both PFS (median, 48.2 months vs 20.8 months; $p = 0.011$) and OS (median not reached in either group, but there was a 34% reduction in risk of death for BV-CHP; $p = 0.0244$). BV-CHP was FDA approved for frontline treatment of CD30+ PTCL in 2018.

Chimeric Antigen Receptor T Cell Therapy Targeting CD30

Chimeric antigen receptor T cells (CAR-T) are a type of adoptive cellular immunotherapy where a patient's own T cells are genetically reengineered to kill cancer cells by recognizing specific tumor-associated antigens. The chimeric antigen receptor (CAR) itself is a protein construct consisting of an antigen-binding single-chain variable fragment (scFv) derived from a monoclonal antibody, fused via a hinge and transmembrane regions to an intracellular portion containing activation and co-stimulatory domains [83]. The majority of CAR endodomains are comprised of a CD3ζ activation subunit originating from the T cell receptor (TCR) along with a co-stimulatory CD28 or 41BB domain derived from T cell co-stimulatory receptors [83–85]. Initially, the first iterations of CAR-T only possessed the CD3ζ domain. These first-generation CAR-T showed disappointing results in early clinical trials secondary to minimal persistence in vivo, which was thought to be due to lack of a co-stimulatory signal [86, 87]. Physiologically, if normal T cells come across an antigen recognized by their TCR but have no co-stimulatory signal provided from CD80 or CD86, the T cells become anergic and stop proliferating [83, 88]. Due to these clinical findings, the second and subsequent generations of CAR-T have had co-stimulatory endodomains incorporated along with the CD3ζ chain, which have significantly enhanced in vivo proliferation and persistence, and also increased their clinical efficacy [89–91] (Fig. 3.1).

The gene encoding the full CAR construct is transferred into normal patient-derived autologous T cells ex vivo usually via a replication-incompetent retroviral or lentiviral vector, where the CAR gene is incorporated into the T cell genome [88, 92]. These newly transduced CAR-T cells are then grown and expanded in culture ex vivo for 2–4 weeks before being reintroduced back into the patient. Prior to reintroduction, the patient receives a lymphodepleting conditioning chemotherapy regimen to reduce the presence of inhibitory regulatory T cells as well as decrease other cellular elements competing for cytokines [93]. Overall, CAR-T cells combine the

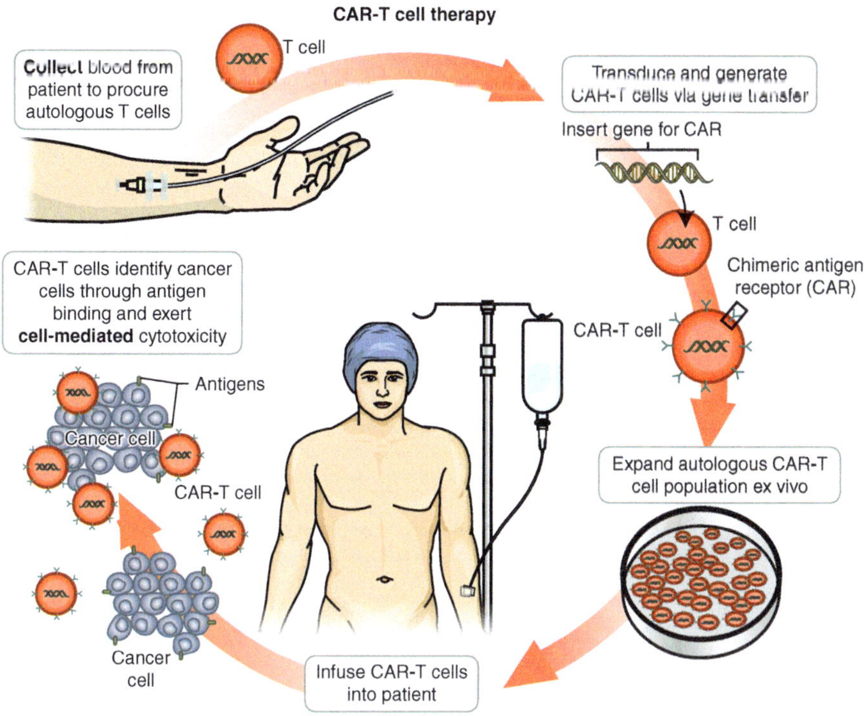

Fig. 3.1 CAR-T cell production. The general process for chimeric antigen receptor T cell (CAR-T cell) production and clinical application into patients. The general process takes approximately 2–4 weeks from the collection of blood from the patient to the reintroduction of the finished CAR-T cell product back into the patient

antigen-binding ability of monoclonal antibodies with the tumoricidal faculties and self-renewal property of T cells. They possess a major advantage over normal T cells in that they eradicate tumor cells independently of the major histocompatibility complex (MHC), which is commonly downregulated or is defective within tumor cells. They also possess the added advantage over allogenic stem cell transplants in that CAR-T cells are a completely autologous system of immunotherapy, thereby largely circumventing potential graft versus host disease risk (Fig. 3.2).

Clinical experience with CAR-T is predominantly with CD19-directed CAR-T therapy in ALL or B cell NHL, since CD19 is an attractive target due to its expression being relegated to B cells and not expressed in other normal human tissues elsewhere. However, since CD30 is universally expressed in HL, ALCL, certain DLBCL subtypes, T cell, and NK/T cell lymphomas, CAR-T directed against it has risen as a potential avenue for therapy. The aforementioned success of brentuximab also further strengthened the viability of such a CD30-targeted approach with CAR-T immunotherapy. Preclinical studies with EBV-specific cytotoxic lymphocytes (EBV-CTLs) being transduced to also express CD30-targeting CAR

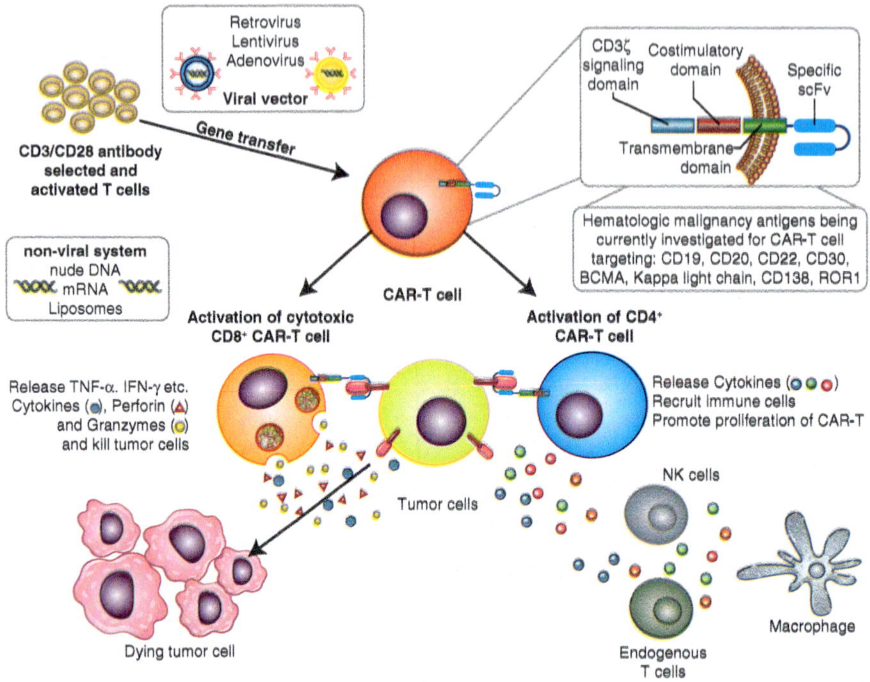

Fig. 3.2 CAR-T cell engineering. Molecular schemata of CAR-T cell generation. (**a**) T cells separated from the blood of the patient are first activated with CD3/CD28 antibodies in culture. (**b**) The gene containing the CAR construct is then transferred into the T cells via a viral vector, usually utilizing either lentivirus or retrovirus. Nonviral vectors with transposon or mRNA electroporation are occasionally used as well. (**c**) After genetic transfer of the CAR construct gene, T cells are able to express the CAR construct on their cell surface. The CAR construct contains an extracellular antigen-binding scFv fragment derived from a monoclonal antibody, which then connects to intracellular signaling domains via a transmembrane domain. Second-generation and more modern CAR-T cell iterations contain at least 1 co-stimulatory domain in addition to the CD3ζ signaling domain. (**d**) A mixture of CD4 and CD8 CAR-T cells are generated through the molecular reengineering process, each of which engages in tumor cytotoxicity either directly or indirectly

(CD30.CAR) showed great efficacy in eradicating autologous EBV+ cHL cells through their native TCR and EBV-/CD30+ HL cells through the CD30.CAR in a xenograft murine model [94].

These promising findings eventually led to a phase I dose escalation study in which seven patients with relapsed/refractory cHL and two patients with relapsed/refractory ALCL were infused with autologous CD30.CAR-T containing the CD28 endodomain [95]. Six of the cHL patients and one ALCL patient had previous brentuximab exposure prior to the CD30.CAR trial. There were three dose levels, from 0.2×10^8 to 2×10^8 CD30.CAR-T/m^2. Genomic quantitative PCR (qPCR), used to detect the persistence of the infused CD30.CAR-T, showed that the CD30.CAR-T cells reached a peak after 1 week post-infusion with a subsequent slow decline over the ensuing 4–5 weeks. However, six patients continued to have detectable CD30.

CAR-T 6 months post-infusion. Out of the seven relapsed/refractory cHL patients, two patients demonstrated CR lasting greater than 2 years, with one of those patients in continued CR after 2.5 years. Three other patients had transient stable disease (SD) lasting at least 6 weeks. Of the two relapsed/refractory ALCL patients, one had a CR lasting 9 months after receiving four infusions of CD30.CAR-T cells. There were no toxicities reported that were deemed attributable to the CAR-T cells, including no reports of cytokine release syndrome. Of note, none of the patients received lymphodepleting conditioning chemotherapy, which may have contributed to the lack of overall adverse events and also the lower number of overall responses.

Another phase I trial enrolled 18 relapsed/refractory patients, 17 of whom had cHL and 1 had cutaneous ALCL [96]. Five of these patients were brentuximab refractory. They received CD30.CAR-T with a 41BB endodomain at intended total doses varying from 1×10^7 to 3×10^7 CAR-T/kg. The patients received one of three forms of conditioning chemotherapy regimens of either fludarabine-cyclophosphamide, gemcitabine-mustargen-cyclophosphamide, or nab-paclitaxel-cyclophosphamide. qPCR was again used to detect the persistence of CD30.CAR-T, which showed similar peak levels of CAR-T cells at 6–9 days and decreasing to negligible levels 4–8 weeks post-infusion. In total, seven patients achieved a PR and six had SD with a median PFS of 6 months. Two of the PR patients who had received a second infusion of CD30.CAR-T had ongoing PR after 12+ months. No statistical difference was detected between the three different conditioning chemotherapy regimens, though all three regimens caused varying levels of cytopenias in all patients. One patient had grade 3 toxicity with liver transaminase abnormalities, and one patient had grade 4 cardiac toxicity felt to be more due to receiving a high dose of cumulative anthracycline in the past. The most common CAR-T-related adverse events were nausea and vomiting (28%), urticarial-like rash (11%), followed by breathlessness, psychiatric disturbances, and pneumonitis (all ~6%). These adverse events mostly occurred 1–3 weeks post-infusion. The levels of various cytokines were also measured, such as TNFα, IL2, IL4, IL6, and IL12. While there was a significant increase in TNFα and IL12 1-week post-infusion of CAR-T, it did not correlate with the observed clinical responses of patients. The other cytokines did not show any dramatic change in levels.

Several CD30.CAR-T clinical trials are underway currently to further investigate its efficacy (Table 3.1). While the published results are suboptimal to date, they do offer optimism as a potential avenue for treating relapsed/refractory CD30+ disease. Preclinical studies investigating how to augment efficacy show promise in improving the functionality of CD30.CAR-T. Since almost 40% of Hodgkin patients express EBV-associated antigens on their RS tumor cells, the aforementioned technique of altering EBV-CTLs to express a concurrent CD30.CAR alongside the native EBV antigen-targeting TCR could be a modality in improving the treatment of cHL [94]. Another innovative approach by the same research group tested methods of improving the homing mechanisms of CD30.CAR-T. RS cells are known to produce the chemokines CCL17 (also known as thymus- and activation-regulated chemokine or TARC) and CCL22 (also known as macrophage-derived chemokine or MDC). CCL17 and CCL22 attract Th2 cells and Tregs via binding to their chemokine receptor CCR4,

Table 3.1 Ongoing CD30.CAR trials. A list of ongoing clinical trials both in the United States and internationally with CD30-targeting CAR-T cell therapy

ClinicalTrial.gov identifier	Study title	Lymphoma subtypes included in trial	Institution/location
NCT03049449	T Cells Expressing a Fully Human Anti-CD30 CAR for CD30-Expressing Lymphomas	$CD30^+$ HL, ALCL, and NHL	National Cancer Institute, Bethesda, MD, USA
NCT02917083	CD30 CAR-T Cells, Relapsed CD30-Expressing Lymphoma (RELY-30)	$CD30^+$ HL, ALCL, and NHL	Baylor College of Medicine; Houston Methodist Hospital; Texas Children's Hospital, Houston, TX, USA
NCT02274584	CAR-T cells Targeting CD30-Positive Lymphomas (4SCAR30273)	$CD30^+$ HL, ALCL, and NHL	University of Florida, Gainesville, USA; Peking University Cancer Hospital, Beijing, China
NCT02690545	Study of CD30 CAR-T Cell Therapy for Relapsed/Refractory $CD30^+$ HL and $CD30^+$NHL	$CD30^+$ HL, ALCL, and NHL	Lineberger Comprehensive Cancer Center at University of North Carolina at Chapel Hill, NC, USA
NCT02663297	Administration of T Lymphocytes for Prevention of Relapse of $CD30^+$ Lymphomas After High-Dose Therapy and Autologous Stem Transplantation	$CD30^+$ HL, $CD30^+$ NHL, or $CD30^+$ lymphoproliferative disorders	Lineberger Comprehensive Cancer Center, University of North Carolina at Chapel Hill, USA
NCT02958410	Study of CD30-Targeted CAR-T Cells in Lymphoid Malignancies	$CD30^+$ HL, ALCL, and NHL	Southwest Hospital of Third Military Medical University, Chongqing, China
NCT02259556	CD30-Directed CAR-T Cell (CART30) Therapy in Patients with Relapsed and/or Refractory CD30-Positive Lymphomas	$CD30^+$ HL, ALCL and NHL	Chinese PLA General Hospital, Beijing, China
NCT03383965	A Clinical Study of CD30 Targeted CAR-T in Treating CD30-Expressing Lymphomas	$CD30^+$ HL, ALCL, and NHL	Weifang People's Hospital Weifang, Shandong, China

where these cells then help to create an immunosuppressive tumor microenvironment around the RS cells. Conversely, cytotoxic CD8+ effector cells lack CCR4, resulting in a chemokine receptor mismatch and inability to traffic across the CCL17/CCL22 gradient. This paucity of tumoricidal cellular elements within Hodgkin lymphoma sites contributes to the hampered inflammatory immune response to HL. Preclinical experiments have also examined reengineering CD30.CAR-T cells to forcibly express

CCR4. These modified CCR4-CD30.CAR-T demonstrated enhanced migration to tumor sites and augmented tumor cytotoxicity in mice engrafted with human HL [97]. Incorporating these mechanisms, along with the exploration of additional cellular processes, could help boost and improve CD30.CAR-T efficacy.

PD-1 Checkpoint Inhibitors

PD-1 is an inhibitory receptor expressed by activated T cells on the cell surface [98]. It has two ligands, PD-L1 and PD-L2, which are highly overexpressed in several solid tumors and hematological malignancies. The chromosomal locus 9p24.1 contains the genes for PD-L1 and PD-L2. Studies show cHL RS cells possessing aberrations in the PD-1/PD-L1 pathway, exhibiting copy number gains of 9p24.1 which correlated with increased PD-L1/L2 expression in RS cells [25, 26]. In addition, the same 9p24.1 locus contains the gene for JAK2, and increased JAK2 expression has been shown to generate increased PD-L1/L2 expression as well [25]. Furthermore, tumor-associated macrophages can accumulate at lymphoma sites and also upregulate their PD-L1 expression, synergistically enriching immunosuppression within the tumor microenvironment [27]. As a result, studies have begun investigating PD-1 checkpoint inhibition, primarily with pembrolizumab and nivolumab. They are both anti-PD-1, humanized IgG4, PD-1 blocking antibodies which have FDA approval for use in solid malignancies such as melanoma and non-small cell lung cancers.

Nivolumab was first examined in a phase I report with relapsed/refractory cHL patients. The ORR in 23 patients was 87% with a CR rate of 17% [28]. A subsequent single-arm phase II study with 80 patients who had also previously failed both auto-SCT and brentuximab treatments showed an ORR 66% with CR rate of 8.8% at a median follow-up of 8.9 months [29]. PFS and OS at 6 months were 77% and 99%, respectively, with an estimated median duration of response of 7.8 months.

Not surprisingly, pembrolizumab has displayed similar levels of efficacy as nivolumab in cHL studies. A phase II trial with 210 relapsed/refractory patients demonstrated ORR of 69% with a CR rate of 22.4% [30]. On subgroup analysis, patients who had relapsed after auto-SCT and BV treatments showed an ORR of 74% and CR rate of 22%. Patients who were ineligible for auto-SCT but received BV had ORR and CR rates of 64% and 25%, respectively. Those who had received an auto-SCT but no BV had ORR and CR rates of 70% and 20%, respectively. The estimated 9-month PFS and OS rates were 63% and 98%, respectively.

Based on the preceding promising results, further trials are underway to implement these checkpoint inhibitors. One ongoing phase III trial is comparing the combination of nivolumab and BV to BV alone in relapsed/refractory patients who are either post-auto-SCT or transplant ineligible (NCT03138499). Another phase III study in progress is investigating pembrolizumab in comparison to BV in relapsed/refractory cHL patients (NCT02684292). Currently, checkpoint inhibition with nivolumab or pembrolizumab is FDA approved in the relapsed/refractory setting and especially represents a viable treatment alternative for patients who have failed auto-SCT and/or BV (Fig. 3.3).

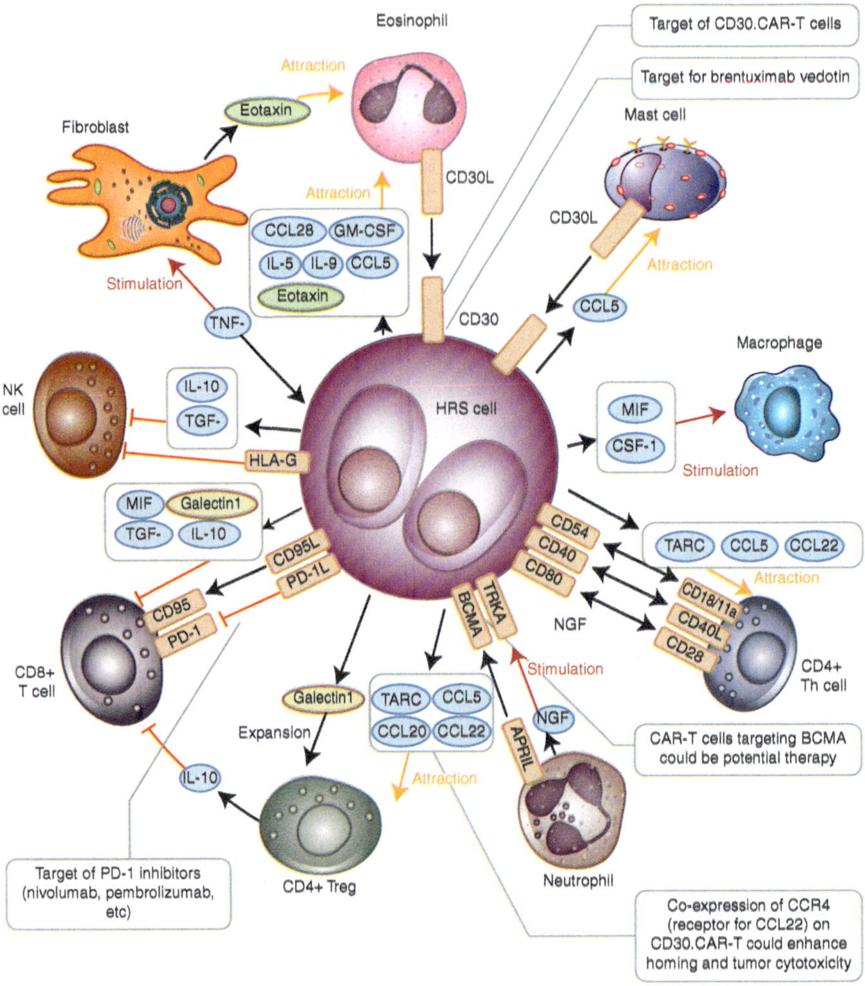

Fig. 3.3 Immunosuppression and immune targets in Hodgkin lymphoma. Hodgkin Reed-Sternberg (HRS) cells employ a variety of immunosuppressive mechanisms within the tumor microenvironment, including cytokine secretion and inhibitory cell surface marker expression. Some of these mechanisms and markers can be targeted by CAR-T cells or other immunotherapies

Conclusion

cHL and ALCL are generally associated with a very good prognosis and high cure rate with frontline therapy. Salvage chemotherapy with auto-SCT offers additional, high chance of cure in the minority of patients that do relapse or are refractory. However, until recently there were very limited treatments for patients with multiple relapsed/refractory disease, with available options only providing very short-term disease control and inevitable relapse. With the advent of new biologic and cellular immunotherapies targeting CD30 like brentuximab and CAR-T, there has been a significant expansion in the treatment armament for these diseases. Clinical trials with these agents have shown great promise and, in the case of brentuximab, have already been approved for use in patients for both frontline and second-line treatments. CD30-directed immunotherapy has also expanded beyond use in cHL and ALCL to other NHL subtypes that occasionally also positively express CD30. With such a potentially broad spectrum of relapsed/refractory lymphoma to treat, CD30-directed immunotherapy can have extensive clinical utility and tangible long-term efficacy and represent a very viable modality for exerting excellent disease control and potential cure for these patients in the very near future.

References

1. Stein H, Mason D, Gerdes J, et al. The expression of the Hodgkin's disease associated antigen Ki-1 in reactive and neoplastic lymphoid tissue: evidence that Reed-Sternberg cells and histiocytic malignancies are derived from activated lymphoid cells. Blood. 1985;66(4):848–58.
2. Horie R, Watanabe T. CD30: expression and function in health and disease. Semin Immunol. 1998;10(6):457–70.
3. Hodgkin Lymphoma [Internet]. National Cancer Institute, Bethesda. Available from: https://seer.cancer.gov/statfacts/html/hodg.html.
4. Grufferman S, Cole P, Smith PG, Lukes RJ. Hodgkin's disease in siblings. N Engl J Med. 1977;296(5):248–50.
5. Cozen W, Katz J, Mack TM. Risk patterns of Hodgkin's disease in Los Angeles vary by cell type. Cancer Epidemiol Biomark Prev. 1992;1(4):261.
6. Swerdlow SH, Campo E, Harris NL, Jaffe ES, et al. WHO classification of tumours of haematopoietic and lymphoid tissues. In: Press I, editor. . Lyon: International Agency for Research on Cancer; 2008.
7. Gopas J, Stern E, Zurgil U, Ozer J, et al. Reed-Sternberg cells in Hodgkin's lymphoma present features of cellular senescence. Cell Death Dis. 2016;7(11):e2457.
8. Schmitz R, Stanelle J, Hansmann ML, Küppers R. Pathogenesis of classical and lymphocyte–predominant Hodgkin lymphoma. Annu Rev Pathol. 2009;4:151–74.
9. Marafioti T, Hummel M, Foss HD, Laumen H, et al. Hodgkin and Reed-Sternberg cells represent an expansion of a single clone originating from a germinal center B-cell with functional immunoglobulin gene rearrangements but defective immunoglobulin transcription. Blood. 2000;95(4):1443–50.
10. Stein H, Marafioti T, Foss HD, Laumen H, et al. Down-regulation of BOB.1/OBF.1 and Oct2 in classical Hodgkin disease but not in lymphocyte predominant Hodgkin disease correlates with immunoglobulin transcription. Blood. 2001;97(2):496–501.
11. Hjalgrim H, Engels E. Infectious aetiology of Hodgkin and non-Hodgkin lymphomas: a review of the epidemiological evidence. J Intern Med. 2008;264(6):537–48.
12. Anagnostopoulos I, Herbst H, Niedobitek G, Stein H. Demonstration of monoclonal EBV genomes in Hodgkin's disease and Ki-1- positive anaplastic large cell lymphoma by combined Southern blot and in situ hybridization. Blood. 1989;74(2):810–6.
13. Bechtel D, Kurth J, Unkel C, Küppers R. Transformation of BCR-deficient germinal-center B cells by EBV supports a major role of the virus in the pathogenesis of Hodgkin and posttransplantation lymphomas. Blood. 2005;106(13):4345–50.
14. Kilger E, Kieser A, Baumann M, Hammerschmidt W. Epstein-Barr virus-mediated B-cell proliferation is dependent upon latent membrane protein 1, which simulates an activated CD40 receptor. EMBO J. 1998;17(6):1700–9.

15. Joos S, Küpper M, Ohl S, von Bonin F, et al. Genomic imbalances including amplification of the tyrosine kinase gene JAK2 in CD30+ Hodgkin cells. Cancer Res. 2000;60(3):549–52.
16. Martin-Subero JI, Gesk S, Harder L, Sonoki T, et al. Recurrent involvement of the REL and BCL11A loci in classical Hodgkin lymphoma. Blood. 2002;99(4):1474–7.
17. Bargou RC, Emmerich F, Krappman D, Bommert K, et al. Constitutive nuclear factor-kappaB-RelA activation is required for proliferation and survival of Hodgkin's disease tumor cells. J Clin Invest. 1997;100(12):2961–9.
18. Otto C, Giefing M, Massow A, Vater I, et al. Genetic lesions of the TRAF3 and MAP3K14 genes in classical Hodgkin lymphoma. Br J Haematol. 2012;157(6):702–8.
19. Schmitz R, Hansmann M, Bohle V, Martin-Subero JI, et al. TNFAIP3 (A20) is a tumor suppressor gene in Hodgkin lymphoma and primary mediastinal B cell lymphoma. J Exp Med. 2009;206(5):981–9.
20. Weniger MA, Melzner I, Menz CK, Wegener S, et al. Mutations of the tumor suppressor gene SOCS-1 in classical Hodgkin lymphoma are frequent and associated with nuclear phospho-STAT5 accumulation. Oncogene. 2006;25(18):2679–84.
21. Gajewski TF, Schreiber H, Fu YX. Innate and adaptive immune cells in the tumor microenvironment. Nat Immunol. 2013;14(10):1014–22.
22. Baitsch L, Fuertes-Marraco S, Legat A, Meyer C, Speiser DE. The three main stumbling blocks for anticancer T cells. Trends Immunol. 2012;33(7):364–72.
23. Ishida T, Ishii T, Inagaki A, et al. Specific recruitment of CC chemokine receptor 4-positive regulatory T cells in Hodgkin lymphoma fosters immune privilege. Cancer Res. 2006;66:5716–22.
24. van den Berg A, Visser L, Poppema S. High expression of the CC chemokine TARC in Reed-Sternberg cells: a possible explanation for the characteristic T-cell infiltrate in Hodgkin's lymphoma. Am J Pathol. 1999;154:1685–91.
25. Green MR, Monti S, Rodig SJ, Juszczynski P, et al. Integrative analysis reveals selective 9p24.1 amplification, increased PD-1 ligand expression, and further induction via JAK2 in nodular sclerosing Hodgkin lymphoma and primary mediastinal large B-cell lymphoma. Blood. 2010;116(17):3268–77.
26. Roemer MG, Advani R, Ligon AH, Natkunam Y, et al. PD-L1 and PD-L2 genetic alterations define classical Hodgkin lymphoma and predict outcome. J Clin Oncol. 2016;34(23):2690–7.
27. Carey CD, Gusenleitner D, Lipschitz M, Roemer MGM, et al. Topological analysis reveals a PD-L1 associated immuno-pretective niche for Reed-Sternberg cells in Hodgkin lymphoma. Blood. 2017;130:2420–30.
28. Ansell SM, Lesokhin A, Borrello I, Halwani A, et al. PD-1 blockade with nivolumab in relapsed or refractory Hodgkin's lymphoma. N Engl J Med. 2015;372(4):311–9.
29. Younes A, Santoro A, Shipp M, Zinzani PL, et al. Nivolumab for classical Hodgkin's lymphoma after failure of both autologous stem-cell transplantation and brentuximab vedotin: a multicentre, multicohort, single-arm phase 2 trial. Lancet Oncol. 2016;17(9):1283–94.
30. Chen R, Zinzani P, Fanale MA, Armand P, et al. Phase II study of the efficacy and safety of pembrolizumab for relapsed/refractory classic Hodgkin lymphoma. J Clin Oncol. 2017;35(19):2125–32.
31. Atkinson K, Austin D, McElwain TJ, Peckham MJ. Alcohol pain in Hodgkin's disease. Cancer. 1976;37:895–9.
32. El-Galaly TC, d'Amore F, Mylam KJ, et al. Routine bone marrow biopsy has little or no therapeutic consequence for positron emission tomography/computed tomography-staged treatment-naïve patients with Hodgkin lymphoma. J Clin Oncol. 2012;30(36):4508–14.
33. Cheson BD. Role of functional imaging in the management of lymphoma. J Clin Oncol. 2011;29(19):1844–54.
34. Cheson BD, Fisher R, Barrington SF, et al. Recommendations for initial evaluation, staging, and response assessment of Hodgkin and non-Hodgkin lymphoma: the Lugano classification. J Clin Oncol. 2014;32(27):3059–68.
35. Hoppe RT, Advani R, Ai WZ, et al. Hodgkin lymphoma, version 2.2015. J Natl Compr Canc Netw. 2015;13(5):554–86.

36. Tubiana M, Henry-Amar M, Carde P, et al. Toward comprehensive management tailored to prognostic factors of patients with clinical stages I and II in Hodgkin's disease: the EORTC Lymphoma Group controlled clinical trials: 1964–1987. Blood. 1989;73(1):47–56.
37. Panel NCCNA. Hodgkin lymphoma: NCCN. 2017. Available from: https://www.nccn.org/professionals/physician_gls/pdf/hodgkins.pdf.
38. Hasenclever D, Diehl V. A prognostic score for advanced Hodgkin's disease. International prognostic factors project on advanced Hodgkin's disease. N Engl J Med. 1998;339(21):1506–14.
39. Gallamini A, Hutchings M, Rigacci L, et al. Early interim 2-[18F]fluoro-2-deoxy-D-glucose positron emission tomography is prognostically superior to international prognostic score in advanced-stage Hodgkin's lymphoma: a report front a joint Italian-Danish study. J Clin Oncol. 2007;25(24):3746–52.
40. Press OW, Li H, Schoder H, Strauss DJ, et al. US intergroup trial of response-adapted therapy for stage III to IV Hodgkin lymphoma using early interim fluorodeoxyglucose–positron emission tomography imaging: Southwest Oncology Group S0816. J Clin Oncol. 2016;34(17):2020–7.
41. Bonnadonna G, Zucali R, Monfardini S, de Lena M, Uslenghi C. Combination chemotherapy of Hodgkin's disease with adriamycin, bleomycin, vinblastine, and imidazole carboxamide versus MOPP. Cancer. 1975;36(1):252–9.
42. Diehl V, Franklin J, Pfreundschuh M, Lathan B, et al. Standard and increased-dose BEACOPP chemotherapy compared with COPP-ABVD for advanced Hodgkin's disease. N Engl J Med. 2003;348(24):2386–95.
43. Ballova V, Rüffer J, Haverkamp H, Pfistner B, et al. A prospectively randomized trial carried out by the German Hodgkin Study Group (GHSG) for elderly patients with advanced Hodgkin's disease comparing BEACOPP baseline and COPP-ABVD (GHSG HD9 study). Ann Oncol. 2005;16(1):124–31.
44. Engert A, Diehl V, Franklin J, Lohri A, et al. Escalated-dose BEACOPP in the treatment of patients with advanced-stage Hodgkin's lymphoma: 10 years of follow-up of the GHSG HD9 study. J Clin Oncol. 2009;27(27):4548–54.
45. Sieniawski M, Reineke T, Nogova L, Josting A, et al. Fertility in male patients with advanced Hodgkin lymphoma treated with BEACOPP: a report of the German Hodgkin Study Group (GHSG). Blood. 2008;111(1):71–6.
46. Armitage JO. Early stage Hodgkin's lymphoma. N Engl J Med. 2008;363(7):653–62.
47. Brenner H, Gondos A, Pulte D. Ongoing improvement in long-term survival of patients with Hodgkin disease at all ages and recent catch-up of older patients. Blood. 2008;111(6):2977–83.
48. Engert A, Plütschow A, Eich HT, Lohri A, et al. Reduced treatment intensity in patients with early-stage Hodgkin's lymphoma. N Engl J Med. 2010;363(7):640–52.
49. Meyer RM, Gospodarowicz M, Connors JM, Pearcey RG, et al. ABVD alone versus radiation-based therapy in limited-stage Hodgkin's lymphoma. N Engl J Med. 2012;366(5):399–408.
50. Eich HT, Diehl V, Görgen H, Pabst T, et al. Intensified chemotherapy and dose-reduced involved-field radiotherapy in patients with early unfavorable Hodgkin's lymphoma: final analysis of the German Hodgkin Study Group HD11 trial. J Clin Oncol. 2010;28(27):4199–206.
51. Viviani S, Zinzani P, Rambaldi A, Brusamolino E, et al. ABVD versus BEACOPP for Hodgkin's lymphoma when high-dose salvage is planned. N Engl J Med. 2011;365(3):203–12.
52. Carde P, Karrasch M, Fortpied C, et al. Eight cycles of ABVD versus four cycles of BEACOPPescalated plus four cycles of BEACOPPbaseline in stage III to IV, international prognostic score >/= 3, high-risk Hodgkin lymphoma: first results of the phase III EORTC 20012 intergroup trial. J Clin Oncol. 2016;34(17):2028–36.
53. Johnson P, Federico M, Kirkwood A, Fosså A, et al. Adapted treatment guided by interim PET-CT scan in advanced Hodgkin's lymphoma. N Engl J Med. 2016;374(25):2419–29.
54. Moskowitz CH, Nimer S, Zelenetz AD, Trippett T, et al. A 2-step comprehensive high-dose chemoradiotherapy second-line program for relapsed and refractory Hodgkin disease: analysis by intent to treat and development of a prognostic model. Blood. 2001;97(3):616–23.

55. Bartlett NL, Niedzwiecki D, Johnson JL, Friedberg JW, et al. Gemcitabine, vinorelbine, and pegylated liposomal doxorubicin (GVD), a salvage regimen in relapsed Hodgkin's lymphoma: CALGB 59804. Ann Oncol. 2007;18(6):1071–9.
56. Kuruvilla J, Nagy T, Pintilie M, Tsang R, et al. Similar response rates and superior early progression-free survival with gemcitabine, dexamethasone, and cisplatin salvage therapy compared with carmustine, etoposide, cytarabine, and melphalan salvage therapy prior to autologous stem cell transplantation for recurrent or refractory Hodgkin lymphoma. Cancer. 2006;106(2):353–60.
57. Santoro A, Mazza R, Pulsoni A, Re A, et al. Bendamustine in combination with gemcitabine and vinorelbine is an effective regimen as induction chemotherapy before autologous stem-cell transplantation for relapsed or refractory Hodgkin lymphoma: final results of a multicenter phase II study. J Clin Oncol. 2016;34(27):3293–9.
58. Brandwein JM, Callum J, Sutcliffe SB, Scott JG, et al. Evaluation of cytoreductive therapy prior to high dose treatment with autologous bone marrow transplantation in relapsed and refractory Hodgkin's disease. Bone Marrow Transplant. 1990;5(2):99.
59. Schmitz N, Pfistner B, Sextro M, Sieber M, et al. Aggressive conventional chemotherapy compared with high-dose chemotherapy with autologous haemopoietic stem-cell transplantation for relapsed chemosensitive Hodgkin's disease: a randomised trial. Lancet Oncol. 2002;359(9323):2065–71.
60. Linch DC, Winfield D, Goldstone AH, McMillan A, et al. Dose intensification with autologous bone-marrow transplantation in relapsed and resistant Hodgkin's disease: results of a BNLI randomised trial. Lancet Oncol. 1993;341(8852):1051–4.
61. Moskowitz CH, Matasar M, Zelenetz AD, Nimer SD, et al. Normalization of pre-ASCT, FDG-PET imaging with second-line, non-cross-resistant, chemotherapy programs improves event-free survival in patients with Hodgkin lymphoma. Blood. 2012;119(7):1665–70.
62. Falini B, Pileri S, Zinzani PL, et al. ALK+ lymphoma: clinico-pathological findings and outcome. Blood. 1999;93(8):2697–706.
63. Surveillance E, and End Results Program. SEER cancer statistics factsheets: anaplastic large cell lymphoma. Bethesda: National Cancer Institute; 2015.
64. Gascoyne RD, Aoun P, Wu D, Chhanabhai M, Skinnider BF, Greiner TC, et al. Prognostic significance of anaplastic lymphoma kinase (ALK) protein expression in adults with anaplastic large cell lymphoma. Blood. 1999;93(11):3913–21.
65. Savage KJ, Harris NL, Vose JM, Ullrich F, Jaffe ES, Connors JM, et al. ALK- anaplastic large-cell lymphoma is clinically and immunophenotypically different from both ALK+ ALCL and peripheral T-cell lymphoma, not otherwise specified: report from the International Peripheral T-Cell Lymphoma Project. Blood. 2008;111(12):5496–504.
66. Sibon D, Fournier M, Brière J, Lamant L, et al. Long-term outcome of adults with systemic anaplastic large-cell lymphoma treated within the Groupe d'Etude des Lymphomes de l'Adulte trials. J Clin Oncol. 2012;30(32):3939–46.
67. Fisher RI, Gaynor E, Dahlberg S, et al. Comparison of a standard regimen (CHOP) with three intensive chemotherapy regimens for advanced non-Hodgkin's lymphoma. N Engl J Med. 1993;328(14):1002–6.
68. Schmitz N, Trümper L, Ziepert M, et al. Treatment and prognosis of mature T-cell and NK-cell lymphoma: an analysis of patients with T-cell lymphoma treated in studies of the German High-Grade Non-Hodgkin Lymphoma Study Group. Blood. 2012;116(18):3418–25.
69. Slack GW, Steidl C, Sehn LH, et al. CD30 expression in de novo diffuse large B-cell lymphoma: a population-based study from British Columbia. Br J Haematol. 2014;167(5):608–17.
70. Sabattini E, Pizzi M, Tabanelli V, et al. CD30 expression in peripheral T-cell lymphomas. Haematologica. 2013;98(8):81–2.
71. Ansell SM, Horwitz S, Engert A, et al. Phase I/II study of an anti-CD30 monoclonal antibody (MDX-060) in Hodgkin's lymphoma and anaplastic large-cell lymphoma. J Clin Oncol. 2007;25(19):2764–9.

72. Younes A, Bartlett N, Leonard JP, et al. Brentuximab vedotin (SGN-35) for relapsed CD30-positive lymphomas. N Engl J Med. 2010;363(19):1812–21.
73. Younes A, Gopal A, Smith SE, et al. Results of a pivotal phase II study of brentuximab vedotin for patients with relapsed or refractory Hodgkin's lymphoma. J Clin Oncol. 2012;30(18):2183–9.
74. Gopal AK, Chen R, Smith SE, et al. Durable remissions in a pivotal phase 2 study of brentuximab vedotin in relapsed or refractory Hodgkin lymphoma. Blood. 2015;125(8):1236–43.
75. Moskowitz CH, Nademanee A, Masszi T, et al. Brentuximab vedotin as consolidation therapy after autologous stem-cell transplantation in patients with Hodgkin's lymphoma at risk of relapse or progression (AETHERA): a randomised, double-blind, placebo-controlled, phase 3 trial. Lancet Oncol. 2015;385(9980):1853–62.
76. Administration UFaD. Brentuximab vedotin information. In: Administration USFaD, editor. Silver Spring: US FDA; 2015.
77. O'Connor OA, Lue J, Sawas A, Amengual JE, et al. Brentuximab vedotin plus bendamustine in relapsed or refractory Hodgkin's lymphoma: an international, multicentre, single-arm, phase 1–2 trial. Lancet Oncol. 2018;19(2):257–66.
78. LaCasce AS, Bociek RG, Sawas A, Caimi P, Agura E, Matous J, et al. Brentuximab vedotin plus bendamustine: a highly active first salvage regimen for relapsed or refractory Hodgkin lymphoma. Blood. 2018;132(1):40–8.
79. Younes A, Connors J, Park SI, Fanale M, et al. Brentuximab vedotin combined with ABVD or AVD for patients with newly diagnosed Hodgkin's lymphoma: a phase 1, open-label, dose-escalation study. Lancet Oncol. 2013;14(13):1348–56.
80. Connors JM, Jurczak W, Straus DJ, Ansell SM, et al. Brentuximab vedotin with chemotherapy for stage III or IV Hodgkin's lymphoma. N Engl J Med. 2018;378(4):331–44.
81. Fanale MA, Horwitz SM, Forero-Torres A, Bartlett NL, Advani RH, Pro B, et al. Five-year outcomes for frontline brentuximab vedotin with CHP for CD30-expressing peripheral T-cell lymphomas. Blood. 2018;131(19):2120–4.
82. Horwitz S, O'Connor OA, Pro B, Illidge T, Fanale M, Advani R, et al. Brentuximab vedotin with chemotherapy for CD30-positive peripheral T-cell lymphoma (ECHELON-2): a global, double-blind, randomised, phase 3 trial. Lancet (London, England). 2019;393(10168):229–40.
83. Dotti G, Gottschalk S, Savoldo B, Brenner M. Design and development of therapies using chimeric antigen receptor-expressing T cells. Immunol Rev. 2014;257(1):107–26.
84. Kochenderfer JN, Feldman S, Zhao Y, Xu H, et al. Construction and preclinical evaluation of an anti-CD19 chimeric antigen receptor. J Immunother. 2009;32(7):689–702.
85. van der Stegen SJ, Hamieh M, Sadelain M. The pharmacology of second-generation chimeric antigen receptors. Nat Rev Drug Discov. 2015;14(7):499–509.
86. Till BG, Jensen M, Wang J, Chen EY, et al. Adoptive immunotherapy for indolent non-Hodgkin lymphoma and mantle cell lymphoma using genetically modified autologous CD20-specific T cells. Blood. 2008;112(6):2261–71.
87. Jensen MC, Popplewell L, Cooper LJ, DiGiusto D, et al. Antitransgene rejection responses contribute to attenuated persistence of adoptively transferred CD20/CD19-specific chimeric antigen receptor redirected T cells in humans. Transplantation. 2010;16(9):1245–56.
88. Geldres C, Savoldo B, Dotti G. Chimeric antigen receptor-redirected T cells return to the bench. Semin Immunol. 2016;28(1):3–9.
89. Kochenderfer JN, Dudley M, Feldman SA, Wilson WH, et al. B-cell depletion and remissions of malignancy along with cytokine-associated toxicity in a clinical trial of anti-CD19 chimeric-antigen-receptor-transduced T cells. Blood. 2012;119(12):2709–20.
90. Brentjens RJ, Riviere I, Park JH, Davila ML, et al. Safety and persistence of adoptively transferred autologous CD19-targeted T cells in patients with relapsed or chemotherapy refractory B-cell leukemias. Blood. 2011;118(18):4817–28.
91. Kalos M, Levine B, Porter DL, Katz S, et al. T cells with chimeric antigen receptors have potent antitumor effects and can establish memory in patients with advanced leukemia. Sci Transl Med. 2011;3(95):95ra73.

92. Brudno JN, Kochenderfer J. Chimeric antigen receptor T-cell therapies for lymphoma. Nat Rev Clin Oncol. 2018;15(1):31–46.
93. Gattinoni L, Finkelstein S, Klebanoff CA, et al. Removal of homeostatic cytokine sinks by lymphodepletion enhances the efficacy of adoptively transferred tumor-specific CD8+ T cells. J Exp Med. 2005;202(7):907–12.
94. Savoldo B, Rooney C, Di Stasi A, Abken H, et al. Epstein Barr virus specific cytotoxic T lymphocytes expressing the anti-CD30zeta artificial chimeric T-cell receptor for immunotherapy of Hodgkin disease. Blood. 2007;110(7):2620–30.
95. Ramos CA, Ballard B, Zhang H, Dakhova O, et al. Clinical and immunological responses after CD30-specific chimeric antigen receptor-redirected lymphocytes. J Clin Invest. 2017;127(9):3462–71.
96. Wang CM, Wu Z, Wang Y, Guo YL, et al. Autologous T cells expressing CD30 chimeric antigen receptors for relapsed or refractory Hodgkin lymphoma: an open-label phase I trial. Clin Cancer Res. 2017;23(5):1156–66.
97. Di Stasi A, De Angelis B, Rooney CM, Zhang L, et al. T lymphocytes coexpressing CCR4 and a chimeric antigen receptor targeting CD30 have improved homing and antitumor activity in a Hodgkin tumor model. Blood. 2009;113(25):6392–402.
98. Baumeister SH, Freeman G, Dranoff G, Sharpe AH. Coinhibitory pathways in immunotherapy for cancer. Annu Rev Immunol. 2016;34:539–73.

Chapter 4
Chronic Lymphocytic Leukemia with Alterations in *TP53*

Catherine C. Coombs

Introduction

Chronic lymphocytic leukemia (CLL) is the most prevalent leukemia in the Western world. In the United States, there are approximately 20,000 new cases diagnosed annually [1]. The disease generally occurs in older individuals with a median age of 70 years and is more commonly seen in men than women. CLL presents heterogeneously, with most patients being diagnosed incidentally after routine blood work demonstrates an elevated white blood cell count. However, other patients can present more dramatically with advanced disease, manifesting as bulky lymphadenopathy, hepatosplenomegaly, symptomatic bone marrow failure, or constitutional symptoms such as fevers, weight loss, or night sweats. The diagnosis of CLL can generally be made from peripheral blood flow cytometry demonstrating a characteristic immunophenotype (CD5+, CD19+, CD23+, with dim CD20) in more than 5000/L clonal B-cells. However, given that mantle cell lymphoma can rarely mimic CLL [2], cytogenetic testing excluding the presence of an (11;14) translocation is necessary for full confirmation. In patients with lymphadenopathy and pathology showing the same immunophenotype as above, but who have less than 5000/L circulating clonal B-cells, the diagnosis would be more accurately called small lymphocytic lymphoma (SLL), which is considered the same disease as CLL. Computed tomography (CT) scans are not routinely indicated in patients with early-stage CLL given that imaging does not improve survival and can detect

C. C. Coombs (✉)
Department of Medicine, Division of Hematology and Oncology, University of North Carolina at Chapel Hill, Chapel Hill, NC, USA
e-mail: Catherine_coombs@med.unc.edu

C. Dittus (ed.), *Novel Therapeutics for Rare Lymphomas*,
https://doi.org/10.1007/978-3-030-25610-4_4

incidental findings leading to costly and risky interventions [3]. In the absence of cytopenias, a bone marrow biopsy and aspirate at the time of diagnosis is not necessary.

Recurrent cytogenetic abnormalities are demonstrated in CLL; the most common aberrations are 13q deletions, trisomy 12, 11q deletions, and 17p deletions (listed from most favorable to least favorable prognostically) [4]. A normal karyotype carries a prognosis intermediate between an isolated 13q deletion(s) and trisomy 12. Demonstration of cytogenetic abnormalities is ideally performed with both fluorescence in situ hybridization (FISH) testing and karyotyping, given that the latter can detect complex karyotypic abnormalities not included in routine CLL FISH panels and which lead to an independent adverse effect on prognosis [5–7]. Stimulation of CLL cells in vitro leads to improved reliability of conventional karyotyping [8]. 17p deletions are only present in 5–10% of patients at initial diagnosis and thus constitute a rare, but clinically important, subset of CLL patients [4, 9].

Recent data also support the utility of molecular testing, with either Sanger-based sequencing or next-generation sequencing, to detect *TP53* mutations that would not be detected on cytogenetic analysis. Detected variants should be cross-referenced with locus-specific databases to ensure pathogenic variants are being reported [10]. *TP53* mutations, in absence of 17p deletions, occur in approximately 5% of treatment-naïve patients [11, 12]. Most commonly, patients have biallelic inactivation of *TP53*, usually with a 17p deletion on one allele and a *TP53* mutation on the other allele, though monoallelic inactivation carries a similarly poor prognostic impact [12, 13]. Even small *TP53*-mutated subclones present at the time of diagnosis have been linked with poorer survival [14, 15].

TP53 aberrations, as detected both by conventional cytogenetic and molecular testing, are significantly more common in the relapsed/refractory setting and may be present in up to half of patients [16]. This emphasizes the need to repeat both cytogenetic and molecular testing at the time of each new therapy in patients who did not have previously documented *TP53* aberrations. These changes arise due to clonal evolution leading to the acquisition of new abnormalities [17, 18] and/or outgrowth of small, previously undetectable clones [19].

IGHV mutation testing and B2-microglobulin are useful tests to send at time of diagnosis, as these can allow for calculation of the patient's CLL International Prognostic Index (CLL-IPI) score (Table 4.1). This is a prognostic model that stratifies patients into one of four risk groups (low, intermediate, high, and very high), developed based on 3472 treatment-naïve patients and validated by other groups [20–22]. Prognosis for patients in the lowest-risk group is excellent, with 93% of patients being alive at 5 years, compared to 23% for patients in the highest-risk group. The survival estimates from this model were generated from data in a pre-novel small-molecule inhibitor setting, so the model may overestimate the impact on survival for adverse features in setting of newer, effective therapies [23]. Note that presence of a *TP53* aberration places a patient at a minimum in the high-risk group given the weight assigned to presence of a 17p deletion or *TP53* mutation [20].

Prior to recent introduction of novel small-molecule inhibitors, which will be discussed at length in this chapter, treatment outcomes for *TP53*-aberrant CLL have

Table 4.1 CLL International Prognostic Index (CLL-IPI) score

Variable	Adverse factor	Points
Age	>65	1
Clinical stage	Rai I–IV or Binet B–C	1
B_2-microglobulin	>3.5 mg/L	2
IGHV mutation status	Unmutated (<2% difference with germline)	2
Deletion of 17p and/or *TP53* mutation	Present	4
Risk	**Score**	**5-year OS (%)**
Low	0–1	93.2
Intermediate	2–3	79.3
High	4–6	63.3
Very high	7–10	23.3

OS overall survival

been dismal. Standard cytotoxic chemotherapy and chemoimmunotherapy in patients with *TP53*-aberrant CLL are associated with low overall response rates (ORR), near absent attainment of complete remission (CR), short progression-free survival (PFS), and poor overall survival (OS) [24–26].

Non-cytotoxic Treatment Approaches

Agents Available Prior to Novel Small-Molecule Inhibitors

Alemtuzumab

Alemtuzumab, a humanized monoclonal antibody against CD52, was first noted to demonstrate activity in *TP53*-aberrant CLL as a monotherapy in a single patient [27] and in a series of patients [28], suggesting a mechanism of action independent of *TP53*. This was followed by a phase 3 study (CAM307) comparing alemtuzumab to chlorambucil in 297 relapsed/refractory CLL patients, where it showed an improved ORR among the 21 patients with 17p deletions [64% (7/11) vs. 20% (2/10)], although this was not statistically significant for this small subset ($p = 0.08$) [29]. Alemtuzumab has also been combined with rituximab in both the upfront and relapsed/refractory settings, though with a paucity of *TP53*-aberrant patients in these studies [30, 31]. One frontline patient had a partial response (PR) followed by Richter's transformation and death, while another achieved a minimal residual disease (MRD)-negative CR. The one relapsed patient with 17p deletion had a PR. Alemtuzumab has significant toxicities including, though not limited to, infusion-related events, neutropenia, and cytomegalovirus (CMV) reactivation [29–32].

High-Dose Steroids plus Rituximab

The combination of high-dose methylprednisone and rituximab achieved an impressive ORR (96%) when studied in the frontline setting [33]. However, only one patient in this study had a 17p deletion, achieving a PR. The single 17p-deleted patient in a study of relapsed/refractory CLL did not respond [34], though another relapsed/refractory study enrolled one 17p patient, who achieved a nodular PR [35]. Overall, with the paucity of 17p patients treated with this regimen, it is unlikely to play an extensive role in the therapeutic armamentarium in light of multiple effective novel small-molecule inhibitors.

Lenalidomide

Lenalidomide is an immunomodulatory agent that has been studied extensively in CLL. In the frontline setting, single-agent lenalidomide was associated with an increased risk of death when compared to chlorambucil, leading to discontinuation of the phase 3 study (the ORIGIN trial) [36]. In the relapsed/refractory setting, it has been studied in combination with rituximab, demonstrating an ORR of 66%, with a 53% ORR (8/15) in patients with 17p deletions [37]. In a pooled series of 208 patients on lenalidomide-based trials (both frontline and relapsed/refractory), Strati et al. demonstrated that among patients who discontinued lenalidomide due to toxicity (43 out of 208 patients), prolonged responses can be seen with median time to next treatment of 40 months (despite median time of lenalidomide exposure of 11 months), suggesting that this agent may lead to sustained responses [37]. However, only 3 of the 43 patients reviewed had 17p deletions [37]. Lenalidomide can be associated with tumor lysis syndrome (TLS) and tumor flare reactions, in addition to hematologic toxicity, which is most significant at higher doses [38]. Further, a recent study demonstrated a worse ORR to lenalidomide-based regimens in patients with *TP53* aberrations [39].

Novel Small-Molecule Inhibitors

Following several pivotal clinical trials, the CLL field has potent novel small-molecule inhibitors available for both frontline treatment and the treatment of relapsed/refractory disease, with multiple Food and Drug Administration (FDA) approvals in the last few years. Specifically, ibrutinib, a first-in-class oral covalent inhibitor of Bruton's tyrosine kinase (BTK), was approved for patients with relapsed/refractory disease in February 2014 and in patients with 17p deletions in the frontline setting in July 2014. The approval was extended to all patients with CLL, regardless of age or line of treatment, in March 2016. Idelalisib, an oral, selective small-molecule inhibitor of the delta isoform of phosphatidylinositol 3-kinase (PI3Kδ), was FDA approved for treatment of relapsed/refractory CLL in combination with rituximab in July 2014. Lastly, venetoclax, an oral small molecule inhibitor of B-cell lymphoma 2 (BCL2), was FDA approved for the treatment of relapsed/refractory CLL in patients with 17p deletions in April 2016. In June 2018, the FDA granted regular approval to venetoclax for patients with or without 17p, who have received at least one prior therapy. The details of the studies leading to these FDA approvals, in addition to ongoing studies, will be the subject of the remainder of this chapter.

Frontline Approaches

Ibrutinib

The BTK inhibitor ibrutinib is the only novel small-molecule inhibitor that has been FDA approved for the frontline treatment of CLL. The initial FDA approval for frontline use only included patients with 17p deletions, though this has subsequently been extended to all patients. Ibrutinib was first examined in the frontline setting in a phase 1b/2 study enrolling untreated elderly patients (>65 years of age) [40]. Of the 29 treatment-naïve patients, 2 had 17p deletions, both of whom had a response to ibrutinib [40]. A phase 2 study using ibrutinib was conducted in patients with *TP53* aberrations, the majority having 17p deletions ($n = 47$) and 4 having *TP53* mutations in the absence of 17p deletions [41]. Ninety-seven percent (32 of 33 evaluable patients) of the treatment-naïve patients attained a response; most responses were PRs or PRs with lymphocytosis [41]. PR with lymphocytosis is a common response in patients with CLL receiving kinase inhibitors and is not a sign of treatment failure [42, 43].

The RESONATE-2 trial, which led to the FDA approval in CLL for all patients, was a phase 3 study comparing ibrutinib to chlorambucil in treatment-naïve patients age 65 and older [44]. Notably, the trial did not enroll patients with 17p deletions, given the known inefficacy of chlorambucil in this population. This trial demonstrated an improved progression-free survival (PFS), ORR, and overall survival (OS) for ibrutinib as compared to chlorambucil.

Ibrutinib toxicity includes diarrhea (seen in 42% of ibrutinib patients in RESONATE-2), atrial fibrillation (seen in 10–16% of patients) [45, 46], bleeding (most often grade 2 or less though can be severe) [47], rash [48], hypertension [49], and rarely ventricular arrhythmias [50].

Ibrutinib has also been combined with chemoimmunotherapy, and there is an ongoing clinical trial combining ibrutinib with fludarabine, cyclophosphamide, and rituximab (FCR) chemotherapy in the frontline setting (NCT02251548). Notably, this trial excludes patients with 17p deletions, likely due to the fact that such patients are often refractory to FCR.

Idelalisib

Idelalisib, a PI3Kδ-inhibitor, has been studied in the frontline setting as well. A phase 2 study of idelalisib plus rituximab in patients 65 and older showed promising efficacy, especially in patients with *TP53* aberrations (100% ORR) [51]. However, further development of this drug in the frontline setting led to concerns regarding increased risks for multiple adverse events, including immune-mediated hepatotoxicity, pneumonitis, and colitis [52]. As a result, this drug is not currently recommended in the frontline setting, and its development in the frontline setting is not currently being pursued.

Venetoclax

The BCL2 inhibitor venetoclax is actively being studied in the frontline setting, though no completed studies have been published at time of this chapter. One study, CLL14, has published the findings from a lead-in phase administering venetoclax and obinutuzumab to 13 previously untreated CLL patients (2 with *TP53* aberrations) with significant comorbid conditions [53]. ORR at 3 months was 100% and 92% rate of peripheral blood MRD negativity at 3 months post completion of treatment. The regimen was tolerated well except with one patient with a grade 4 infusion-related reaction that discontinued study treatment [53].

Relapsed/Refractory Approaches

Ibrutinib

In patients who have not already received frontline ibrutinib, this agent is highly effective in the relapsed/refractory setting. Ibrutinib demonstrated a 71% ORR in a phase 1b/2 trial, with responses occurring in 68% (19/28) of patients with 17p deletions [54]. The PFS and OS at 26 months were 57% and 70%, respectively. Based on these findings, a phase 2 study of ibrutinib was conducted, enrolling 144 relapsed patients, all with 17p deletions (RESONATE-17) [55]. This study showed a 64% ORR at median follow-up of 11.5 months and 83% at 27.6 months. A phase 3, open-label, randomized study (RESONATE) was conducted to compare ibrutinib to ofatumumab in patients with previously treated CLL, where ibrutinib demonstrated improved PFS, OS, and ORR compared to ofatumumab [54].

With 5 years of follow-up for trials enrolling both treatment-naïve elderly patients and patients with *TP53* aberrations, the depth of response has increased over time, and the majority of patients remain progression-free. Specifically, Ahn et al. reported a 58.2% 5-year PFS for patients with *TP53* aberrations; 16 of 50 patients were relapsed/refractory and had a more rapid progression than the treatment-naïve *TP53* patients [56]. Similarly, O'Brien et al. reported a 92% 5-year PFS among treatment-naïve patients and 44% in relapsed/refractory patients, with a median PFS of 26 months in patients with 17p deletions (*TP53* mutation status not reported) [49].

Idelalisib

Idelalisib was examined as a monotherapy in a phase 1 trial of 54 heavily pretreated CLL patients, 24% of whom had *TP53* aberrations, and produced a 72% ORR, with most responses being PRs and PRs with lymphocytosis [57]. Subsequently, a phase 3 randomized study was performed in relapsed CLL patients with significant coexisting medical comorbidities, comparing rituximab with idelalisib to rituximab with placebo [58]. The idelalisib arm outperformed the placebo arm with respect to PFS (not reached vs. 5.5 months, $p < 0.001$), ORR (81% vs. 13%, $p < 0.001$), and OS at 12 months (92% vs. 80%, $p = 0.02$) [58]. The PFS benefit of idelalisib was seen in the 96 patients with 17p deletions and/or *TP53* mutations [HR for disease progression or death = 0.12 (CI of 0.05–0.32)] [58]. A phase 3 randomized study was conducted to compare idelalisib with bendamustine and rituximab (BR) to BR alone in relapsed CLL patients who were candidates for intensive chemotherapy [59]. The idelalisib arm demonstrated superior PFS (20.8 months vs. 11.1 months), (hazard ratio [HR] 0.33, 95% CI 0.25–0.44; $p < 0.0001$) though with an increased number of infections, serious adverse reactions, and deaths in the idelalisib arm [59]. The improved response rate was seen in the 137 patients with *TP53* aberrations, with median PFS for idelalisib arm of 11.3 months vs. 8.3 months for the BR arm (HR, 0.47; 95% CI, 0.31, 0.72; $p < 0.0001$) [59]. Idelalisib has also been studied in combination with ofatumumab, demonstrating improved median PFS when compared to ofatumumab alone (16.3 months vs. 8.0 months, adjusted HR 0.27, 95% CI 0.19–0.39, $p < 0.0001$) [60]. Recent recommendations suggest patients getting treated with idelalisib-containing regimens should receive prophylaxis against *Pneumocystis jirovecii* pneumonia and be monitored for CMV reactivation.

Venetoclax

The phase 1 study evaluating venetoclax monotherapy in relapsed CLL patients led to an encouraging 79% ORR, with a 71% ORR and 16% CR rate in patients with 17p deletions [61]. However, TLS was a significant toxicity in this study, occurring in 10 of 56 patients (18%). TLS led to serious clinical sequelae in two patients: one required emergent hemodialysis for renal failure (after a single 50 mg dose) and another experienced sudden death (on 2nd day of stepping up to 1200 mg dose) [61].

An open-label phase 2 study of venetoclax was conducted in relapsed CLL patients with 17p deletions, which demonstrated a 79% ORR and an 8% CR/CRi rate [62]. Venetoclax has also been studied in combination with rituximab, with an 86% ORR and 51% CR rate [63]. Further, 20 of 25 of the patients attaining a CR achieved MRD negativity on bone marrow biopsies [63]. There was one death from TLS in this study after a patient was administered starting dose of 50 mg. Subsequently, patients began receiving 20 mg as a starting dose [63]. As a result of these studies, a ramp-up protocol has been designed with administration recommendations based upon the patient's TLS risk, as measured by baseline computed tomography (CT) and circulating absolute lymphocyte count (Table 4.2). Venetoclax appears to be effective in patients who have progressed on both ibrutinib and idelalisib [64, 65].

A phase 3 trial compared the efficacy of venetoclax plus rituximab (VR) to BR (MURANO trial). The VR regimen comprises the traditional 5-week venetoclax ramp-up period followed by six cycles of rituximab and then 2 years of venetoclax

Table 4.2 Tumor lysis syndrome (TLS) risk stratification and monitoring recommendations for patients initiating venetoclax [105]

Tumor burden assessment		
Low risk	All nodes <5 cm and ALC <25 × 10^9/L	
Medium risk*	Any node 5–10 cm or ALC ≥25 × 10^9/L	
High risk	Any node >10 cm or	
	Any node >5 cm and ALC ≥25 × 10^9/L	
Prophylaxis/monitoring recommendations		
Low risk	Oral hydration (1.5–2 L/day) and allopurinol	Pre-dose: TLS labs prior to every dose
		Post-dose: TLS labs 6–8 and 24 h post the 20 and 50 mg doses
Medium risk	Oral hydration (1.5–2 L/day) and allopurinol	Pre-dose: TLS labs prior to every dose
	*If a patient has a creatinine clearance of <80 mL/min, consider following "high-risk" recommendations for prophylaxis and hospital monitoring for the 20 and 50 mg doses	Post-dose: TLS labs 6–8 and 24 h post the 20 and 50 mg doses
High risk	Oral hydration (1.5–2 L/day) and IV hydration with 150–200 mL/h, as tolerated	Pre-dose: TLS labs prior to every dose
	Allopurinol and consider rasburicase if the baseline uric acid level is elevated	Post-dose instructions depend on dose level: Inpatient monitoring for the 20 and 50 mg doses Post-dose: TLS labs at 4, 8, 12, and 24 h Outpatient monitoring for subsequent dose levels Post-dose: TLS labs at 6–8 and 24 h

*A subset of patients with medium TLS risk should be treated as "high risk" if their creatinine clearance is <80

TLS labs include potassium, uric acid, phosphorus, calcium, and creatinine. Any baseline abnormalities should be corrected prior to proceeding with treatment

ALC absolute lymphocyte count, *IV* intravenous, *TLS* tumor lysis syndrome

monotherapy. Findings demonstrated that VR was superior to BR with respect to 2-year PFS (HR for progression or death, 0.17; 95% CI, 0.11–0.25; $p < 0.001$), with a high rate of MRD negativity among VR-treated patients compared to BR (62.4% vs. 13.3%, respectively, for patients achieving MRD negativity in peripheral blood at the 9-month time point) [66]. Notably, VR was superior for patients with 17p deletions and/or *TP53* mutations with median PFS not reached for both groups, compared to 15.4 months and 12.9 months for the 17p-deleted patients and *TP53*-mutated patients receiving BR, respectively [66, 67]. Based upon the MURANO study, in June 2018, the FDA granted regular approval for venetoclax for patients with and without 17p deletions, who have received at least one prior therapy. In Europe, venetoclax's approval is wider, indicated as a frontline therapy for patients with *TP53* aberrations who are unsuitable for a B-cell receptor pathway inhibitor and to patients in the relapsed setting regardless of *TP53* status.

How to Best Sequence Novel Small-Molecule Inhibitors in the Relapsed Setting

With the availability of multiple effective novel agents, a natural question that has arisen is how to best sequence these therapies [68]. Ibrutinib is the only novel small-molecule inhibitor indicated in the frontline setting at this time, but what is the best approach for patients who progress on, or are intolerant to, ibrutinib? Both retrospective and prospective data have indicated an excellent response to venetoclax following ibrutinib therapy [64, 69]. The response rate for idelalisib following ibrutinib seems lower, though numbers are too small to draw firm conclusions (venetoclax ORR of 79% versus idelalisib ORR of 46%, PFS HR 0.6 with $p = 0.06$) [69]. In absence of an appropriate clinical trial, my approach for *TP53*-aberrant CLL includes treatment with ibrutinib in the frontline setting. In the setting of progression on ibrutinib, I generally select a venetoclax-based regimen, preferably VR given the high response rate, general tolerability, and limited treatment course with this approach. Venetoclax monotherapy has a high response rate, but the current treatment paradigm includes indefinite therapy rather than a limited treatment course. Further details regarding treatment approaches are outlined in Figs. 4.1 and 4.2.

Selected Early-Phase Agents in Development

Though ibrutinib, venetoclax, and idelalisib have revolutionized the CLL field, patients can still progress and/or develop intolerance to these agents, necessitating consideration of alternative therapies. Though ibrutinib has shown a relatively low discontinuation rate within its clinical trials [70], real-world studies have demonstrated a higher rate of discontinuation (42%), most often due to toxicity/intolerance [71]. Another study showed a 51% rate of discontinuation

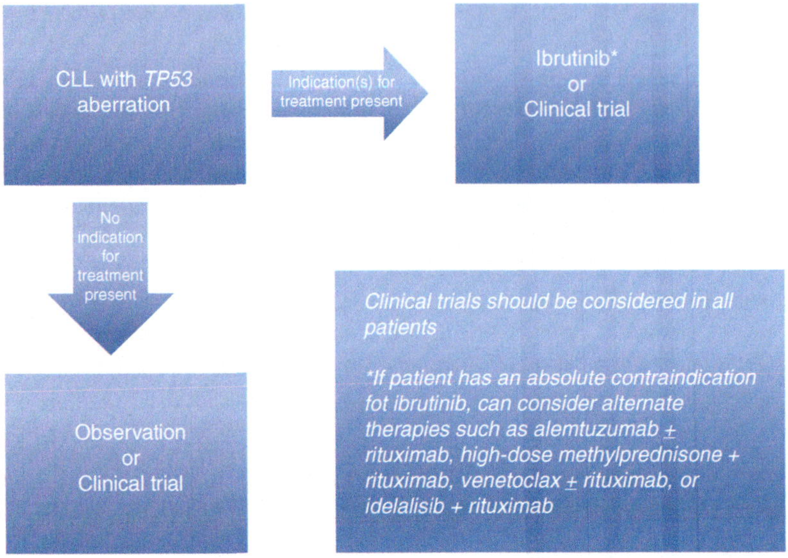

Fig. 4.1 Recommended treatment approach for untreated CLL patients with *TP53* aberrations

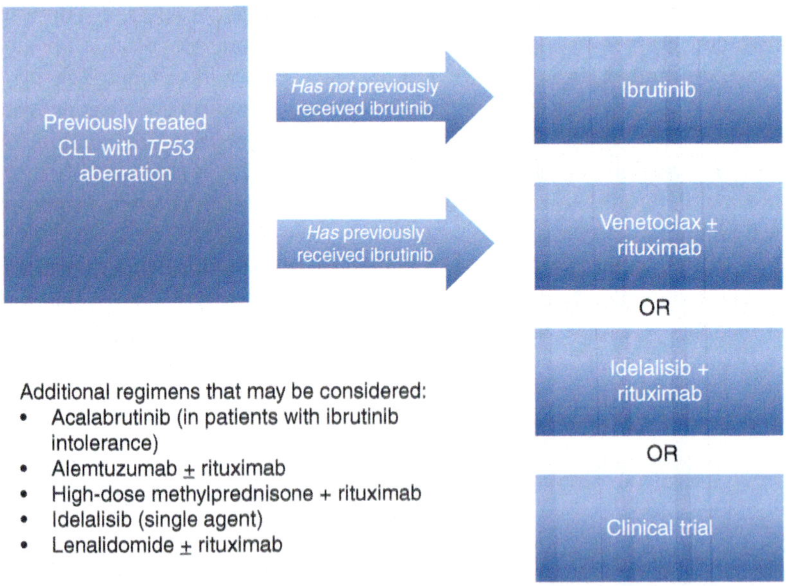

Fig. 4.2 Recommended treatment approach for previously treated CLL patients with *TP53* aberrations

due to toxicity upon reviewing patients treated with ibrutinib or idelalisib [72]. Outcomes following ibrutinib discontinuation are generally poor, with the poorest outcomes among patients who discontinue due to Richter's transformation as opposed to disease progression or intolerance [73, 74]. Ibrutinib resistance has been linked to acquired mutations in *BTK* and *PLCG2*, as demonstrated by multiple studies [75–77]. Mechanisms of idelalisib resistance have not yet been described in the literature. The mechanism behind venetoclax resistance is more variable based on limited studies to date. In a cohort of eight patients, acquired mutations in *BTG1* and *CDKN2A/B* were identified in two and three patients, respectively [78].

Newer BTK Inhibitors

Acalabrutinib

Acalabrutinib is a more selective, irreversible second-generation inhibitor of BTK that was designed to improve on the safety and efficacy of ibrutinib, given that it does not irreversibly target alternative kinases such as ITK, EGFR, and TEC. It was studied in a phase 1–2 trial in patients with relapsed CLL and led to a 95% ORR, with 85% PR and 10% PR with lymphocytosis, with a 100% ORR in patients with 17p deletions [79]. The safety profile of this agent is encouraging with no episodes of grade ≥3 bleeding and 3% of patients with atrial fibrillation in an updated analysis [80]. The agent is currently only FDA approved for mantle-cell lymphoma. A randomized, open-label non-inferiority phase 3 study comparing acalabrutinib to ibrutinib (NCT02477696) in previously treated CLL patients is currently active, but no results have been reported. An additional phase 3 study comparing acalabrutinib to investigator's choice of idelalisib with rituximab or bendamustine with rituximab, in previously treated CLL patients, is currently recruiting (NCT02970318).

ONO/GS-4059/Tirabrutinib

ONO/GS-4059/tirabrutinib is a selective BTK inhibitor, which has been tested in patients with relapsed/refractory B-cell lymphoid malignancies in a phase 1 study; 8 of 25 CLL patients had 17p deletion, and another 4 had a *TP53* mutation in absence of 17p deletion. There was a 96% ORR in the evaluable CLL patients [81]. There was one treatment-related grade 3 bleeding event among the CLL patients. Tirabrutinib is being further developed in combination with other agents including idelalisib, obinutuzumab, and entospletinib (NCT02968563, NCT02457598, and NCT02983617).

Newer PI3K Inhibitors

Duvelisib is a novel oral dual PI3K-δ and γ inhibitor that has been studied in multiple hematologic cancers, including CLL. In the phase 1 study of this compound, a 56% ORR was noted among the 55 relapsed/refractory CLL patients, including one CR [82]. Its toxicity profile appears similar to idelalisib. The drug continues to be developed, and we are currently awaiting results from a phase 3 trial comparing it to ofatumumab in relapsed/refractory CLL (NCT02004522, patients must be naïve to PI3K and BTK inhibitors).

SYK Inhibitors

Entospletinib (GS-9973) is an oral selective inhibitor of spleen tyrosine kinase (SYK), which is constitutively activated and essential for cell proliferation and survival in multiple B-cell malignancies. This agent was studied in a phase 2 trial including 41 relapsed/refractory CLL patients (ten of whom had 17p deletions or *TP53* mutations) and demonstrated a 24-week PFS of 70% (median PFS of 13.8 months) and an ORR of 61% (predominantly PRs, no CRs), with response not being statistically significantly lower among patients with 17p deletions and *TP53* mutations [83]. This study has completed enrollment though final results have not yet been reported (NCT01799889). Entospletinib has also been combined with idelalisib, though this combination was limited by a high incidence of pneumonitis (18% patients), most of which were severe [84].

CAR-T Cells

Chimeric antigen receptor-modified T-cells (CAR-T) have been an active area of clinical research for many cancer types, including CLL [85–87]. A phase 1/2 open-label clinical trial of anti-CD19 CAR-T cells in refractory CLL was performed by Turtle et al., demonstrating an ORR of 74% including 21% CR rate in a highly pretreated cohort, which included 14 patients with 17p deletions [88]. Similar findings including an ORR of 57% were obtained in a smaller study of 14 patients [89]. Toxicity of CAR-T cells can be severe, including cytokine-release syndrome and neurotoxicity [90–92].

Allogeneic Hematopoietic Stem Cell Transplantation

In this era of effective novel small-molecule inhibitors, allogeneic hematopoietic stem cell transplantation (alloHSCT) has been utilized less frequently [93, 94], including in patients with *TP53* aberrations [95]. AlloHSCT can be an effective and reasonably safe approach for younger patients with high-risk disease, including patients with *TP53* aberrations. Ten-year follow-up from CLL3X, a trial from the German CLL group [96], evaluating reduced-intensity conditioning alloHSCT in patients with HR-CLL has recently been reported [97]. This demonstrated sustained disease control in a subset of patients, with 34% disease-free survival rate at 10 years, though with a significant rate of non-relapse mortality (20%) [97]. Patients with *TP53* aberrations did not fare worse than patients without *TP53* abnormalities [97].

Richter's transformation, the transformation of CLL most often to a diffuse large B-cell lymphoma, carries a poor prognosis though patients can achieve long-term survival following alloHSCT [98]. Richter's syndrome may be more common in patients with poor-risk genetic features including 17p deletion, mutations in *TP53* and *NOTCH1*, and complex karyotype [99, 100].

Ongoing Clinical Trials Utilizing Novel Small-Molecule Inhibitors

Treatment of Asymptomatic CLL

Prior work has suggested that early treatment for patients with asymptomatic CLL does not improve survival, which is why the standard approach is close observation until an indication for treatment develops [101]. However, in the setting of less toxic, novel small-molecule inhibitors, this paradigm is being revisited (NCT0251855 and NCT01351896 are active but not recruiting, with additional studies currently in various stages of development) [102].

Current Clinical Trials Including Patients with TP53-Aberrant CLL

There are many clinical trials combining novel small-molecule inhibitors in both the frontline and relapsed/refractory setting, though the most commonly utilized combinations generally include ibrutinib, venetoclax, and/or obinutuzumab (Table 4.3). Preclinical work is suggestive of synergy between ibrutinib and venetoclax, with BTK inhibition leading to increased mitochondrial BCL-2 dependency [103, 104]. In absence of an available clinical trial, suggestions for treatment approaches for the frontline and relapsed/refractory setting are outlined in Figs. 4.1 and 4.2, respectively.

Table 4.3 Trials utilizing novel small-molecule inhibitor combinations in the (a) frontline and (b) relapsed/refractory settings

Trial	Agents	Schedule	Population	Status[a]
(a)				
Captivate NCT02910583	Ibrutinib Venetoclax	Ibrutinib monotherapy for first 3 cycles followed by combination treatment for at least 12 cycles If MRD negative: treatment is followed by either ongoing ibrutinib or ibrutinib placebo capsules If MRD positive: treatment is followed by continuous combination therapy with ibrutinib and venetoclax or ibrutinib only	Ages 18–70	Active, not recruiting
NCT02756897	Ibrutinib Venetoclax	Ibrutinib monotherapy for three cycles. At start of cycle 4, venetoclax is added as a weekly escalation. The combination continues for an additional 24 cycles	Ages 18 and older High-risk CLL (17p or 11q deletion, mutated *TP53*, unmutated IGHV, or age ≥65)	Recruiting
NCT03128879	Ibrutinib Venetoclax	Patients who have already been on ibrutinib for at least 12 months can enroll on study, where venetoclax is added as a weekly escalation while continuing ibrutinib	Ages 18 and older High-risk CLL (17p and 11q deletions, TP53 mutation, or complex karyotype) have a known ibrutinib resistance mutation without progression on ibrutinib or have not achieved B2-microglobulin normalization after a year on ibrutinib. Patients must have received at least 12 months of ibrutinib and have measurable disease	Recruiting
CLL2-GiVe NCT02758665	Ibrutinib Venetoclax Obinutuzumab	Obinutuzumab is administered for cycles 1–6. Ibrutinib is given for cycles 1–15. Venetoclax is given in cycles 1–12, introduced in escalating doses. The full dose of venetoclax (400 mg) is administered for cycles 3–12	Ages 18 and older, there are arms for both physically fit and unfit patients Patients must have 17p deletion and/or *TP53* mutation	Recruiting
(b)				
NCT02756897	Ibrutinib Venetoclax	Ibrutinib monotherapy for three cycles. At start of cycle 4, venetoclax introduced by a weekly escalation. The combination continues for an additional 24 cycles	Ages 18 and older Relapsed and/or refractory to at least one prior therapy No prior ibrutinib or venetoclax	Recruiting

Bloodwise TAP Clarity study ISCRTN13751862	Ibrutinib Venetoclax	8 weeks of ibrutinib monotherapy followed by venetoclax introduced by a weekly escalation. Patients continue on the combination for the same duration of time that it takes them to achieve MRD negativity	Relapsed within 3 years of FCR or BR or had 17p deletion and failed at least one line of therapy	Active, not recruiting[b]
NCT02427451	Ibrutinib Venetoclax Obinutuzumab	Patients receive obinutuzumab on day 1 for up to eight cycles. Cycle 2, ibrutinib is added. Cycle 3, venetoclax is initiated. Treatment continues up to 14 cycles in absence of disease progression or toxicity	Ages 18 and older Received at least one prior therapy Cannot have known BTK mutation or CLL refractory to or progressed during ibrutinib	Active, not recruiting
NCT03422393	Ibrutinib Venetoclax	Patients receive either 420, 560, or 840 mg of ibrutinib in addition to introduction of increasing doses of venetoclax	Ages 18 and older Patients must have been on ibrutinib monotherapy and experienced disease progression. Primary ibrutinib resistance is excluded	Not yet recruiting
NCT03045328	Ibrutinib Venetoclax	Patients receive ibrutinib on week 1, day 1. Venetoclax begins on week 9, day 1, and continues until week 61, day 7	Ages 18 and older No prior treatment with ibrutinib or venetoclax	Recruiting
NCT03226301	Ibrutinib Venetoclax	Patients receive ibrutinib for two cycles followed by venetoclax, which is initiated as a weekly ramp-up beginning in cycle 3 and continued through cycle 15. MRD-positive patients continue on ibrutinib monotherapy until progression/relapsed. MRD-negative patients are randomized to either continuous ibrutinib monotherapy or observation. For patients who relapse on observation period, treatment is reinitiated with ibrutinib and venetoclax for 12 cycles	Ages 18 and older Refractory to or in relapse after initial therapy No prior treatment with ibrutinib or venetoclax	Recruiting

Studies excluding patients with 17p deletions and/or TP53 mutations are not listed
MRD minimal residual disease, *BTK* Bruton's tyrosine kinase
[a]Clinical trial status was obtained from https://www.clinicaltrials.gov on March 21, 2018
[b]This study is not listed on clinicaltrials.gov though the abstract presented at the 2017 American Society of Hematology meeting indicated that all planned 50 CLL patients had been enrolled

Conclusions

The introduction of novel small-molecule inhibitors, including ibrutinib, idelalisib, and venetoclax, has changed the treatment landscape for CLL patients with *TP53* aberrations. This subset of CLL patients previously had few, if any, effective options but now has the choice of several effective agents. The prognosis of patients with *TP53* aberrations is likely improved as compared to what is predicted using the CLL-IPI model; their specific prognosis may be more clearly elucidated by incorporation of patients treated with such agents into newer prognostic models. At this time, novel agents are continued indefinitely, provided that the patient's disease is responding and the agent is being tolerated without significant toxicity. Ongoing research will help determine the role of combination therapy with novel agents, most promisingly ibrutinib and venetoclax, with many ongoing trials utilizing attainment of MRD negativity as a benchmark by which treatment discontinuation can be evaluated.

References

1. SEER Cancer Stat Facts: Chronic Lymphocytic Leukemia (CLL). 2017.
2. Ondrejka SL, Lai R, Smith SD, Hsi ED. Indolent mantle cell leukemia: a clinicopathological variant characterized by isolated lymphocytosis, interstitial bone marrow involvement, kappa light chain restriction, and good prognosis. Haematologica. 2011;96(8):1121–7.
3. Hicks LK, Bering H, Carson KR, Haynes AE, Kleinerman J, Kukreti V, et al. Five hematologic tests and treatments to question. Blood. 2014;124(24):3524–8.
4. Dohner H, Stilgenbauer S, Benner A, Leupolt E, Krober A, Bullinger L, et al. Genomic aberrations and survival in chronic lymphocytic leukemia. N Engl J Med. 2000;343(26):1910–6.
5. Puiggros A, Collado R, Calasanz MJ, Ortega M, Ruiz-Xiville N, Rivas-Delgado A, et al. Patients with chronic lymphocytic leukemia and complex karyotype show an adverse outcome even in absence of TP53/ATM FISH deletions. Oncotarget. 2017;8(33):54297–303.
6. Dubuc AM, Davids MS, Pulluqi M, Pulluqi O, Hoang K, Hernandez-Sanchez JM, et al. FISHing in the dark: how the combination of FISH and conventional karyotyping improves the diagnostic yield in CpG-stimulated chronic lymphocytic leukemia. Am J Hematol. 2016;91(10):978–83.
7. Jaglowski SM, Ruppert AS, Heerema NA, Bingman A, Flynn JM, Grever MR, et al. Complex karyotype predicts for inferior outcomes following reduced-intensity conditioning allogeneic transplant for chronic lymphocytic leukaemia. Br J Haematol. 2012;159(1):82–7.
8. Buhmann R, Kurzeder C, Rehklau J, Westhaus D, Bursch S, Hiddemann W, et al. CD40L stimulation enhances the ability of conventional metaphase cytogenetics to detect chromosome aberrations in B-cell chronic lymphocytic leukaemia cells. Br J Haematol. 2002;118(4):968–75.
9. Dewald GW, Brockman SR, Paternoster SF, Bone ND, O'Fallon JR, Allmer C, et al. Chromosome anomalies detected by interphase fluorescence in situ hybridization: correlation with significant biological features of B-cell chronic lymphocytic leukaemia. Br J Haematol. 2003;121(2):287–95.
10. Malcikova J, Tausch E, Rossi D, Sutton LA, Soussi T, Zenz T, et al. ERIC recommendations for TP53 mutation analysis in chronic lymphocytic leukemia-update on methodological approaches and results interpretation. Leukemia. 2018;32:1070–80.
11. Malcikova J, Smardova J, Rocnova L, Tichy B, Kuglik P, Vranova V, et al. Monoallelic and biallelic inactivation of TP53 gene in chronic lymphocytic leukemia: selection, impact on survival, and response to DNA damage. Blood. 2009;114(26):5307–14.

12. Zenz T, Krober A, Scherer K, Habe S, Buhler A, Benner A, et al. Monoallelic TP53 inactivation is associated with poor prognosis in chronic lymphocytic leukemia: results from a detailed genetic characterization with long-term follow-up. Blood. 2008;112(8):3322–9.
13. Zenz T, Eichhorst B, Busch R, Denzel T, Habe S, Winkler D, et al. TP53 mutation and survival in chronic lymphocytic leukemia. J Clin Oncol. 2010;28(29):4473–9.
14. Rossi D, Khiabanian H, Spina V, Ciardullo C, Bruscaggin A, Fama R, et al. Clinical impact of small TP53 mutated subclones in chronic lymphocytic leukemia. Blood. 2014;123(14):2139–47.
15. Landau DA, Carter SL, Stojanov P, McKenna A, Stevenson K, Lawrence MS, et al. Evolution and impact of subclonal mutations in chronic lymphocytic leukemia. Cell. 2013;152(4):714–26.
16. Zenz T, Habe S, Denzel T, Mohr J, Winkler D, Buhler A, et al. Detailed analysis of p53 pathway defects in fludarabine-refractory chronic lymphocytic leukemia (CLL): dissecting the contribution of 17p deletion, TP53 mutation, p53-p21 dysfunction, and miR34a in a prospective clinical trial. Blood. 2009;114(13):2589–97.
17. Shanafelt TD, Witzig TE, Fink SR, Jenkins RB, Paternoster SF, Smoley SA, et al. Prospective evaluation of clonal evolution during long-term follow-up of patients with untreated early-stage chronic lymphocytic leukemia. J Clin Oncol. 2006;24(28):4634–41.
18. Malcikova J, Stano-Kozubik K, Tichy B, Kantorova B, Pavlova S, Tom N, et al. Detailed analysis of therapy-driven clonal evolution of TP53 mutations in chronic lymphocytic leukemia. Leukemia. 2015;29(4):877–85.
19. Knittel G, Rehkamper T, Korovkina D, Liedgens P, Fritz C, Torgovnick A, et al. Two mouse models reveal an actionable PARP1 dependence in aggressive chronic lymphocytic leukemia. Nat Commun. 2017;8(1):153.
20. International CLL-IPI Working Group. An international prognostic index for patients with chronic lymphocytic leukaemia (CLL-IPI): a meta-analysis of individual patient data. Lancet Oncol. 2016;17(6):779–90.
21. Gentile M, Shanafelt TD, Rossi D, Laurenti L, Mauro FR, Molica S, et al. Validation of the CLL-IPI and comparison with the MDACC prognostic index in newly diagnosed patients. Blood. 2016;128(16):2093–5.
22. Molica S, Shanafelt TD, Giannarelli D, Gentile M, Mirabelli R, Cutrona G, et al. The chronic lymphocytic leukemia international prognostic index predicts time to first treatment in early CLL: independent validation in a prospective cohort of early stage patients. Am J Hematol. 2016;91(11):1090–5.
23. Boddu P, Ferrajoli A. Prognostic factors in the era of targeted therapies in CLL. Curr Hematol Malig Rep. 2018;13:78–90.
24. Hallek M, Fischer K, Fingerle-Rowson G, Fink AM, Busch R, Mayer J, et al. Addition of rituximab to fludarabine and cyclophosphamide in patients with chronic lymphocytic leukaemia: a randomised, open-label, phase 3 trial. Lancet. 2010;376(9747):1164–74.
25. Dohner H, Fischer K, Bentz M, Hansen K, Benner A, Cabot G, et al. p53 gene deletion predicts for poor survival and non-response to therapy with purine analogs in chronic B-cell leukemias. Blood. 1995;85(6):1580–9.
26. el Rouby S, Thomas A, Costin D, Rosenberg CR, Potmesil M, Silber R, et al. p53 gene mutation in B-cell chronic lymphocytic leukemia is associated with drug resistance and is independent of MDR1/MDR3 gene expression. Blood. 1993;82(11):3452–9.
27. Stilgenbauer S, Dohner H. Campath-1H-induced complete remission of chronic lymphocytic leukemia despite p53 gene mutation and resistance to chemotherapy. N Engl J Med. 2002;347(6):452–3.
28. Lozanski G, Heerema NA, Flinn IW, Smith L, Harbison J, Webb J, et al. Alemtuzumab is an effective therapy for chronic lymphocytic leukemia with p53 mutations and deletions. Blood. 2004;103(9):3278–81.
29. Hillmen P, Skotnicki AB, Robak T, Jaksic B, Dmoszynska A, Wu J, et al. Alemtuzumab compared with chlorambucil as first-line therapy for chronic lymphocytic leukemia. J Clin Oncol. 2007;25(35):5616–23.
30. Faderl S, Ferrajoli A, Wierda W, O'Brien S, Lerner S, Keating MJ. Alemtuzumab by continuous intravenous infusion followed by subcutaneous injection plus rituximab in the treatment of patients with chronic lymphocytic leukemia recurrence. Cancer. 2010;116(10):2360–5.

31. Frankfurt O, Ma S, Gordon L, Winter JN, Horowitz JM, Rademaker A, et al. Phase II study of alemtuzumab-rituximab therapy in previously untreated patients with chronic lymphocytic leukemia: short- and long-term outcomes. Leuk Lymphoma. 2015;56(2):315–23.
32. Keating MJ, Flinn I, Jain V, Binet JL, Hillmen P, Byrd J, et al. Therapeutic role of alemtuzumab (Campath-1H) in patients who have failed fludarabine: results of a large international study. Blood. 2002;99(10):3554–61.
33. Castro JE, James DF, Sandoval-Sus JD, Jain S, Bole J, Rassenti L, et al. Rituximab in combination with high-dose methylprednisolone for the treatment of chronic lymphocytic leukemia. Leukemia. 2009;23(10):1779–89.
34. Dungarwalla M, Evans SO, Riley U, Catovsky D, Dearden CE, Matutes E. High dose methylprednisolone and rituximab is an effective therapy in advanced refractory chronic lymphocytic leukemia resistant to fludarabine therapy. Haematologica. 2008;93(3):475–6.
35. Castro JE, Sandoval-Sus JD, Bole J, Rassenti L, Kipps TJ. Rituximab in combination with high-dose methylprednisolone for the treatment of fludarabine refractory high-risk chronic lymphocytic leukemia. Leukemia. 2008;22(11):2048–53.
36. Chanan-Khan A, Egyed M, Robak T, Martinelli de Oliveira FA, Echeveste MA, Dolan S, et al. Randomized phase 3 study of lenalidomide versus chlorambucil as first-line therapy for older patients with chronic lymphocytic leukemia (the ORIGIN trial). Leukemia. 2017;31(5):1240–3.
37. Strati P, Ferrajoli A, Wierda WG, Jain N, Thompson PA, O'Brien SM, et al. Sustained long-lasting responses after lenalidomide discontinuation in patients with chronic lymphocytic leukemia. Leukemia. 2018;32:2278–81.
38. Chanan-Khan A, Miller KC, Musial L, Lawrence D, Padmanabhan S, Takeshita K, et al. Clinical efficacy of lenalidomide in patients with relapsed or refractory chronic lymphocytic leukemia: results of a phase II study. J Clin Oncol. 2006;24(34):5343–9.
39. Takahashi K, Hu B, Wang F, Yan Y, Kim E, Vitale C, et al. Clinical implications of cancer gene mutations in patients with chronic lymphocytic leukemia treated with lenalidomide. Blood. 2018;131:1820–32.
40. O'Brien S, Furman RR, Coutre SE, Sharman JP, Burger JA, Blum KA, et al. Ibrutinib as initial therapy for elderly patients with chronic lymphocytic leukaemia or small lymphocytic lymphoma: an open-label, multicentre, phase 1b/2 trial. Lancet Oncol. 2014;15(1):48–58.
41. Farooqui MZ, Valdez J, Martyr S, Aue G, Saba N, Niemann CU, et al. Ibrutinib for previously untreated and relapsed or refractory chronic lymphocytic leukaemia with TP53 aberrations: a phase 2, single-arm trial. Lancet Oncol. 2015;16(2):169–76.
42. Woyach JA, Smucker K, Smith LL, Lozanski A, Zhong Y, Ruppert AS, et al. Prolonged lymphocytosis during ibrutinib therapy is associated with distinct molecular characteristics and does not indicate a suboptimal response to therapy. Blood. 2014;123(12):1810–7.
43. Herman SE, Niemann CU, Farooqui M, Jones J, Mustafa RZ, Lipsky A, et al. Ibrutinib-induced lymphocytosis in patients with chronic lymphocytic leukemia: correlative analyses from a phase II study. Leukemia. 2014;28(11):2188–96.
44. Burger JA, Tedeschi A, Barr PM, Robak T, Owen C, Ghia P, et al. Ibrutinib as initial therapy for patients with chronic lymphocytic leukemia. N Engl J Med. 2015;373(25):2425–37.
45. Brown JR, Moslehi J, O'Brien S, Ghia P, Hillmen P, Cymbalista F, et al. Characterization of atrial fibrillation adverse events reported in ibrutinib randomized controlled registration trials. Haematologica. 2017;102(10):1796–805.
46. Wiczer TE, Levine LB, Brumbaugh J, Coggins J, Zhao Q, Ruppert AS, et al. Cumulative incidence, risk factors, and management of atrial fibrillation in patients receiving ibrutinib. Blood Adv. 2017;1(20):1739–48.
47. Lipsky AH, Farooqui MZ, Tian X, Martyr S, Cullinane AM, Nghiem K, et al. Incidence and risk factors of bleeding-related adverse events in patients with chronic lymphocytic leukemia treated with ibrutinib. Haematologica. 2015;100(12):1571–8.
48. Iberri DJ, Kwong BY, Stevens LA, Coutre SE, Kim J, Sabile JM, et al. Ibrutinib-associated rash: a single-centre experience of clinicopathological features and management. Br J Haematol. 2018;180(1):164–6.

49. O'Brien S, Furman RR, Coutre S, Flinn IW, Burger JA, Blum K, et al. Single-agent ibrutinib in treatment-naive and relapsed/refractory chronic lymphocytic leukemia: a 5-year experience. Blood. 2018;131(17):1910–9.
50. Lampson BL, Yu L, Glynn RJ, Barrientos JC, Jacobsen ED, Banerji V, et al. Ventricular arrhythmias and sudden death in patients taking ibrutinib. Blood. 2017;129(18):2581–4.
51. O'Brien SM, Lamanna N, Kipps TJ, Flinn I, Zelenetz AD, Burger JA, et al. A phase 2 study of idelalisib plus rituximab in treatment-naive older patients with chronic lymphocytic leukemia. Blood. 2015;126(25):2686–94.
52. Lampson BL, Kasar SN, Matos TR, Morgan EA, Rassenti L, Davids MS, et al. Idelalisib given front-line for treatment of chronic lymphocytic leukemia causes frequent immune-mediated hepatotoxicity. Blood. 2016;128(2):195–203.
53. Fischer K, Al-Sawaf O, Fink AM, Dixon M, Bahlo J, Warburton S, et al. Venetoclax and obinutuzumab in chronic lymphocytic leukemia. Blood. 2017;129(19):2702–5.
54. Byrd JC, Brown JR, O'Brien S, Barrientos JC, Kay NE, Reddy NM, et al. Ibrutinib versus ofatumumab in previously treated chronic lymphoid leukemia. N Engl J Med. 2014;371(3):213–23.
55. O'Brien S, Jones JA, Coutre SE, Mato AR, Hillmen P, Tam C, et al. Ibrutinib for patients with relapsed or refractory chronic lymphocytic leukaemia with 17p deletion (RESONATE-17): a phase 2, open-label, multicentre study. Lancet Oncol. 2016;17(10):1409–18.
56. Ahn IE, Farooqui MZH, Tian X, Valdez J, Sun C, Soto S, et al. Depth and durability of response to ibrutinib in CLL: 5-year follow-up of a phase II study. Blood. 2018;131:2357–66.
57. Brown JR, Byrd JC, Coutre SE, Benson DM, Flinn IW, Wagner-Johnston ND, et al. Idelalisib, an inhibitor of phosphatidylinositol 3-kinase p110delta, for relapsed/refractory chronic lymphocytic leukemia. Blood. 2014;123(22):3390–7.
58. Furman RR, Sharman JP, Coutre SE, Cheson BD, Pagel JM, Hillmen P, et al. Idelalisib and rituximab in relapsed chronic lymphocytic leukemia. N Engl J Med. 2014;370(11):997–1007.
59. Zelenetz AD, Barrientos JC, Brown JR, Coiffier B, Delgado J, Egyed M, et al. Idelalisib or placebo in combination with bendamustine and rituximab in patients with relapsed or refractory chronic lymphocytic leukaemia: interim results from a phase 3, randomised, double-blind, placebo-controlled trial. Lancet Oncol. 2017;18(3):297–311.
60. Jones JA, Robak T, Brown JR, Awan FT, Badoux X, Coutre S, et al. Efficacy and safety of idelalisib in combination with ofatumumab for previously treated chronic lymphocytic leukaemia: an open-label, randomised phase 3 trial. Lancet Haematol. 2017;4(3):e114–e26.
61. Roberts AW, Davids MS, Pagel JM, Kahl BS, Puvvada SD, Gerecitano JF, et al. Targeting BCL2 with venetoclax in relapsed chronic lymphocytic leukemia. N Engl J Med. 2016;374(4):311–22.
62. Stilgenbauer S, Eichhorst B, Schetelig J, Coutre S, Seymour JF, Munir T, et al. Venetoclax in relapsed or refractory chronic lymphocytic leukaemia with 17p deletion: a multicentre, open-label, phase 2 study. Lancet Oncol. 2016;17(6):768–78.
63. Seymour JF, Ma S, Brander DM, Choi MY, Barrientos J, Davids MS, et al. Venetoclax plus rituximab in relapsed or refractory chronic lymphocytic leukaemia: a phase 1b study. Lancet Oncol. 2017;18(2):230–40.
64. Jones JA, Mato AR, Wierda WG, Davids MS, Choi M, Cheson BD, et al. Venetoclax for chronic lymphocytic leukaemia progressing after ibrutinib: an interim analysis of a multicentre, open-label, phase 2 trial. Lancet Oncol. 2018;19(1):65–75.
65. Coutre S, Choi M, Furman RR, Eradat H, Heffner L, Jones JA, et al. Venetoclax for patients with chronic lymphocytic leukemia who progressed during or after idelalisib therapy. Blood. 2018;131:1704–11.
66. Seymour J, Kipps T, Eichhorst B, Hillmen P, Rosario J, Assouline S, et al. Venetoclax-rituximab in relapsed or refractory chronic lymphocytic leukemia. N Engl J Med. 2018;378(12):1107–20.
67. Seymour J, Kipps T, Eichhorst B, Hillmen P, D'Rozario J, Assouline S, et al. Venetoclax plus rituximab is superior to bendamustine plus rituximab in patients with relapsed/refractory chronic lymphocytic leukemia – results from pre-planned interim analysis of the randomized phase 3 Murano study. Am Soc Hematol Meet. 2017;130:LBA-2.

68. Davids MS. How should we sequence and combine novel therapies in CLL? Hematology Am Soc Hematol Educ Program. 2017;2017(1):346–53.
69. Mato AR, Hill BT, Lamanna N, Barr PM, Ujjani CS, Brander DM, et al. Optimal sequencing of ibrutinib, idelalisib, and venetoclax in chronic lymphocytic leukemia: results from a multicenter study of 683 patients. Ann Oncol. 2017;28(5):1050–6.
70. Maddocks KJ, Ruppert AS, Lozanski G, Heerema NA, Zhao W, Abruzzo L, et al. Etiology of ibrutinib therapy discontinuation and outcomes in patients with chronic lymphocytic leukemia. JAMA Oncol. 2015;1(1):80–7.
71. Mato AR, Nabhan C, Thompson MC, Lamanna N, Brander DM, Hill B, et al. Toxicities and outcomes of 621 ibrutinib-treated chronic lymphocytic leukemia patients in the United States: a real-world analysis. Haematologica. 2018;103(5):874–9.
72. Mato AR, Nabhan C, Barr PM, Ujjani CS, Hill BT, Lamanna N, et al. Outcomes of CLL patients treated with sequential kinase inhibitor therapy: a real world experience. Blood. 2016;128(18):2199–205.
73. Jain P, Thompson PA, Keating M, Estrov Z, Ferrajoli A, Jain N, et al. Long-term outcomes for patients with chronic lymphocytic leukemia who discontinue ibrutinib. Cancer. 2017;123(12):2268–73.
74. Jain P, Keating M, Wierda W, Estrov Z, Ferrajoli A, Jain N, et al. Outcomes of patients with chronic lymphocytic leukemia after discontinuing ibrutinib. Blood. 2015;125(13):2062–7.
75. Ahn IE, Underbayev C, Albitar A, Herman SE, Tian X, Maric I, et al. Clonal evolution leading to ibrutinib resistance in chronic lymphocytic leukemia. Blood. 2017;129(11):1469–79.
76. Woyach JA, Ruppert AS, Guinn D, Lehman A, Blachly JS, Lozanski A, et al. BTK(C481S)-mediated resistance to ibrutinib in chronic lymphocytic leukemia. J Clin Oncol. 2017;35(13):1437–43.
77. Woyach JA, Furman RR, Liu TM, Ozer HG, Zapatka M, Ruppert AS, et al. Resistance mechanisms for the Bruton's tyrosine kinase inhibitor ibrutinib. N Engl J Med. 2014;370(24):2286–94.
78. Herling CD, Abedpour N, Weiss J, Schmitt A, Jachimowicz RD, Merkel O, et al. Clonal dynamics towards the development of venetoclax resistance in chronic lymphocytic leukemia. Nat Commun. 2018;9(1):727.
79. Byrd JC, Harrington B, O'Brien S, Jones JA, Schuh A, Devereux S, et al. Acalabrutinib (ACP-196) in relapsed chronic lymphocytic leukemia. N Engl J Med. 2016;374(4):323–32.
80. Byrd J, Wierda W, Schuh A, Devereux S, Chaves J, Brown J, et al. Acalabrutinib monotherapy in patients with relapsed/refractory chronic lymphocytic leukemia: updated results from the phase 1/2 ACE-CL-001 study. Am Soc Hematol Meet. 2017;130:498.
81. Walter HS, Rule SA, Dyer MJ, Karlin L, Jones C, Cazin B, et al. A phase 1 clinical trial of the selective BTK inhibitor ONO/GS-4059 in relapsed and refractory mature B-cell malignancies. Blood. 2016;127(4):411–9.
82. Flinn IW, O'Brien S, Kahl B, Patel M, Oki Y, Foss FF, et al. Duvelisib, a novel oral dual inhibitor of PI3K-delta,gamma, is clinically active in advanced hematologic malignancies. Blood. 2018;131(8):877–87.
83. Sharman J, Hawkins M, Kolibaba K, Boxer M, Klein L, Wu M, et al. An open-label phase 2 trial of entospletinib (GS-9973), a selective spleen tyrosine kinase inhibitor, in chronic lymphocytic leukemia. Blood. 2015;125(15):2336–43.
84. Barr PM, Saylors GB, Spurgeon SE, Cheson BD, Greenwald DR, O'Brien SM, et al. Phase 2 study of idelalisib and entospletinib: pneumonitis limits combination therapy in relapsed refractory CLL and NHL. Blood. 2016;127(20):2411–5.
85. Xia AL, Wang XC, Lu YJ, Lu XJ, Sun B. Chimeric-antigen receptor T (CAR-T) cell therapy for solid tumors: challenges and opportunities. Oncotarget. 2017;8(52):90521–31.
86. Park JH, Geyer MB, Brentjens RJ. CD19-targeted CAR T-cell therapeutics for hematologic malignancies: interpreting clinical outcomes to date. Blood. 2016;127(26):3312–20.
87. Porter DL, Levine BL, Kalos M, Bagg A, June CH. Chimeric antigen receptor-modified T cells in chronic lymphoid leukemia. N Engl J Med. 2011;365(8):725–33.
88. Turtle CJ, Hay KA, Hanafi LA, Li D, Cherian S, Chen X, et al. Durable molecular remissions in chronic lymphocytic leukemia treated with CD19-specific chimeric antigen receptor-modified T cells after failure of ibrutinib. J Clin Oncol. 2017;35(26):3010–20.

89. Porter DL, Hwang WT, Frey NV, Lacey SF, Shaw PA, Loren AW, et al. Chimeric antigen receptor T cells persist and induce sustained remissions in relapsed refractory chronic lymphocytic leukemia. Sci Transl Med. 2015;7(303):303ra139.
90. Porter D, Frey N, Wood PA, Weng Y, Grupp SA. Grading of cytokine release syndrome associated with the CAR T cell therapy tisagenlecleucel. J Hematol Oncol. 2018;11(1):35.
91. Frey N. Cytokine release syndrome: who is at risk and how to treat. Best Pract Res Clin Haematol. 2017;30(4):336–40.
92. Neelapu SS, Tummala S, Kebriaei P, Wierda W, Gutierrez C, Locke FL, et al. Chimeric antigen receptor T-cell therapy – assessment and management of toxicities. Nat Rev Clin Oncol. 2018;15(1):47–62.
93. Dreger P, Schetelig J, Andersen N, Corradini P, van Gelder M, Gribben J, et al. Managing high-risk CLL during transition to a new treatment era: stem cell transplantation or novel agents? Blood. 2014;124(26):3841–9.
94. Kharfan-Dabaja MA, Kumar A, Hamadani M, Stilgenbauer S, Ghia P, Anasetti C, et al. Clinical practice recommendations for use of allogeneic hematopoietic cell transplantation in chronic lymphocytic leukemia on behalf of the guidelines Committee of the American Society for Blood and Marrow Transplantation. Biol Blood Marrow Transplant. 2016;22(12):2117–25.
95. Montserrat E, Dreger P. Treatment of chronic lymphocytic leukemia with del(17p)/TP53 mutation: allogeneic hematopoietic stem cell transplantation or BCR-signaling inhibitors? Clin Lymphoma Myeloma Leuk. 2016;16(Suppl):S74–81.
96. Dreger P, Dohner H, Ritgen M, Bottcher S, Busch R, Dietrich S, et al. Allogeneic stem cell transplantation provides durable disease control in poor-risk chronic lymphocytic leukemia: long-term clinical and MRD results of the German CLL study group CLL3X trial. Blood. 2010;116(14):2438–47.
97. Kramer I, Stilgenbauer S, Dietrich S, Bottcher S, Zeis M, Stadler M, et al. Allogeneic hematopoietic cell transplantation for high-risk CLL: 10-year follow-up of the GCLLSG CLL3X trial. Blood. 2017;130(12):1477–80.
98. Tsimberidou AM, O'Brien S, Khouri I, Giles FJ, Kantarjian HM, Champlin R, et al. Clinical outcomes and prognostic factors in patients with Richter's syndrome treated with chemotherapy or chemoimmunotherapy with or without stem-cell transplantation. J Clin Oncol. 2006;24(15):2343–51.
99. Strati P, Keating MJ, O'Brien SM, Ferrajoli A, Burger J, Faderl S, et al. Outcomes of first-line treatment for chronic lymphocytic leukemia with 17p deletion. Haematologica. 2014;99(8):1350–5.
100. Rossi D. Richter's syndrome: novel and promising therapeutic alternatives. Best Pract Res Clin Haematol. 2016;29(1):30–9.
101. Dighiero G, Maloum K, Desablens B, Cazin B, Navarro M, Leblay R, et al. Chlorambucil in indolent chronic lymphocytic leukemia. French cooperative group on chronic lymphocytic leukemia. N Engl J Med. 1998;338(21):1506–14.
102. Langerbeins P, Bahlo J, Rhein C, Cramer P, Pflug N, Fischer K, et al. The CLL12 trial protocol: a placebo-controlled double-blind phase III study of ibrutinib in the treatment of early-stage chronic lymphocytic leukemia patients with risk of early disease progression. Future Oncol. 2015;11(13):1895–903.
103. Deng J, Isik E, Fernandes SM, Brown JR, Letai A, Davids MS. Bruton's tyrosine kinase inhibition increases BCL-2 dependence and enhances sensitivity to venetoclax in chronic lymphocytic leukemia. Leukemia. 2017;31(10):2075–84.
104. Cervantes-Gomez F, Lamothe B, Woyach JA, Wierda WG, Keating MJ, Balakrishnan K, et al. Pharmacological and protein profiling suggests venetoclax (ABT-199) as optimal partner with ibrutinib in chronic lymphocytic leukemia. Clin Cancer Res. 2015;21(16):3705–15.
105. Venetoclax: risk assessment, prophylaxis, and monitoring measures for TLS. https://www.venclextahcp.com/venclexta-dosing-regimen/tumor-lysis-syndrome-risk-assessment.html.

Chapter 5
Mantle Cell Lymphoma

Daniel R. Reed and Craig A. Portell

Introduction

Mantle cell lymphoma (MCL) is a mature B-cell subtype of non-Hodgkin's lymphoma (NHL). It is characterized by the t(11,14) (q13q32) translocation leading to the fusion of cyclin D1 to the immunoglobulin heavy-chain gene locus and overproduction of cyclin D1 [1]. MCL is a rare disease and represents 6% of all NHL diagnoses. Caucasian males are the highest represented demographic group diagnosed, with an average age of onset of 67. Overall, the incidence of this disease also appears to be increasing, especially in the elderly population [2, 3]. MCL is classified as either classical, indolent, or blastoid with all three representing different presentations, biology, and clinical course and response to treatment. In general, it is an incurable lymphoma, but there has been significant progress in the treatment of patients, leading to improved outcomes. In this chapter, we will review the presentation and clinical course of MCL, as well as frontline and relapsed treatment modalities. We will then review exciting research into novel targets and combination therapy.

Clinical Presentation

Presentations of MCL vary according to underlying classification of the disease. Patients with conventional disease usually present to their physician with symptoms of lymphadenopathy or early satiety and abdominal pain secondary to hepatosplenomegaly [4]. B symptoms (night sweats, fevers, weight loss) are also common clinical presentations in MCL. Extra-nodal sites are very common in MCL, and

D. R. Reed · C. A. Portell (✉)
Division of Hematology/Oncology, University of Virginia, Charlottesville, VA, USA
e-mail: Drr3d@hscmail.mcc.virginia.edu; Cp4ys@hscmail.mcc.virginia.edu

C. Dittus (ed.), *Novel Therapeutics for Rare Lymphomas*,
https://doi.org/10.1007/978-3-030-25610-4_5

there is a predilection for the gastrointestinal (GI) tract, particularly the colon, which can lead to patients presenting with obstructive symptoms, dysphagia, and odynophagia. Of note, upper and lower endoscopies in asymptomatic patients have demonstrated a high incidence of involvement of MCL in the GI tract [5, 6]. Alternatively, MCL can be discovered after evaluation of an asymptomatic patient with lymphocytosis on a CBC which is a common presentation with indolent disease. Blastoid variant MCL has a varied presentation but usually is associated with night sweats, weight loss, fever, diffuse lymphadenopathy, and sometimes, neurologic symptoms secondary to central nervous system (CNS) involvement.

Diagnosis

An excisional lymph node biopsy is the preferred biopsy method, but a core needle biopsy is sometimes necessary and can provide a diagnosis of MCL. Fine needle aspiration is inadequate for diagnosing any lymphoma. Biopsy of involved tissue, such as a bone marrow or GI tract biopsy, can sometimes be used to obtain a diagnosis. MCL histology is described as small lymphoid cells with irregular nuclear contours and a cleaved appearance. There are four distinct histologic variants of MCL: small cell, marginal zone-like, blastoid, and pleomorphic variants. Classical MCL is classified as wild-type IGHV and is characterized by the expression of SOX11.

Leukemic non-nodal MCL is a separate classification characterized by IGHV mutated status and B cells not expressing SOX11 [7, 8]. The immunophenotype of MCL is defined by expression of CD20, CD19, IgM, IgD, and CD5. They are negative for CD23 and positive for FMC7 distinguishing them from chronic lymphocytic lymphoma (CLL). Fluorescence in situ hybridization (FISH) demonstrates t(11,14)(q13q32) that defines overexpression of cyclin D1 through the fusion of the immunoglobulin heavy-chain enhancer region to CCND1 leading to unregulated cell cycle activation. Cyclin D1 negative disease is rare, but has been described with the overexpression of CCND2 or CCND3 and is usually SOX-11+ [9].

Staging/Workup

Clinical evaluation for staging includes peripheral blood CBC, LDH, beta-2 microglobulin, and CT neck, chest, abdomen, and pelvis. PET is often used in staging MCL with a goal to identify extra-nodal disease; however, its established role is not clearly defined. CNS involvement is rare, and, therefore, a diagnostic lumbar puncture is only obtained if clinically indicated, such as when neurologic symptoms are present. Blastoid histology subtype, Ki67 > 30%, and high MIPI (>6) have been shown to be high-risk factors for CNS involvement with around 25% incidence in 2 years [10, 11]. Bone marrow biopsy is not imperative for staging, but should be considered if there is peripheral blood involvement or cytopenias. Most MCL is stage

IV when diagnosed, usually coinciding with peripheral blood or bone marrow (BM) involvement. However, in situ MCL has been recently described, but this is a rare presentation of disease and should only be considered after full workup, including BM biopsy and EGD/colonoscopy with random biopsies even if asymptomatic [12].

Prognosis

MCL is a heterogeneous disease with variations and pathologic characteristics that have been found to influence prognosis. The Mantle Cell Lymphoma International Prognostic Index (MIPI) and MIPI-B with Ki-67 index are the most widely known and used models for prognosis and risk stratification [13, 14]. Recently the MCL2 trial was updated to reflect the improvement in overall survival (OS) to 12.7 years reflecting the impact of novel therapies and approaches to this disease [15]. Increasing knowledge regarding the impact of tumor biology has contributed to defining prognosis. In a multivariate analysis, TP53 point mutation status, most often associated with blastoid morphologies, was found to be an adverse prognostic indicator with an OS of only 1.8 years and a relapse rate of 50% within 1 year of treatment and a smaller benefit for consolidative therapy with autologous stem cell transplantation [16].

Conventional Treatment Approach

There are a small number of low-risk (low MIPI score) patients that can be observed without need for treatment. Martin and colleagues demonstrated in a retrospective analysis that patients with low IPI scores and stage I or II disease undergoing deferred treatment did not have a worse OS compared to those who received intensive induction [17]. Cohen et al. demonstrated that patients with a leukemic presentation and lack of B symptoms were associated with increased likelihood of deferred therapy and provided an independent predictor of OS for all patients in the study [18]. These patients usually present with only a leukemic phase, some degree of splenomegaly, and no adenopathy. Abrisqueta et al. found an improvement in median OS in asymptomatic MCL patients compared to the early treatment group, 72 versus 52.5 months, respectively, $p = 0.041$ reinforcing the safety of observation versus treatment in the asymptomatic patient [19].

Most patients present with advanced, symptomatic, or high tumor burden disease which necessitates treatment. Fitness and age are used for initial treatment decisions. We will discuss intensive approaches for younger, fit patients and less intensive approaches for older, unfit patients separately:

Young and Fit Patients: The standard of care for initial treatment of young (<65 years old) patients, without significant comorbidities, is intensive induction chemo-immunotherapy followed by consolidative autologous stem cell transplant.

Several induction regimens have been examined over the years, and there are several clinical trials aimed to evaluate the best induction regimen. While there is no standard of care currently, regimens containing high-dose cytarabine have been demonstrated to have the best overall and progression-free survival. In the recently updated European MCL Younger trial, six cycles of alternating R-CHOP/R-DHAP (rituximab, cyclophosphamide, doxorubicin, vincristine, prednisone/rituximab, dexamethasone, high-dose cytarabine, and cisplatin) followed by a high-dose-containing cytarabine conditioning regimen and autologous stem cell transplant (ASCT) demonstrated a significant improvement in time to treatment failure with a median 9.1 years compared to the median of 3.9 years observed in the control group of six cycles of R-CHOP then ASCT [20]. The NORDIC Lymphoma Group MCL2 trial investigated rituximab with R-maxi-CHOP alternating with high-dose cytarabine followed by ASCT. In the most recent 15-year update of the NORDIC trial, OS was reported at 12.7 and PFS was 8.5 years, and 40% of patients remained in first remission [15]. The University of Texas MD Anderson Cancer Center (MD Anderson) reported on a regimen of R-hyperCVAD, and the median OS was 10.7 years; however there was an increased risk of myelodysplastic syndrome and treatment-related acute myeloid leukemia as well as a decrease in mobilization for stem cell collection for ASCT seen in SWOG 1106 trial [21, 22]. Therefore, the regimen has not been widely adopted.

The role of frontline ASCT for consolidation has been considered standard of care and shown to improve OS in patients who achieve complete remission (CR) after induction [23]. Further, ASCT use in the frontline setting leads to improved OS compared to the relapsed/refractory setting [24]. What is not known is if all MCL patients, who are candidates for induction, benefit from ASCT in the frontline setting. The role of ASCT is currently being investigated for minimal residual disease (MRD) negative patients though the US cooperative groups (NCT03267433). In patients with remission after an induction regimen of R-DHAP and consolidative autologous transplant, the LyMA trial demonstrated that maintenance rituximab, 375 mg/m^2 administered every 2 months for 3 years after transplantation, increased overall, progression-free, and event-free survival [24]. Oxaliplatin is often replaced for cisplatin in this regimen (R-DHAX) and has been shown to have decreased renal toxicity, and no impact on overall survival compared to R-DHAP [25–27].

Elderly Patients: For patients who are not candidates for stem cell transplant and intensive induction, bendamustine and rituximab (BR) is considered a standard of care. Several chemotherapy regimens have been investigated including R-CHOP and R-FC; however, none have been shown to be superior to BR in terms of toxicity and efficacy [28, 29]. The role of maintenance rituximab after BR induction in this patient population is still to be determined with Rummel et al. evaluating patients with 2 years of maintenance rituximab after BR induction versus observation showing no statistically significant difference in progression-free survival PFS [30]. For an intermediate intensity approach, 40 patients received the combination of rituximab, bendamustine, and cytarabine in a phase II study that demonstrated an ORR of 100% with 70% achieving a CR and a 2-year PFS of 95% for untreated patients [31]. The R-BAC500 trial in Italy explored the combination of BR backbone with low-dose cytarabine as an induction therapy in elderly patients and showed a 2-year PFS of 81% and OS of

Table 5.1 Novel target/combination trials

Novel target or combination	Indication	Study name	Clinical trial identifier
Bortezomib, cytarabine, and dexamethasone	RR MCL	BATMAN	NCT02840539
Ixazomib and ibrutinib	RR MCL	PrE0404	NCT03323151
Ibrutinib and bortezomib	RR MCL		NCT02356458
Ibrutinib and venetoclax	RR MCL	SYMPATICO	NCT03112174
Obinutuzumab and ibrutinib	RR MCL	OAsIs	NCT02558816
BGB-3111	RR MCL		NCT03206970
Bendamustine, rituximab, ibrutinib and venetoclax	RR MCL		NCT03295240
BR and acalabrutinib	Front line, NI		NCT02972840
Ibrutinib and pembrolizumab	RR MCL CLL		NCT03153202
CART-19	RR MCL		NCT02081937
Bendamustine and obinutuzumab	Front line, NI		NCT03311126
Enzalutamide	RR MCL		NCT02489123
BCL201 and Idelalisib	RR MCL Fol		NCT02603445
INCB050465	RR MCL	CITADEL-205	NCT03235544
Alisertib, bortezomib and rituximab	RR NHL and MCL		NCT01695941
TGR-1202 and ibrutinib	RR MCL & CLL		NCT02268851
Cirmtuzumab and Ibrutinib	RR MCL CLL		NCT03088878
Onalespib	RR NHL		NCT02572453
JCAR017	RR NHL	TRANSCEND-001	NCT02631044
Nivolumab and lenalidomide	RR NHL		NCT03015896
ONC201	RR NHL		NCT02420795
ACY 1215	RR NHL HL		NCT02091063
Romidepsin and 5-azacitidine	RR NHL		NCT01998035
Pralatrexate and romidepsin	RR NHL		NCT01947140

FL NI front line non-intensive, *RR MCL* relapsed/refractory mantle cell lymphoma, *R NHL* relapsed/refractory non-Hodgkin's lymphoma, multiple histologies, *CLL* chronic lymphocytic lymphoma, *HL* Hodgkin's lymphoma, *Fol* follicular lymphoma

85%. In addition to known therapies, several novel agents and combination of novel agents with chemotherapy are in clinical trials for patients who are not candidates for stem cell transplant or intensive induction chemotherapy (Table 5.1).

Frontline Novel Agents With or Without Chemotherapy

Novel agents are being explored in the frontline setting predominantly in patients who are not candidates for stem cell transplant. Adjustments to known chemotherapy regimens are being studied to reduce toxicity. Kahl et al. investigated a modified hyperCVAD regimen without methotrexate and cytarabine and with rituximab maintenance which demonstrated an impressive overall response rate (ORR) of 85% and a 2-year reported OS of 82% [32]. The proteasome inhibitor bortezomib is being added to this modified hyperCVAD regimen (VcR-CVAD) showing an improved ORR of 90% and a 6-year OS of 70% [33].

In patients who are candidates for transplant, novel agents are being evaluated in standard induction regimens. In efforts to reduce the toxicity but maintain the efficacy of the hyperCVAD regimen pioneered by MD Anderson, the phase II WINDOW I trial (NCT02427620) is evaluating frontline use of ibrutinib and rituximab as part one of an induction and then use of R-hyperCVAD in part 2 which has demonstrated ORR of 100% in part 1 with all patients obtaining CR after part 2 with primary end points not reached at this time [34]. Bendamustine and rituximab is also being investigated in frontline patients who are candidates for transplant. After BR, patients received rituximab and high-dose cytarabine if they had no evidence of progressive disease; they then went on to get ASCT. Most patients, 96%, obtained a CR and 93% achieved MRD after BR/RC. After ASCT, a 96% PFS was observed with a median follow-up of 13 months [35]. There will need to be a cooperative group effort to evaluate these novel therapies in comparison.

In addition, since the activity of bendamustine and rituximab has been shown to be effective in patients treated with a non-intensive approach, several trials are investigating using this backbone regimen to add additional targeted agents. The SHINE trial (NCT01776840) is a pending phase III study evaluating BR plus ibrutinib vs BR plus placebo that has finished enrollment but has not been reported. The ACE-LY-308 trial (NCT02972840) is investigating the combination of acalabrutinib, a second-generation Bruton's tyrosine kinase (BTK) inhibitor, with BR backbone versus a placebo BR and is currently actively enrolling patients. Preliminary results of LENA-BERIT (NCT00963534), which studied the combination of lenalidomide and BR, reported a median PFS of 42 months and were significant for increased rate of opportunistic infections, neutropenia, and secondary malignancies [36]. The proteasome inhibitor bortezomib has been shown to be active in the frontline treatment of MCL when combined with rituximab, doxorubicin, cyclophosphamide, and prednisone (VR-CAP) in the LYM-3002 study. This study showed a median progression-free survival of 16.1 months in the R-CHOP arm and 30.7 months in the VR-CAP arm [37]. SWOG S0601 evaluated bortezomib in addition to R-CHOP induction and bortezomib maintenance for patients with, at least, stable disease which demonstrated a PFS of 28% and OS of 66% with one of the most common non-hematologic toxicities being grade 1 or 2 sensory neuropathy (57%) during induction and maintenance [38]. BR is being combined with bortezomib during induction and lenalidomide during maintenance in a US intergroup study (E1411) (NCT01415752) and has also finished enrollment, but results are pending.

Lenalidomide, an immune modulator agent, has demonstrated success with induction therapies in MCL. When combined with rituximab, in a non-chemotherapy regimen, Ruan et al. demonstrated a 92% response rate with a median progression-free survival that had not been reached and a 2-year OS of 97% [39]. This combination was relatively well-tolerated, with low rates of grade 3 and 4 toxicities. In addition, lenalidomide is being investigated in the frontline setting in combination with rituximab and ibrutinib (NCT032307).

Novel Agents in Relapsed/Refractory MCL

Multi-agent chemotherapy has not been able to show a superior response rate compared to targeted therapy in the relapsed or refractory setting of MCL. Allogeneic stem cell transplant in patients with relapsed or refractory disease has shown promising results in selected patient populations with OS at 5 years of between 73% and 62%; however, patient survival is limited by a high-transplant-related mortality reported at 24% in 5 years [40, 41]. Further, not all patients are eligible for allogeneic stem cell transplant particularly given the generally advanced age at diagnosis in MCL.

The B-cell receptor (BCR) complex has been demonstrated to play an important role in the survival and proliferation of MCL [42]. Targeting BTK, a vital mediator in the BCR pathway, has been the focus of research in relapsed refractory MCL [43]. Ibrutinib, an irreversible BTK inhibitor that binds to the phosphorylation activation site of BTK, has shown an ORR of 68% and 2-year PFS of about 30%, giving it FDA approval in relapsed/refractory R/R MCL [44]. Time to response has been shown to range from 2 to 5 months and improves with longer drug exposure [45]. A recent pooled analysis of the SPARK, RAY, and PCYC-1104 and CAN3001 trials, all studies involving single-agent ibrutinib in R/R MCL, with 3.5 years of follow-up, showed a median PFS of 13 months and OS of 37% at 5 years. Further, the benefit of ibrutinib is seen primarily when it is used in earlier lines of therapy [46]. This benefit has been confirmed in several other retrospective analyses [47–50]. Around one third of patients develop primary resistance to ibrutinib with a median response rate of 1.5 years [45]. Failure of ibrutinib has been shown to portend poor prognosis, and patients are less likely to respond to salvage chemotherapy [51]. Ibrutinib is, overall, well-tolerated with the most common adverse effects being diarrhea, fatigue, and cough. More serious adverse events include bleeding and atrial fibrillation. Rule and colleagues showed the cumulative incidence of hemorrhage was 7.3%, and the incidence of atrial fibrillation was 5.9%, which decreased over the observed time in their pooled analysis [46, 52].

The most recent BTK inhibitor to receive FDA approval is the second-generation agent acalabrutinib [53]. Use of this agent has demonstrated less frequent atrial fibrillation and bleeding/thrombocytopenia with improved response rates compared to ibrutinib across trials [44, 54]. It does seem as though patients in the ibrutinib trial, though, had higher risk disease and a higher proportion of refractory patients. Finally, new novel BTK inhibitors tirabrutinib (ONO-GS 4059) and zanubrutinib (BGB-3111) are in early clinical trials and showing promise [55, 56].

After activation of BTK, downstream signaling leads to activation of mTOR (mammalian target of rapamycin) and NF-KB (nuclear factor kappa-light-chain-enhancer of activated B cells) through PI3K/AKT/mTOR pathway [57].

Temsirolimus, an mTOR inhibitor, has been demonstrated to be active in MCL with an ORR of 22% and duration of response (DOR) of 7.1 months in a phase III study [58]. When combined with rituximab, temsirolimus has an improved ORR of 59% including a high response for rituximab refractory patients [59]. Temsirolimus was shown to be inferior in PFS (14.6 months versus 6.2 months) and poorly tolerated compared to ibrutinib [60], making its utility as a single agent less exciting.

Through activation of AKT pathway, BTK activation leads to NF-KB activity. Immunomodulators have multiple effects, but one includes inhibiting NF-KB by limiting translocation into the nucleus [61]. Lenalidomide, an immunomodulator agent, as a single agent has been shown to be effective in R/R MCL. In the EMERGE study, single-agent lenalidomide was shown to have an ORR of 28% with DOR of 16.6 months and PFS of 4 months with patients who were heavily pretreated [62]. The SPRINT trial compared lenalidomide to investigator's choice of chemotherapy and showed an improved of PFS for lenalidomide (median 8.6 months versus 5.4 months) [63]. In the MAGNIFY trial, lenalidomide, when combined with rituximab, was shown to have an ORR of 54% in patients with relapsed MCL [64]. In patients who previously failed ibrutinib, MCL-004, an observational study analyzing outcomes of patients on lenalidomide either monotherapy or in combination with other agents, showed an ORR of 29% and median DOR of 20 weeks [65]. In addition, when combined with bendamustine and rituximab, lenalidomide was shown to have median PFS of 20 months and OS of 67% at 24 months [66].

Bortezomib is a proteasome inhibitor with multiple effects including inhibiting proteins that regulate the cell cycle, inducing apoptosis and cell death, and has been shown to be active in MCL [61]. The phase II PINNACLE trial evaluated bortezomib in the relapsed refractory setting of patients with MCL and demonstrated an ORR of 33% with a median DOR of 9.2 months and OS of 23.5 months [67]. When combined with CHOP, bortezomib was shown to be effective with an ORR of 82.6% and median OS of 35.6 months compared to patients who just received CHOP alone (11.8 months) [68].

Further down the signaling pathway of the BCR is phosphoinositide 3-kinase (PI3K) which has been shown to contribute to the survival and proliferation of MCL [69]. Idelalisib is an oral agent that inhibits the delta isoform of PI3K and has shown to have an ORR of 40% in an early phase I study in MCL [70]. A second PI3K inhibitor, copanlisib, which has both alpha and delta inhibitions, demonstrated efficacy in early phase II trial with an ORR of 63.5% [71].

Venetoclax, an inhibitor of the anti-apoptotic protein B-cell lymphoma 2 (BCL-2), demonstrated a high response rate in MCL of 75% and CR of 21% with median PFS of 14 months and an OS at 12 months of 82%. Patients had response durations up to 2.5 years [72]. Tam et al. combined venetoclax and ibrutinib in a phase II study for patients with R/R MCL which demonstrated an impressive ORR of 71% within 16 weeks with 63% of patients obtaining a complete remission.

The 8-month survival was estimated at 81% and was generally well-tolerated, with fatigue and diarrhea being the most common side effect [73].

MCL is characterized by the balanced translocation (11,14) leading to increase in cyclin D1 expression suggesting that inhibition of this pathway would be a rea-

Table 5.2 Novel agents in R/R Mcl with response and survival data

Agent	Study size (*n*)	Median age	Median # preceding treatments (*n*)	ORR (%)	CR (%)	PFS (months)	OS (months)
Ibrutinib	115	68	3	68	21	13.9	NR
Acalabrutinib	124	68	2	81	40	NR	NR
Temsirolimus	162	67	3	22	2	4.8	12.8
Lenalidomide	134	67	4	28	7.5	4.0	19
Bortezomib	155	65	1	32	8	6.5	23.5
Idelalisib	40	69	4	40	5	3.7	NR
Venetoclax	28	72	3	75	21	14	NR

ORR objective response rate %, *CR* complete response %, *PFS* progression-free survival in months, *OS* overall survival in months, *NR* not reached at time of study publication

sonable target by drugs. Palbociclib, an oral CDK 4/6 inhibitor currently approved in metastatic estrogen receptor-positive breast cancer, has been shown to have a relatively low ORR of 18% in MCL patients as single agent [74]. Other CDK inhibitors are in development to be studied in MCL [75]. In patients who failed at least one line of therapy in relapse, ibrutinib and palbociclib provided 8 out of 18 patients with a CR and demonstrated a PFS of 68% in 1 year [76]. AT7519M, a CDK inhibitor targeting multiple kinases, demonstrated an ORR of 27% in MCL [77]. Novel agents in current clinical practice for R/R MCL are outlined in Table 5.2.

Finally, chimeric antigen receptor-activated T-cell (CAR-T) cell therapy is being investigated in MCL but currently only in the relapsed/refractory setting, and role of this treatment is yet to be determined in this disease [78, 79].

Recommended Treatment Approach for Frontline and Relapsed/Refractory Disease

The recommendation of a clinical trial is always important in a disease like MCL where standard of care therapies do not provide cures. While there is no standard induction treatment for MCL, high-dose cytarabine is an imperative component of frontline regimens. At our institution, for patients who are candidates for intensive therapy, we prefer treatment with four cycles of R-DHAX with oxaliplatin in place of cisplatin. This regimen has been shown to have improved renal tolerance versus cisplatin without difference in survival [25–27]. The patients are then consolidated with autologous stem cell transplant with 3 years of maintenance rituximab per the LyMA trial. For patients who are not candidates for intensive therapy, we prefer a combination of bendamustine and rituximab if no clinical trial is available. In more frail patients, we consider lenalidomide-rituximab or combination rituximab, bendamustine, and cytarabine for a more intermediate intensity approach.

At the time of relapse, a clinical trial should be the first treatment choice offered. Otherwise, a BTK inhibitor should be used given the high response early in the treatment paradigm. The choice between ibrutinib and acalabrutinib depends on patient comorbidities and characteristics. Unfortunately, ibrutinib failure is common, and subsequent lines of therapy should include other novel agents including lenalidomide and venetoclax. Other agents can also be considered, as outlined in this chapter and seen in Table 5.1.

References

1. Jares P, Colomer D, Campo E. Genetic and molecular pathogenesis of mantle cell lymphoma: perspectives for new targeted therapeutics. Nat Rev Cancer. 2007;7(10):750–62.
2. Zhou Y, Wang H, Fang W, Romaguer JE, Zhang Y, Delasalle KB, et al. Incidence trends of mantle cell lymphoma in the United States between 1992 and 2004. Cancer. 2008;113(4):791–8.
3. Epperla N, Hamadani M, Fenske TS, Costa LJ. Incidence and survival trends in mantle cell lymphoma. Br J Haematol. 2017;181:703–6.
4. Swerdlow SH, Williams ME. From centrocytic to mantle cell lymphoma: a clinicopathologic and molecular review of 3 decades. Hum Pathol. 2002;33(1):7–20.
5. Romaguera JE, Medeiros LJ, Hagemeister FB, Fayad LE, Rodriguez MA, Pro B, et al. Frequency of gastrointestinal involvement and its clinical significance in mantle cell lymphoma. Cancer. 2003;97(3):586–91.
6. Kim JH, Jung HW, Kang KJ, Min BH, Lee JH, Chang DK, et al. Endoscopic findings in mantle cell lymphoma with gastrointestinal tract involvement. Acta Haematol. 2012;127(3):129–34.
7. Swerdlow SH, Campo E, Pileri SA, Harris NL, Stein H, Siebert R, et al. The 2016 revision of the World Health Organization classification of lymphoid neoplasms. Blood. 2016;127(20):2375–90.
8. Fernandez V, Salamero O, Espinet B, Sole F, Royo C, Navarro A, et al. Genomic and gene expression profiling defines indolent forms of mantle cell lymphoma. Cancer Res. 2010;70(4):1408–18.
9. Narurkar R, Alkayem M, Liu D. SOX11 is a biomarker for cyclin D1-negative mantle cell lymphoma. Biomark Res. 2016;4:6.
10. Cheah CY, George A, Gine E, Chiappella A, Kluin-Nelemans HC, Jurczak W, et al. Central nervous system involvement in mantle cell lymphoma: clinical features, prognostic factors and outcomes from the European mantle cell lymphoma network. Ann Oncol. 2013;24(8):2119–23.
11. Chin CK, Cheah CY. How I treat patients with aggressive lymphoma at high risk of CNS relapse. Blood. 2017;130(7):867–74.
12. Karube K, Scarfo L, Campo E, Ghia P. Monoclonal B cell lymphocytosis and "in situ" lymphoma. Semin Cancer Biol. 2014;24:3–14.
13. Hoster E, Dreyling M, Klapper W, Gisselbrecht C, van Hoof A, Kluin-Nelemans HC, et al. A new prognostic index (MIPI) for patients with advanced-stage mantle cell lymphoma. Blood. 2008;111(2):558–65.
14. Geisler CH, Kolstad A, Laurell A, Raty R, Jerkeman M, Eriksson M, et al. The mantle cell lymphoma international prognostic index (MIPI) is superior to the international prognostic index (IPI) in predicting survival following intensive first-line immunochemotherapy and autologous stem cell transplantation (ASCT). Blood. 2010;115(8):1530–3.
15. Eskelund CW, Kolstad A, Jerkeman M, Raty R, Laurell A, Eloranta S, et al. 15-year follow-up of the second Nordic mantle cell lymphoma trial (MCL2): prolonged remissions without survival plateau. Br J Haematol. 2016;175(3):410–8.
16. Eskelund CW, Dahl C, Hansen JW, Westman M, Kolstad A, Pedersen LB, et al. TP53 mutations identify younger mantle cell lymphoma patients who do not benefit from intensive chemoimmunotherapy. Blood. 2017;130(17):1903–10.

17. Martin P, Chadburn A, Christos P, Weil K, Furman RR, Ruan J, et al. Outcome of deferred initial therapy in mantle-cell lymphoma. J Clin Oncol. 2009;27(8):1209–13.
18. Cohen JB, Han X, Jemal A, Ward EM, Flowers CR. Deferred therapy is associated with improved overall survival in patients with newly diagnosed mantle cell lymphoma. Cancer. 2016;122(15):2356–63.
19. Abrisqueta P, Scott DW, Slack GW, Steidl C, Mottok A, Gascoyne RD, et al. Observation as the initial management strategy in patients with mantle cell lymphoma. Ann Oncol. 2017;28(10):2489–95.
20. Hermine O, Hoster E, Walewski J, Bosly A, Stilgenbauer S, Thieblemont C, et al. Addition of high-dose cytarabine to immunochemotherapy before autologous stem-cell transplantation in patients aged 65 years or younger with mantle cell lymphoma (MCL younger): a randomised, open-label, phase 3 trial of the European mantle cell lymphoma network. Lancet. 2016;388(10044):565–75.
21. Chihara D, Cheah CY, Westin JR, Fayad LE, Rodriguez MA, Hagemeister FB, et al. Rituximab plus hyper-CVAD alternating with MTX/Ara-C in patients with newly diagnosed mantle cell lymphoma: 15-year follow-up of a phase II study from the MD Anderson Cancer Center. Br J Haematol. 2016;172(1):80–8.
22. Chen RW, Li H, Bernstein SH, Kahwash S, Rimsza LM, Forman SJ, et al. RB but not R-HCVAD is a feasible induction regimen prior to auto-HCT in frontline MCL: results of SWOG study S1106. Br J Haematol. 2017;176(5):759–69.
23. Dreyling M, Lenz G, Hoster E, Van Hoof A, Gisselbrecht C, Schmits R, et al. Early consolidation by myeloablative radiochemotherapy followed by autologous stem cell transplantation in first remission significantly prolongs progression-free survival in mantle-cell lymphoma: results of a prospective randomized trial of the European MCL network. Blood. 2005;105(7):2677–84.
24. Le Gouill S, Thieblemont C, Oberic L, Moreau A, Bouabdallah K, Dartigeas C, et al. Rituximab after autologous stem-cell transplantation in mantle-cell lymphoma. N Engl J Med. 2017;377(13):1250–60.
25. Lacout C, De Vries M, Seegers-Thepot V, Clavert A, Farhi J, Mercier M, et al. R-DHA-Oxaliplatin versus R-DHA-cisplatin regimen in B-cell Nhl's treatment: a eight years retrospective study. Blood. 2015. American Society of Hematology;126(23):3959.
26. Lignon J, Sibon D, Madelaine I, Brice P, Franchi P, Briere J, et al. Rituximab, dexamethasone, cytarabine, and oxaliplatin (R-DHAX) is an effective and safe salvage regimen in relapsed/refractory B-cell non-Hodgkin lymphoma. Clin Lymphoma Myeloma Leuk. 2010;10(4):262–9.
27. Le Gouill S, Thieblemont C, Oberic L, Bouabdallah K, Gyan E, Damaj G, et al. R-DHA-Oxaliplatin before autologous stem cell transplantation prolongs PFS and OS as compared to R-DHA-carboplatin and R-DHA-cisplatin in patients with mantle cell lymphoma, a subgroup analysis of the LyMa trial. Blood. 2017. American Society of Hematology;130(Suppl 1):1496.
28. Kluin-Nelemans HC, Hoster E, Hermine O, Walewski J, Trneny M, Geisler CH, et al. Treatment of older patients with mantle-cell lymphoma. N Engl J Med. 2012;367(6):520–31.
29. Flinn IW, van der Jagt R, Kahl BS, Wood P, Hawkins TE, Macdonald D, et al. Randomized trial of bendamustine-rituximab or R-CHOP/R-CVP in first-line treatment of indolent NHL or MCL: the BRIGHT study. Blood. 2014;123(19):2944–52.
30. Rummel MJ, Knauf W, Goerner M, Soeling U, Lange E, Hertenstein B, et al. Two years rituximab maintenance vs. observation after first-line treatment with bendamustine plus rituximab (B-R) in patients with mantle cell lymphoma: first results of a prospective, randomized, multicenter phase II study (a subgroup study of the StiL NHL7-2008 MAINTAIN trial). J Clin Oncol. 2016;34(15):7503.
31. Visco C, Finotto S, Zambello R, Paolini R, Menin A, Zanotti R, et al. Combination of rituximab, bendamustine, and cytarabine for patients with mantle-cell non-Hodgkin lymphoma ineligible for intensive regimens or autologous transplantation. J Clin Oncol. 2013;31(11):1442–9.
32. Kahl BS, McGovern J, Blank J, Jaslowski A, Bayer G, Bottner WA, et al. Phase II study of modified hyper-CVAD with rituximab maintenance for previously untreated mantle

cell lymphoma: a Wisconsin oncology network study. Blood. 2004. American Society of Hematology;104(11):1388.
33. Chang JE, Carmichael LL, Kim K, Peterson C, Yang DT, Traynor AM, et al. VcR-CVAD induction chemotherapy followed by maintenance rituximab produces durable remissions in mantle cell lymphoma: a Wisconsin oncology network study. Clin Lymphoma Myeloma Leuk. 2018;18(1):e61–7.
34. Wang ML, Lee H, Thirumurthi S, Chuang H, Hagemeister F, Westin J, et al. Ibrutinib rituximab followed by reduced chemo-immunotherapy consolidation in young, newly diagnosed mantle cell lymphoma patients: a window of opportunity to reduce chemo. Hematol Oncol. 2017;35:142–3.
35. Armand P, Redd R, Bsat J, Mayuram S, Giardino A, Fisher DC, et al. A phase 2 study of rituximab-bendamustine and rituximab-Cytarabine for transplant-eligible patients with mantle cell lymphoma. Br J Haematol. 2016;173(1):89–95.
36. Albertsson-Lindblad A, Kolstad A, Laurell A, Raty R, Gronbaek K, Sundberg J, et al. Lenalidomide-bendamustine-rituximab in patients older than 65 years with untreated mantle cell lymphoma. Blood. 2016;128(14):1814–20.
37. Robak T, Huang H, Jin J, Zhu J, Liu T, Samoilova O, et al. Bortezomib-based therapy for newly diagnosed mantle-cell lymphoma. N Engl J Med. 2015;372(10):944–53.
38. Till BG, Li H, Bernstein SH, Fisher RI, Burack R, Rimsza LM, et al. Phase II trial of R-CHOP plus Bortezomib induction therapy followed by bortezomib maintenance for previously untreated mantle cell lymphoma: SWOG 0601. Blood. 2014. American Society of Hematology;124(21):149.
39. Ruan J, Martin P, Shah B, Schuster SJ, Smith SM, Furman RR, et al. Lenalidomide plus rituximab as initial treatment for mantle-cell lymphoma. N Engl J Med. 2015;373(19):1835–44.
40. Kruger WH, Hirt C, Basara N, Sayer HG, Behre G, Fischer T, et al. Allogeneic stem cell transplantation for mantle cell lymphoma – final report from the prospective trials of the east German Study Group Haematology/Oncology (OSHO). Ann Hematol. 2014;93(9):1587–97.
41. Tessoulin B, Ceballos P, Chevallier P, Blaise D, Tournilhac O, Gauthier J, et al. Allogeneic stem cell transplantation for patients with mantle cell lymphoma who failed autologous stem cell transplantation: a national survey of the SFGM-TC. Bone Marrow Transplant. 2016;51(9):1184–90.
42. Saba NS, Liu D, Herman SE, Underbayev C, Tian X, Behrend D, et al. Pathogenic role of B-cell receptor signaling and canonical NF-kappaB activation in mantle cell lymphoma. Blood. 2016;128(1):82–92.
43. Cinar M, Hamedani F, Mo Z, Cinar B, Amin HM, Alkan S. Bruton tyrosine kinase is commonly overexpressed in mantle cell lymphoma and its attenuation by ibrutinib induces apoptosis. Leuk Res. 2013;37(10):1271–7.
44. Wang ML, Rule S, Martin P, Goy A, Auer R, Kahl BS, et al. Targeting BTK with ibrutinib in relapsed or refractory mantle-cell lymphoma. N Engl J Med. 2013;369(6):507–16.
45. Wang ML, Blum KA, Martin P, Goy A, Auer R, Kahl BS, et al. Long-term follow-up of MCL patients treated with single-agent ibrutinib: updated safety and efficacy results. Blood. 2015;126(6):739–45.
46. Rule S, Dreyling M, Goy A, Hess G, Auer R, Kahl BS, et al. Median 3.5-year follow-up of ibrutinib treatment in patients with relapsed/refractory mantle cell lymphoma: a pooled analysis. Blood. 2017. American Society of Hematol;130(Suppl 1):151.
47. Stefoni V, Sottotetti F, Gotti M, Spina M, Volpetti S, Ferrero S, et al. Multicenter retrospective observational study to assess the clinical characteristics and the outcome of patients with relapsed or refractory mantle cell non-Hodgkin's lymphoma treated in Italy according to the ibrutinib named patient program. Blood. 2016. American Society of Hematology;128(22):2985.
48. Tucker DL, Naylor G, Kruger A, Hamilton MS, Follows G, Rule SA. Ibrutinib is a safe and effective therapy for systemic mantle cell lymphoma with central nervous system involvement – a multi-centre case series from the United Kingdom. Br J Haematol. 2017;178(2):327–9.

49. Epperla N, Hamadani M, Cashen AF, Ahn KW, Oak E, Kanate AS, et al. Predictive factors and outcomes for ibrutinib therapy in relapsed/refractory mantle cell lymphoma-a "real world" study. Hematol Oncol. 2017;35(4):528–35.
50. Rule S, Dreyling M, Goy A, Hess G, Auer R, Kahl B, et al. Outcomes in 370 patients with mantle cell lymphoma treated with ibrutinib: a pooled analysis from three open-label studies. Br J Haematol. 2017;179(3):430–8.
51. Cheah CY, Chihara D, Romaguera JE, Fowler NH, Seymour JF, Hagemeister FB, et al. Patients with mantle cell lymphoma failing ibrutinib are unlikely to respond to salvage chemotherapy and have poor outcomes. Ann Oncol. 2015;26(6):1175–9.
52. Kunk PR, Mock J, Devitt ME, Palkimas S, Sen J, Portell CA, et al. Major bleeding with ibrutinib: more than expected. Blood. 2016American Society of Hematology;128(22):3229.
53. Wu J, Zhang M, Liu D. Acalabrutinib (ACP-196): a selective second-generation BTK inhibitor. J Hematol Oncol. 2016;9:21.
54. Wang M, Rule S, Zinzani PL, Goy A, Casasnovas O, Smith SD, et al. Acalabrutinib in relapsed or refractory mantle cell lymphoma (ACE-LY-004): a single-arm, multicentre, phase 2 trial. Lancet. 2017;391:659–67.
55. Walter HS, Rule SA, Dyer MJ, Karlin L, Jones C, Cazin B, et al. A phase 1 clinical trial of the selective BTK inhibitor ONO/GS-4059 in relapsed and refractory mature B-cell malignancies. Blood. 2016;127(4):411–9.
56. Tam CS, Simpson D, Opat S, Kim WS, Wang M, Cull G, et al. Safety and activity of the highly specific BTK inhibitor BGB-3111 in patients with indolent and aggressive non Hodgkin's lymphoma. Blood. 2017. American Society of Hematology;130(Suppl 1):152.
57. Majchrzak A, Witkowska M, Smolewski P. Inhibition of the PI3K/Akt/mTOR signaling pathway in diffuse large B-cell lymphoma: current knowledge and clinical significance. Molecules. 2014;19(9):14304–15.
58. Hess G, Herbrecht R, Romaguera J, Verhoef G, Crump M, Gisselbrecht C, et al. Phase III study to evaluate temsirolimus compared with investigator's choice therapy for the treatment of relapsed or refractory mantle cell lymphoma. J Clin Oncol. 2009;27(23):3822–9.
59. Ansell SM, Tang H, Kurtin PJ, Koenig PA, Inwards DJ, Shah K, et al. Temsirolimus and rituximab in patients with relapsed or refractory mantle cell lymphoma: a phase 2 study. Lancet Oncol. 2011;12(4):361–8.
60. Dreyling M, Jurczak W, Jerkeman M, Silva RS, Rusconi C, Trneny M, et al. Ibrutinib versus temsirolimus in patients with relapsed or refractory mantle-cell lymphoma: an international, randomised, open-label, phase 3 study. Lancet. 2016;387(10020):770–8.
61. Pham LV, Tamayo AT, Yoshimura LC, Lo P, Ford RJ. Inhibition of constitutive NF-kappa B activation in mantle cell lymphoma B cells leads to induction of cell cycle arrest and apoptosis. J Immunol. 2003;171(1):88–95.
62. Goy A, Sinha R, Williams ME, Kalayoglu Besisik S, Drach J, Ramchandren R, et al. Single-agent lenalidomide in patients with mantle-cell lymphoma who relapsed or progressed after or were refractory to bortezomib: phase II MCL-001 (EMERGE) study. J Clin Oncol. 2013;31(29):3688–95.
63. Arcaini L, Lamy T, Walewski J, Belada D, Mayer J, Radford J, et al. Prospective subgroup analyses of the randomized MCL-002 (SPRINT) study: lenalidomide versus investigator's choice in relapsed or refractory mantle cell lymphoma. Br J Haematol. 2018;180(2):224–35.
64. Andorsky DJ, Yacoub A, Bitran JD, Melear J, Brooks HD, Foon KA, et al. MAGNIFY: phase IIIb randomized study of lenalidomide plus rituximab (R^2) followed by lenalidomide vs. rituximab maintenance in subjects with relapsed/refractory follicular, marginal zone, or mantle cell lymphoma. Blood. 2016. American Society of Hematology;128(22):1798.
65. Wang M, Schuster SJ, Phillips T, Lossos IS, Goy A, Rule S, et al. Observational study of lenalidomide in patients with mantle cell lymphoma who relapsed/progressed after or were refractory/intolerant to ibrutinib (MCL-004). J Hematol Oncol. 2017;10:171. https://doi.org/10.1186/s13045-017-0537-5.

66. Zaja F, Ferrero S, Stelitano C, Ferrari A, Salvi F, Arcari A, et al. Second-line rituximab, lenalidomide, and bendamustine in mantle cell lymphoma: a phase II clinical trial of the Fondazione Italiana Linfomi. Haematologica. 2017;102(5):e203–6.
67. Goy A, Bernstein SH, Kahl BS, Djulbegovic B, Robertson MJ, de Vos S, et al. Bortezomib in patients with relapsed or refractory mantle cell lymphoma: updated time-to-event analyses of the multicenter phase 2 PINNACLE study. Ann Oncol. 2009;20(3):520–5.
68. Furtado M, Johnson R, Kruger A, Turner D, Rule S. Addition of bortezomib to standard dose chop chemotherapy improves response and survival in relapsed mantle cell lymphoma. Br J Haematol. 2015;168(1):55–62.
69. Dal Col J, Zancai P, Terrin L, Guidoboni M, Ponzoni M, Pavan A, et al. Distinct functional significance of Akt and mTOR constitutive activation in mantle cell lymphoma. Blood. 2008;111(10):5142–51.
70. Kahl BS, Spurgeon SE, Furman RR, Flinn IW, Coutre SE, Brown JR, et al. A phase 1 study of the PI3K delta inhibitor idelalisib in patients with relapsed/refractory mantle cell lymphoma (MCL). Blood. 2014;123(22):3398–405.
71. Dreyling M, Morschhauser F, Bouabdallah K, Bron D, Cunningham D, Assouline SE, et al. Phase II study of copanlisib, a PI3K inhibitor, in relapsed or refractory, indolent or aggressive lymphoma. Ann Oncol. 2017;28(9):2169–78.
72. Davids MS, Roberts AW, Seymour JF, Pagel JM, Kahl BS, Wierda WG, et al. Phase I first-in-human study of venetoclax in patients with relapsed or refractory non-Hodgkin lymphoma. J Clin Oncol. 2017;35(8):826–33.
73. Tam CSL, Roberts AW, Anderson MA, Dawson S, Hicks RJ, Burbury K, et al. Combination ibrutinib (Ibr) and venetoclax (Ven) for the treatment of mantle cell lymphoma (MCL): primary endpoint assessment of the phase 2 AIM study. J Clin Oncol. 2017;35(15):7520.
74. Leonard JP, LaCasce AS, Smith MR, Noy A, Chirieac LR, Rodig SJ, et al. Selective CDK4/6 inhibition with tumor responses by PD0332991 in patients with mantle cell lymphoma. Blood. 2012;119(20):4597–607.
75. Cassaday RD, Goy A, Advani S, Chawla P, Nachankar R, Gandhi M, et al. A phase II, single-arm, open-label, multicenter study to evaluate the efficacy and safety of P276-00, a cyclin-dependent kinase inhibitor, in patients with relapsed or refractory mantle cell lymphoma. Clin Lymphoma Myeloma Leuk. 2015;15(7):392–7.
76. Martin P, Blum K, Bartlett NL, Park SI, Maddocks KJ, Ruan J, et al. A phase I trial of ibrutinib plus palbociclib in patients with previously treated mantle cell lymphoma. Blood. 2016. American Society of Hematology;128(22):150.
77. Seftel MD, Kuruvilla J, Kouroukis T, Banerji V, Fraser G, Crump M, et al. The CDK inhibitor AT7519M in patients with relapsed or refractory chronic lymphocytic leukemia (CLL) and mantle cell lymphoma. A phase II study of the Canadian Cancer Trials Group. Leuk Lymphoma. 2017;58(6):1358–65.
78. Chen W, Du X, Luo C, Zhang Q, Wang M. Anti-CD19 chimeric antigen receptor T cells improve responses to chemotherapy-refractory mantle cell lymphoma: a case report. Blood. 2016. American Society of Hematology;128(22):5393.
79. Abramson JS, Palomba L, Gordon LI, Lunning M, Arnason J, Forero-Torres A, et al. Transcend NHL 001: immunotherapy with the CD19-directed CAR T-cell product JCAR017 results in high complete response rates in relapsed or refractory B-cell non-Hodgkin lymphoma. Blood. 2016. American Society of Hematology;128(22):4192.

Chapter 6
Current and Emerging Treatment Strategies for Primary Mediastinal B-Cell Lymphoma

Christin B. DeStefano, Kieron Dunleavy, and Catherine Lai

Introduction

Primary mediastinal B-cell lymphoma (PMBCL) is an aggressive subtype of non-Hodgkin lymphoma (NHL) arising from thymic B-lymphocytes. PMBCL shares clinical and biologic features with classic nodular sclerosing Hodgkin lymphoma (HL). First reported in a 1980 case series, PMBCL was first recognized as a distinct clinicopathologic entity in the 2001 World Health Organization lymphoma classification [1]. Herein is an overview of the epidemiology, pathogenesis, standard management, and emerging treatment strategies for PMBCL.

Epidemiology

PMBCL is rare, representing 2.4% of all NHLs [2]. Based on a surveillance, epidemiology, and end results (SEER) analysis, the age-adjusted incidence is 0.4 per million-person years, which has been steadily increasing over the past decade for unclear reasons [3]. The majority of PMBCL patients are young women in their third to fourth decade of life [3]. Despite females being more commonly affected than males, hormonal factors do not appear to play a role in the risk or pathogenesis

C. B. DeStefano
Uniformed Services University, Bethesda, MD, USA
e-mail: christin.destefano@us.af.mil

K. Dunleavy
George Washington University Hospital, Washington, DC, USA
e-mail: kdunleavy@mfa.gwu.edu

C. Lai (✉)
MedStar Georgetown University Hospital, Washington, DC, USA
e-mail: Catherine.lai@gunet.georgetown.edu

C. Dittus (ed.), *Novel Therapeutics for Rare Lymphomas*,
https://doi.org/10.1007/978-3-030-25610-4_6

of PMBCL [4]. Aside from gender, the only other known risk factor is inheritance of a germline mutation in the MLL gene (5533C>A) [5].

Clinical Presentation

Most patients will present with constitutional symptoms and a symptomatic bulky anterior mediastinal mass, resulting in chest discomfort, cough, and dyspnea [6]. Superior vena cava syndrome and pleural and pericardial effusions are not uncommon, and in advanced cases, patients can have a pericardial tamponade [7]. Patients with bulky disease ($\geq$10 cm in diameter) can present with tumor lysis syndrome. Bone marrow and subdiaphragmatic involvement are unusual but can sometimes occur at initial presentation [8]. Relapsed PMBCL is often extranodal and may involve organs such as the liver, gastrointestinal tract, kidneys, ovaries, and central nervous system.

Pathology and Gene Expression

PMBCL is comprised of medium to large B-lymphocytes morphologically resembling centroblasts, centrocytes, and less commonly immunoblasts. Morphologically, PMBCL is similar to HL in that there is a background of sclerosis and occasional Reed-Sternberg cells [8]. However, unlike HL, which has a characteristic immunophenotype of being strongly CD15 and CD30 positive with weak to negative expression of B-cell markers, PMBCL is characterized by negative CD15, patchy or weak CD30, and strong expression of common B-cell antigens including CD20 and CD79a. PMBCL is also distinct from mediastinal gray zone lymphoma, which has morphological and immunohistochemical features in between PMBCL and HL. Factors that drive thymic B-cell formation toward one entity over the others are not completely understood [9]. Gene expression studies have revealed an overlap in more than one third of overexpressed genes between PMBCL and HL, including PD-L2 [10]. In addition to overlapping gene expression, PMBCL and HL share dysregulated JAK-STAT and NF-kB signaling pathways and an "immune privilege" phenotype evidenced by downregulation of MHC class I/II and upregulation of PD-L1 through 9p.24 amplifications, which result in reduced immunogenicity and "immune privilege" [11–15].

Diagnosis

The differential for an anterior mediastinal mass is broad and includes PMBCL, other types of NHL, HL, thymoma, thymic carcinoma, thymic cysts, germ cell tumors to include teratoma, and ectopic thyroid tissue. Therefore, to confirm the diagnosis of PMBCL, a tissue biopsy is required. An excisional or core needle biopsy may not be possible because of the location or may not be diagnostic due to fibrosis and/or necrosis. Therefore, a surgical biopsy obtained through mediastinoscopy or thoracoscopy may be necessary in certain situations.

Staging

The Lugano classification includes recommendations for staging and response assessments of all NHLs [16]. Compared to Ann Arbor which is descriptive and can only be used for staging, Lugano incorporates fluorodeoxyglucose (FDG) positron emission tomography (PET)/CT scan into the initial evaluation and response criteria. As PMBCL rarely involves the bone marrow, a biopsy is not needed to complete staging. Irrespective of whether the disease burden is limited or extensive, all patients are treated with advanced stage treatment strategies.

Work-Up

As with all aggressive NHLs, the work-up requires a complete history and physical, laboratory studies including complete blood count (CBC) with differential, complete metabolic panel (CMP), lactate dehydrogenase (LDH), tumor lysis labs, HIV testing, and viral hepatitis serologies, as well as a FDG-PET/CT scan. Central nervous system (CNS) involvement is also rare, and brain imaging should only be considered if neurologic deficits are present. All patients will need an echocardiogram prior to receiving an anthracycline-containing regimen.

Prognosis

The prognosis of PMBCL is excellent, with a 5-year relative survival of 86% based on the SEER-18 database [17]. Unlike other NHLs, the international prognostic index is not prognostic for PMBCL in the rituximab era [18]. However, age above 38 years, the presence of pleural or pericardial effusions, the presence of constitutional symptoms, and a poor performance status are prognostic and associated with inferior outcomes in certain studies [7]. A negative end-of-treatment PET scan is also prognostic and identifies patients at very low risk of relapse. Patients with relapsed or refractory PMBCL do poorly and have outcomes inferior to that of relapsed or refractory DLBCL. Thus, optimization of frontline treatment is paramount.

Frontline Management

PMBCL patients tend to tolerate therapy well due to their young age, and as with many other aggressive lymphomas, PMBCL is highly curable. Because relapsed/refractory PMBCL portends a dismal prognosis, it is imperative to offer an optimal frontline treatment strategy that balances the benefits of treatment intensity with the risks of late and long-term treatment toxicities. Published studies on the frontline management of PMBCL are limited to single arm studies, retrospective studies, or subgroup analyses of larger studies for NHL and are listed in Table 6.1. Although PMBCL was first described nearly 40 years ago, due to its rarity, there are yet to be any prospective randomized controlled trials to guide management [19]. Despite the paucity of studies, R-CHOP chemotherapy (rituximab with cyclophosphamide, doxorubicin, vincristine, and prednisone) with consolidative mediastinal radiotherapy has historically been a standard approach.

Before rituximab gained approval with CHOP, multiple studies assessed the impact of treatment intensity on outcomes for PMBCL and found that dose-intensity correlated with better treatment outcomes. For example, high-intensity regimens such as MACOP or VACOP-B (methotrexate with leucovorin rescue or etoposide with doxorubicin, cyclophosphamide, vincristine, prednisone, and bleomycin) and ProMACE-CytaBOM (cyclophosphamide, doxorubicin, etoposide, bleomycin, vincristine, methotrexate, and prednisone) produce better response rates and long-term survival than CHOP for PMBCL [20–22]. Similarly, when compared to CHOP, high-dose chemotherapy followed by autologous stem cell rescue (HDC/ASCR) has produced superior rates of complete responses (CR), 75% vs. 61%; 10-year progression free survival (PFS), 78% vs. 35%; and 10-year overall survival (OS), 77% vs. 44% [22].

The approval of rituximab for NHL closed the efficacy gap between CHOP and higher-intensity regimens. In a subset analysis of patients with PMBCL in the phase III MabThera International Trial (MInT), the incorporation of rituximab to CHOP chemotherapy improved the rates of CR from 54% to 90% ($p = 0.015$), the 3-year event-free survival (EFS) from 52% to 78% ($p = 0.012$), and the 3-year OS from 78% to 89% ($p = 0.158$) while substantially decreasing the rate of progressive disease (PD) from 24% to 2.5% ($p < 0.001$) [23]. In another retrospective study including 80 unselected patients with PMBCL, the addition of rituximab to CHOP-based regimens raised the 10-year PFS from 67% to 95% and the 10-year OS from 72% to 92% [17]. The addition of rituximab to higher-intensity regimens, however, did not improve outcomes. In an Italian retrospective study that included PMBCL patients treated with R-MACOP-B, the CR rate was 80%, and projected 5-year OS rate was 80%, which was not dissimilar to historical controls using MACOP-B in the pre-rituximab era [24]. Likewise, when compared with R-CHOP, R-VACOP-B did not produce better 5-year PFS or OS rates [25]. As a result of these studies, it was generally accepted that incorporation of rituximab into frontline treatment for PMBCL obviates the need for chemotherapy regimens of higher intensity than CHOP.

Table 6.1 Studies for de novo PMBCL

Reference	Study type	# of patients	Regimen	% receiving RT	CR (%)	RFS (%)	OS (%)
Lazzarino et al. [20]	Case series	30	CHOP ± RT	All with CR	36	72[a] (3 years)	36[a] (3 years)
			V/MACOP-B ± RT		73		
Todeschini et al. [21]	Retrospective	138	CHOP ± IFRT	76% with CR	51	39 (5 years)	NR
			V/MACOP-B ± IFRT		80	76 (5 years)	NR
Mazzarotto et al. [25]	Retrospective	53	ProMACE-MOPP, V/ MACOP-B + IFRT	100%	38	93 (5-year)	86 (5-years)
Zinzani et al. [22]	Retrospective	426	CHOP/CHOP-B ± IFRT	All with CR and 84% with PR	61	33 (10 years)	44 (10 years)
			V/MACOP-B/ProMACE CytaBOM ± IFRT		79	67 (10 years)	71 (10 years)
			HDC/ASCR		75	78 (10 years)	77 (10 years)
Savage et al. [7]	Retrospective	153	MACOP-B	39% total	N/A	N/R	87[b] (5 years)
			CHOP		N/A	N/R	71[b] (5 years)
			R-CHOP		N/A	N/R	82 (5 years)
Rieger et al. [23]	Subgroup analysis of prospective phase III study	87	CHOP	67.40%	54	52 (3 years)	78 (3 years)
			R-CHOP	72.80%	80	78 (3 years)	89 (3 years)
Zinzani et al. [24]	Retrospective	45	R + V/MACOP-B + radiotherapy	100%	80	88 (5 years)	80 (5 years)
	Retrospective	95	R-VACOP-B	None	N/A	83[c] (5 years)	97 (5 years)
			R-CHOP21		N/A	69[c] (5 years)	

(continued)

Table 6.1 (continued)

Reference	Study type	# of patients	Regimen	% receiving RT	CR (%)	RFS (%)	OS (%)
			VACOP-B		N/A	62 (5 years)	88 (5 years)
			CHOP21		N/A	20 (5 years)	
Soumerai et al. [28]	Retrospective	63	R-CHOP ± radiotherapy	77%	79	68 (5 years)	79 (5 years)
Vassilakopoulos et al. [27]	Retrospective	76	R-CHOP ± radiotherapy	76%	N/A	81 (5 years)	89 (5 years)
Ahn et al. [29]	Retrospective	21	R-CHOP ± radiotherapy	57%	N/A	79 (3 years)	83 (3 years)
	Subgroup analysis of prospective phase III study	50	R-CHOP14 or 21 ± radiotherapy	58%	43	80 (5 years)	84[d] (5 years)
Dunleavy et al. [34]	Prospective phase II study	51	DA-EPOCH-R	4%	N/A	93 (5 years)	97 (5 years)
Giulino-Roth et al. [44]	Retrospective	156	DA-EPOCH-R	15%	N/A	86 (5 years)	95 (5 years)
Shah et al. [45]	Retrospective	132	DA-EPOCH-R	59%	84	NR	89 (2 years)
			R-CHOP	13%	70	NR	91 (2 years)

NR not reported
[a]Includes total cohort
[b]The difference in survival was only significant between MACOP-B and CHOP
[c]The PFS difference between R-MACOP-B and R-CHOP was nonsignificant
[d]There was a trend toward improved OS with R-CHOP14 > R-CHOP21

Although consolidative involved field radiotherapy played a pivotal role in the management of PMBCL in the pre-rituximab era, currently there are yet to be any studies demonstrating a survival benefit [26, 27]. Additionally, 20–25% of patients will experience a relapse or primary refractory disease after treatment with R-CHOP and consolidative mediastinal radiotherapy [28, 29]. The late and long-term toxicities of irradiation are not inconsequential, including bone marrow toxicity, accelerated coronary artery disease, a heightened risk of breast cancer, thyroid cancer, and therapy-related myeloid neoplasms, some of which can occur up to 40 years after initial treatment [30–32]. Because radiotherapy has long-term risks and does not appear to impact survival, other studies have assessed omission of radiotherapy or the use of imaging to guide end of treatment radiation.

Treatment Response Assessment

The presence of a residual anterior mediastinal mass after treatment is very common and is often due to fibrosis, sclerosis, or necrosis of the initial tumor bulk. However, it can be difficult to discriminate residual disease versus fibrosis with a CT scan alone. Several studies have assessed the role of end-of-treatment PET imaging in PMBCL using the 5-point Deauville scoring system, revealing that this measure is associated with a high negative predictive value for treatment failures. The landmark prospective phase II IELSG 26 study demonstrated that using the liver uptake as a cut-off (Deauville 1–3 vs. 4–5) effectively stratified patients into low and high risk for treatment failure after receiving a rituximab and anthracycline-based treatment regimen, with a 5-year progression-free survival (PFS) of 99% vs. 68% and OS of 100% vs. 83%, respectively [33]. When used after DA-EPOCH-R, end-of-treatment PET imaging is associated with a very good negative predictive value of 100%, further supporting that a negative end-of-treatment PET scan can identify patients at low risk of relapse [34].

Most patients in the IELSG 26 study received mediastinal radiotherapy; therefore it is not clear if treatment can be "de-escalated" with radiotherapy omission based on the results of a negative end-of-treatment PET scan. In a retrospective Canadian study by Savage et al., patients with a positive end-of-treatment PET after R-CHOP received consolidative radiotherapy, whereas those with a negative PET did not. Using risk-adapted radiotherapy consolidation, there was no difference in the 5-year time to progression (78% vs. 83%, $p = 0.735$) or overall survival (88.5% vs. 95%, $p = 0.271$), supporting the notion that radiotherapy omission in low-risk patients can be safe and feasible [35]. This proof of principle is being tested prospectively in the ongoing phase III IELSG-37 study, which omits consolidative radiotherapy among patients who achieve a complete metabolic response on their end-of-treatment PET scan after a rituximab and anthracycline-based regimen (NCT01599559).

False-positive end-of-treatment PET scans can occur about 40% of the time and are often due to inflammation [27]. To mitigate false positives due to rebound thymic uptake, imaging should be obtained 6–8 weeks after receipt of chemotherapy or myeloid growth factor support and 12 weeks after receipt of radiotherapy [36]. Although consensus guidelines recommend a biopsy consideration in the case of a positive end-of-treatment PET scan, this exposes the patient to a potentially unnecessary procedure. There are some data to support the use of serial PET imaging to decipher true refractory disease from false-positive disease, as the former will demonstrate persistent FDG avidity and the latter will improve with time [37, 38].

Management of Relapsed or Refractory PMBCL

There is no accepted standard treatment approach for relapsed/refractory PMBCL. Among those with relapsed or refractory disease, the prognosis is dismal and is inferior to that of relapsed/refractory DLBCL, with an inferior response to salvage chemotherapy (25% vs. 48%, $p = 0.01$) and inferior 2-year overall survival (15% vs. 34%, $p = 0.018$) [39]. High-dose chemotherapy followed by autologous stem cell rescue (HDC/ASCR) might be a good option for patients with late relapses (≥12 months) that demonstrate chemosensitivity but is unlikely to be beneficial for primary refractory or chemorefractory early relapsed disease [40, 41]. Patients who have primary refractory or early relapsed disease have a particularly bleak prognosis with a median survival of approximately 6 months, and better treatments in this population are needed [42]. Allogeneic transplant can be utilized, but limited retrospective data suggest the benefit is minimal and transplant-related mortality high [43]. Published studies on management of relapsed or refractory PMBCL are listed in Table 6.2.

Novel Approaches for Untreated PMBCL

In an attempt to omit mediastinal radiotherapy, the National Cancer Institute (NCI) led a prospective phase II study assessing the efficacy of infusional dose-adjusted etoposide, doxorubicin, and cyclophosphamide with vincristine, prednisone, and rituximab (DA-EPOCH-R) with myeloid growth factor support for untreated PMBCL [33]. Fifty-one patients with median age of 30 and 59% females were enrolled. Many participants in the study had high-risk features – 65% had bulky disease, 53% had extranodal disease, 47% had pleural effusions, and 29% had stage IV disease. All had malignant cells that expressed CD20. After a median follow-up of 63 months, the EFS and OS were 93% and 97%, respectively. Eighteen patients had a positive end-of-treatment PET (defined by the study as Deauville 3–5), of which only three had confirmed residual disease and two of these received mediastinal irradiation. Hospitalization for febrile neutropenia occurred in 13% of the cycles, and there were no episodes of cardiotoxicity. Although not directly compared with R-CHOP and consolidative radiotherapy, the results of this study show that higher-intensity chemoimmunotherapy can have high response rates and also support omission of radiotherapy in frontline treatment. A retrospective study assessed the efficacy of frontline DA-EPOCH-R for PMBCL and included 156

Table 6.2 Studies for R/R PMBCL

Reference	Study type	# of patients	Regimen	CR (%)	RFS (%)	OS (%)
Neelapu et al. [48]	Phase II study	24	Autologous anti-CD19 CAR-T cells	71	NR	NR
Zinzani et al. [50]	Phase Ib study	18	Pembrolizumab	12	NR	NR
Zinzani et al. [50]	Phase II study	15	Brentuximab vedotin	0	NR	NR
Jacobsen et al. [52]	Phase II study	6	Brentuximab vedotin	17	NR	NR
Aoki et al. [40]	Retrospective	44	HDC/ASCR	64	61 (4 years)	70 (4 years)
Avivi et al. [41]	Retrospective	44	HDC/ASCR – chemosensitive disease	NR	64 (3 years)	85 (3 years)
		24	HDC/ASCR – chemorefractory disease	NR	39 (3 years)	41 (3 years)
Khouri et al. [43]	Retrospective	17	Allogeneic transplant	3-year PFS and OS 41% and 46%	41 (3 years)	46 (3 years)

NR not reported, *CAR-T cells* chimeric antigen receptor T cells, *HDC/ASCR* high dose chemotherapy followed by autologous stem cell rescue

adults and children, of whom 14.9% received radiotherapy. The 3-year EFS and OS were 85.9% and 95.4%, respectively, and 75% achieved a negative end-of-treatment PET scan which correlated with an improved EFS [44]. Although DA-EPOCH-R has never been prospectively compared to standard R-CHOP with consolidative radiotherapy, a multicenter retrospective analysis involving 132 patients compared these two frontline treatment approaches and reported that recipients of DA-EPOCH-R were less likely to receive radiotherapy (13% vs. 59%) and had higher CR rates (84% vs. 70%, $p = 0.046$). The 2-year OS rates were similar at 89% for R-CHOP recipients and 91% for DA-EPOCH-R recipients [45]. DA-EPOCH-R is associated with relatively low rates of female infertility in patients under the age of 40, which is important given the patient demographics of this disease [46].

Novel Approaches in the Relapsed and Refractory Setting

Immunotherapy

Given the "immune privilege" phenotype of PMBCL and similarity to classic HL, the role of immunotherapy for the management of PMBCL is currently being explored. Bone marrow transplant is the oldest form of immunotherapy, and new therapies such as chimeric antigen receptor T-cells (CAR-T cells) and checkpoint inhibitors appear promising. Immunotherapy approaches mentioned below are novel, and as such it is unclear how to best combine or sequence these agents with traditional treatment approaches.

CAR-T Cells

CAR-T cells have made dramatic differences for patients with relapsed or refractory acute lymphoblastic leukemia and DLBCL and have recently been granted full food and drug administration (FDA) approval for PMBCL. CAR-T cells are autologously derived cytotoxic T-lymphocytes that are engineered ex vivo to incorporate tumor antigen recognition moieties and T-cell signaling domains [47]. Because PMBCL is characterized by immune exhaustion and expresses the immunogenic CD19 antigen, CAR-T cells have been studied for use in PMBCL. The phase II ZUMA-1 study assessed the efficacy of the autologously derived anti-CD19 CAR-T cells, axicabtagene ciloleucel, and included patients with refractory DLBCL (cohort 1) and PMBCL or transformed follicular lymphoma (cohort 2) [48]. After leukapheresis with CAR-T manufacturing, patients received a fixed low-dose conditioning regimen consisting of fludarabine and cyclophosphamide followed by two million CAR-T cells per kg of body weight. Of the 111 patients included in the study, 8 had PMBCL. The median time from leukapheresis to infusion of CAR-T cells was 17 days. In cohort 2, the overall response rate (ORR) was 83% which included 71% CRs. Responses were not adversely affected by the use of tocilizumab or corticosteroids. At 18 months of follow-up, about half of the patients were still alive. The most common drug-related adverse events were cytopenias, cytokine release syndrome, and neurotoxicity, the latter two of which have issued FDA black box warnings. As a result of the ZUMA-1 study, the FDA granted full approval of axicabtagene ciloleucel for use in relapsed or refractory large B-cell lymphoma, including PMBCL that has been previously treated with at least two lines of systemic therapy.

Checkpoint Inhibitors

The immune privilege phenotype of PMBCL lends an opportunity to be exploited with immune checkpoint inhibitors. Up to 100% of cases of PMBCL are associated with enhanced PD-L1 expression, due to 9p24.1 gains in about half of cases and rearrangements at the PDL1/2 locus in about 20% of cases [49]. The phase Ib keynote-013 study assessed the efficacy of the anti-PD1 antibody pembrolizumab for relapsed/refractory PMBCL [50]. Eighteen patients were enrolled and treated. The median age was 30 and over 70% were female. The patients were heavily pre-treated – with a median of three prior treatments, one third had received prior HDC/ASCR, and nearly two thirds had undergone prior radiotherapy. Sixty-one percent of patients experienced grade 1/2 toxicities, including hypothyroidism, diarrhea, nausea, and fatigue. There were only two grade 3/4 toxicities which included neutropenia and veno-occlusive disease post-allogeneic transplant. The ORR was 41%, which included two patients who achieved a CR. After a median follow-up duration of 11.3 months, the median duration of response had not been reached. A subsequent phase II study confirmed a similar treatment efficacy of pembrolizumab for patients with relapsed/refractory PMBCL resulting in FDA drug approval (NCT02576990).

Anti-CD30 Directed Therapy

Most cases of PMBCL overexpress CD30, and hence there is scientific rationale that CD30-directed therapies may be efficacious. Despite the success of the anti-CD30 antibody-drug complex brentuximab vedotin (BV) for use in classic HL, systemic and primary cutaneous anaplastic large cell lymphoma, and mycosis fungoides, this agent does not have a role as monotherapy for the treatment of PMBCL based on the results of two phase II studies. The first is an Italian study which assessed the safety and efficacy of standard-dosed BV for relapsed/refractory CD30+ PMBCL [51]. Fifteen patients were enrolled. The median age was 29 and the majority were female. The median prior number of treatments was 3, and over half had received HDC/ASCR and radiotherapy. The ORR was 13.3% and consisted of all partial responses that lasted less than 3 months. Forty percent experienced drug-related adverse events, which were comprised of mostly grade 1/2 peripheral neuropathy, atrial fibrillation, transaminitis and anemia. The second study was a phase II trial assessing the efficacy of BV for DLBCL with variable CD30 expression and included six patients with PMBCL [52]. There was only one response to BV which was a CR, producing an ORR of 17%. The discrepancy in the treatment efficacy of BV between PMBCL and other CD30-expressing lymphomas likely has to do with the characteristics of CD30 expression. Although most cases of PMBCL are associated with CD30 overexpression, up to one third do not express CD30 [53]. Among those that do express CD30, the expression is typically at low levels and can be very heterogeneous [54].

Clinical Trials

The ongoing clinical trials for untreated and relapsed/refractory PMBCL are listed in Table 6.3.

Table 6.3 Ongoing clinical studies

Therapy	Study type	Setting	Clinical trial #
Mediastinal radiotherapy	Phase III study	Untreated PMBCL achieving CMR after chemoimmunotherapy	NCT01599559
DA-EPOCH-R	Phase II study	Children and adolescents with untreated PMBCL	NCT01516567
Pembrolizumab	Phase II study	R/R PMBCL	NCT02576990
Autologous anti-CD19 CAR-T cells + durvalumab	Phase I study	R/R NHL including PMBCL	NCT02706405
Autologous anti-CD19 CAR-T cells	Phase I study	R/R DLBCL, PMBCL, grade 3B FL, MCL	NCT2631044
Nivolumab + varlilumab	Phase II study	R/R NHL including PMBCL	NCT03038672
Ibrutinib + pembrolizumab	Phase 1 study	R/R NHL including PMBCL	NCT02950220
Vorinostat + pembrolizumab	Phase I study	R/R NHL including PMBCL	NCT03150329
Gemcitabine/vinorelbine/doxorubicin + PD-1 antibody ± low-dose decitabine	Phase I/II study	R/R PMBCL	NCT03346642
Bendamustine + rituximab + ibrutinib	Phase II study	R/R NHL including PMBCL	NCT02747732
Obinutuzumab + ICE	Phase II study	R/R CD20+ B-cell NHL	NCT02393157
Lenalidomide + R-ICE	Phase I/II study	R/R DLBCL including PMBCL	NCT02628405
Idelalisib + R-ICE	Phase I study	R/R DLBCL and PMBCL	NCT03349346
Tazemetostat	Phase I/II study	R/R B-cell NHL including PMBCL	NCT01897571

R/R relapsed/refractory, *CMR* complete metabolic response, *NHL* non-Hodgkin lymphoma, *DLBCL* diffuse large B-cell lymphoma, *FL* follicular lymphoma, *MCL* mantle cell lymphoma

Consolidative Radiotherapy

To determine whether consolidative mediastinal radiotherapy can be omitted, the ongoing IELSG-37 phase III study (NCT01599559) which opened in 2012 is enrolling patients with a negative end-of-treatment PET/CT scan after receipt of a rituximab-based chemotherapy regimen, including CHOP-14 or CHOP-21, DA-EPOCH, Mega-CHOP, VACOP-B, or MACOP-B. Enrollees are assigned to either observation or 3-D conformal radiotherapy with a total dose of 30 Gy. The primary and secondary endpoints of this study are PFS and OS, respectively. Notably this is the first and only phase III study on PMBCL to date.

Small Molecule Inhibitors

Given their success in indolent and aggressive NHLs, multiple ongoing early phase trials are assessing the efficacy of small molecule inhibitors for treatment of DLBCL including PMBCL. Ongoing studies include various combinations of targeted agents with salvage chemotherapy regimens including the oral Bruton tyrosine kinase inhibitor ibrutinib in combination with bendamustine and rituximab (NCT02747732), the immunomodulatory agent lenalidomide and the PI3K inhibitor idelalisib partnered with salvage R-ICE (NCT02628405, NCT03349346), and lastly the EZH2 histone methyltransferase inhibitor tazemetostat as monotherapy (NCT01897571).

Immunotherapy

A multitude of clinical trials are assessing the feasibility and efficacy of combination therapy utilizing checkpoint inhibitors. An ongoing phase II study evaluates the anti-PD1 antibody nivolumab alongside the co-stimulatory CD27 agonist varlilumab (NCT03038672). Ongoing phase I studies are evaluating potential synergy between pembrolizumab and ibrutinib (NCT02950220) as well as the histone deacetylase inhibitor vorinostat (NCT03150329). The type II glycoengineered anti-CD20 antibody obinutuzumab is partnered with salvage ifosfamide, carboplatin, and etoposide (ICE) chemotherapy in another early phase study for patients with relapsed aggressive lymphoma including PMBCL (NCT02393157). Another phase I/II study in China is assessing gemcitabine, vinorelbine, doxorubicin, and checkpoint inhibition with or without low-dose decitabine priming (NCT03346642).

As checkpoint inhibitors can enhance the longevity of CAR-T cells by dampening their exhaustion in vitro, it is possible that combining these remedies may produce synergistic immune toxicity in vivo [55]. A phase I study at the Fred Hutchinson Cancer Research Center (NCT02706405) will assess the safety and pharmacokinetic profile of autologous anti-CD19 CAR-T cells in combination with the anti-PDL1 antibody durvalumab. In this study, patients with relapsed/refractory NHL including subsets of PMBCL will receive JCAR014 on day 0, followed by durvalumab on day 28, which will continue every 4 weeks for up to 10 doses in the absence of disease progression or unacceptable toxicity. Other clinical trials are exploring CAR-T cells for NHL patients including PMBCL, to include the phase I TRANSCEND-NHL-001 trial which utilizes JCAR017 for relapsed/refractory DLBCL, PMBCL, grade 3B follicular lymphoma, and mantle cell lymphoma (NCT 02631044).

In summary, given the strong immune privilege phenotype of PMBCL, the role of immunotherapy in the relapsed and refractory is becoming increasingly recognized. Combinations and sequences of checkpoint inhibitors and CAR-Ts in addition to small molecule inhibitors and monoclonal antibodies are being assessed in ongoing early phase studies.

Preclinical Studies

Given that enhanced JAK2 signaling plays a role in the pathogenesis of PMBCL, it is possible that JAK2 inhibitors might be efficacious for management. A selective JAK2 inhibitor, fedratinib, was studied in vitro and in vivo for PMBCL and HL [56]. When utilized in cell lines and murine xenograft models, JAK2 inhibition resulted in decreased cell proliferation, increased apoptosis, and increased survival with simultaneous decreased expression of PD-L1. There was an inverse correlation between the effective drug concentration and 9p24.1/JAK2 copy number.

Recommended Treatment Approach

Frontline Management

The two generally accepted frontline treatment approaches consist of 6–8 cycles of DA-EPOCH-R without radiotherapy and R-CHOP with consolidative radiotherapy. The frontline treatment approach should be individualized and incorporate the patient's age, cardiac reserve, candidacy for intensive chemotherapy and radiotherapy, the presence of disease outside of a radiation field, pleural/pericardial effusions, bulky disease, and the patient's desire for fertility. DA-EPOCH-R should be strongly recommended based on the low efficacy of R-CHOP and toxicity of radiotherapy.

Once a management approach has been selected, patients should be monitored for treatment toxicities and response assessment. An interim CT scan after at least two cycles of treatment should be performed to ensure the disease is not progressing on treatment. An end-of-treatment FDG PET/CT should be obtained at least 6–8 weeks following chemotherapy and at least 12 weeks following radiotherapy. If a complete metabolic response is achieved, the patient should enter surveillance, which generally consists of a history, physical exam, and labwork (with or without CT imaging) every 6 months for the first 2 years after treatment completion.

If a residual FDG-avid mass is present on the end-of-treatment PET scan, in the absence of clinical suspicion for refractory disease, it would be reasonable to perform repeat PET imaging at 6–8 weeks to evaluate for resolution. FDG-avid lesions that are falsely positive will improve with time, whereas residual disease will remain PET positive and increase in uptake. If refractory disease is suspected or if repeat PET imaging does not normalize, then a tissue biopsy is needed to confirm presence of lymphoma.

Management of Relapsed or Refractory PMBCL

Since relapsed or refractory PMBCL portends a dismal prognosis, a clinical trial should be strongly considered for all patients. If the patient is not a clinical trial candidate or if a clinical trial is not available, then management strategies employing salvage chemotherapy, radiotherapy, HDC/ASCR, CAR-T cells, checkpoint inhibitors, and allogeneic transplant can be utilized. If not given in the frontline setting, salvage radiotherapy can be curative if the disease is confined to the mediastinum. As relapsed or refractory disease can involve extranodal sites to include the gastrointestinal tract and CNS, careful assessments of any gastrointestinal or neurologic symptoms should ensue.

The treatment approach must take into account the patient's age, burden of disease, likelihood of having chemosensitive disease, fitness for intensive therapy, likelihood of being able to perform proper cell collections HDC/ASCR or CAR-T cells, and general goals of care. The standard approach to relapsed PMBCL in a transplant-eligible patient is salvage chemotherapy to autologous SCT [57]. For transplant-ineligible patients with chemotherapy-sensitive disease, a course of salvage chemotherapy should be pursued. In chemotherapy-resistant patients, a PD-1 inhibitor is reasonable.

Eligible patients who have received at least two prior lines of therapy can consider axicabtagene ciloleucel based on the aforementioned ZUMA-1 trial which revealed excellent response rates surpassing 70% in this population. However, the duration of response is not known, and it would be important to also human leukocyte antigen (HLA) type the patient and refer the patient to an allotransplant center.

Conclusions

PMBCL is a rare and underrepresented subtype of NHL with a predilection for young females in their third or fourth decade of life. Despite nearly 40 years of awareness of this distinct clinicopathologic entity, there are yet to be any randomized phase III trials to guide management, highlighting the importance of clinical trial enrollment. Despite a lack of high-level evidence, the standard de facto treatment has historically consisted of R-CHOP followed by consolidative mediastinal radiotherapy. However, due to late and long-term toxicities of irradiation, higher-intensity treatments with high remission rates omitting radiation such as DA-EPOCH-R should be highly considered. Additionally, end-of-treatment PET scan can stratify patients after chemotherapy and aid in risk-adapted, individualized treatment approaches. Given the immune privilege phenotype of PMBCL, the role of immunotherapy for relapsed or refractory disease has been promising in early studies.

References

1. Jaffe ES, Harris NL, Stein H, et al. World Health Organization classification of tumors. Pathology and genetics of tumours of haematopoietic and lymphoid tissues. Lyon: IARC Press; 2001.
2. The Non-Hodgkin's Lymphoma Classification Project. A clinical evaluation of the International Lymphoma Study Group classification of non-Hodgkin's lymphoma. Blood. 1997;89:3909–18.
3. Liu PP, Wang KF, Xia Y, et al. Racial patterns of patients with primary mediastinal large B-cell lymphoma. Medicine (Baltimore). 2016;95(27):e4054.
4. Romaguera JE, Meilus S, Rodriguez J, et al. Endocrine characterization of primary mediastinal lymphoma. Leuk Lymphoma. 1996;23(5–6):613–5.
5. Saarinen S, Kaasinen E, Karjalainen-Lindsberg ML, et al. Primary mediastinal large B-cell lymphoma segregating in a family: exome sequencing identifies MLL as a candidate predisposition gene. Blood. 2013;121(17):3428–30.
6. Jacobson JO, Aisenberg AC, Lamarre L, et al. Mediastinal large cell lymphoma. An uncommon subset of adult lymphoma curable with combined modality therapy. Cancer. 1988;62:1893.
7. Savage KJ, Al-Rajhi N, Voss N, et al. Favorable outcome of primary mediastinal large B-cell lymphoma in a single institution: the British Columbia experience. Ann Oncol. 2006;17:123.
8. Swerdlow SH, Campo E, Harris NL, et al. World Health Organization classification of tumours of haematopoietic and lymphoid tissues. Lyon: IARC Press; 2008.
9. Dunleavy K, Wilson WH. Primary mediastinal B-cell lymphoma and mediastinal gray zone lymphoma: do they require a unique therapeutic approach? Blood. 2015;125(1):33–9.
10. Rosenwald A, Wright G, Leroy K, et al. Molecular diagnosis of primary mediastinal B cell lymphoma identifies a clinically favorable subgroup of diffuse large B cell lymphoma related to Hodgkin lymphoma. J Exp Med. 2003;198(6):851–62.
11. Savage KL, Monti S, Kutok JL, et al. The molecular signature of mediastinal large B-cell lymphoma differs from that of the other diffuse large B-cell lymphomas and shares features with classical Hodgkin lymphoma. Blood. 2003;102:3871–9.
12. Gunawardana J, Chan FC, Telenius A, et al. Recurrent somatic mutations of PTPN1 in primary mediastinal B cell lymphoma and Hodgkin lymphoma. Nat Genet. 2014;46(4):329–35.
13. Steidl C, Shah SP, Woolcock BW, et al. MHC class II transactivator CIITA is a recurrent gene fusion partner in lymphoid cancers. Nature. 2011;471(7338):377–81.
14. Rimsza LM, Roberts RA, Campo E, et al. Loss of major histocompatibility class II expression in non-immune-privileged site diffuse large B-cell lymphoma is highly coordinated and not due to chromosomal deletions. Blood. 2006;107:1101–7.
15. Twa DD, Chan FC, Ben-Neriah S, et al. Genomic rearrangements involving programmed death ligands are recurrent in primary mediastinal large B-cell lymphoma. Blood. 2014;123:2062–5.
16. Cheson BD, Fisher RI, Barrington SF, et al. Recommendations for initial evaluation, staging, and response assessment of Hodgkin and non-Hodgkin lymphoma: the Lugano classification. J Clin Oncol. 2014;32(27):3059–67.
17. Surveillance, Epidemiology, and End Results (SEER) Program (www.seer.cancer.gov) SEER*Stat Database: Overall Survival – SEER 18, Nov 2016 Sub (1973–2014) – Linked To County Attributes – Total U.S., 1969–2015 Counties, National Cancer Institute, DCCPS, Surveillance Research Program, released April 2017. Accessed 15 Nov 2017.
18. Lisenko K, Dingeldein G, Cremer M, et al. Addition of rituximab to CHOP-like chemotherapy in first line treatment of primary mediastinal B-cell lymphoma. BMC Cancer. 2017;17:359.
19. Lichtenstein AK, Levine A, Taylor CR, et al. Primary mediastinal lymphoma in adults. Am J Med. 1980;68(4):509–14.
20. Lazzarino M, Orlandi E, Paulli M, et al. Primary mediastinal B-cell lymphoma with sclerosis: an aggressive tumor with distinctive clinical and pathologic features. J Clin Oncol. 1993;11(12):2306–13.
21. Todeschini G, Secchi S, Morra E, et al. Primary mediastinal large B-cell lymphoma (PMlBCL): long-term results from a retrospective multicenter Italian experience in 138 patients treated with CHOP or MACOP-B/VACOP-B. Br J Cancer. 2004;90:372–6.

22. Zinzani PL, Martelli M, Bertini M, et al. Induction chemotherapy strategies for primary mediastinal large B-cell lymphoma with sclerosis: a retrospective multinational study on 426 previously untreated patients. Haematologica. 2002;87(12):1258–64.
23. Rieger M, Osterborg A, Pettengell R, et al. Primary mediastinal B-cell lymphoma treated with CHOP-like chemotherapy with or without rituximab: results of the Mabthera International Trial Group study. Ann Oncol. 2011;22:664–70.
24. Zinzani PL, Stefoni V, Finolezzi E, et al. Rituximab combined with MACOP-B or VACOP-B and radiation therapy in primary mediastinal large B-cell lymphoma: a retrospective study. Clin Lymphoma Myeloma. 2009;9(5):381–5.
25. Mazzarotto R, Boso C, Vianello F, et al. Primary mediastinal large B-cell lymphoma: results of intensive chemotherapy regimens (MACOP-B/VACOP-B) plus involved field radiotherapy on 53 patients. A single institution experience. Int J Radiat Oncol Biol Phys. 2007;68(3):823–9.
26. Giri S, Bhatt VR, Pathak R, Bociek G, et al. Role of radiation therapy in primary mediastinal large B-cell lymphoma in rituximab era: a US population-based analysis. Am J Hematol. 2015;90(11):1052–4.
27. Vassilakopoulos TP, Pangalis GA, Katsigiannis A, et al. Rituximab, cyclophosphamide, doxorubicin, vincristine, and prednisone with or without radiotherapy in primary mediastinal large B-cell lymphoma: the emerging standard of care. Oncologist. 2012;17:239–49.
28. Soumerai JD, Hellmann MD, Feng Y, et al. Treatment of primary mediastinal B-cell lymphoma with rituximab, cyclophosphamide, doxorubicin, vincristine and prednisone is associated with a high rate of primary refractory disease. Leuk Lymphoma. 2014;55(3):538–43.
29. Ahn HK, Kim SJ, Yun J, et al. Improved treatment outcome of primary mediastinal large B-cell lymphoma after introduction of rituximab in Korean patients. Int J Hematol. 2010;91(3):456–63.
30. Schaapveld M, Aleman B, van Eggermond A, et al. Second cancer risk up to 40 years after treatment for Hodgkin's lymphoma. N Engl J Med. 2015;373:2499–511.
31. Van Nimwegen FA, Schaapveld M, Cutter DJ. Radiation dose-response relationship for risk of coronary heart disease in survivors of Hodgkin lymphoma. J Clin Oncol. 2016;34(3):235–43.
32. Kamran SC, de Gonzalez AB, Ng A, et al. Therapeutic radiation and the potential risk of second malignancies. Cancer. 2016;122(12):1809–21.
33. Martelli M, Ceriani L, Zucca E, et al. [18F]fluorodeoxyglucose positron emission tomography predicts survival after chemoimmunotherapy for primary mediastinal large B-cell lymphoma: results of the International Extranodal Lymphoma Study Group IELSG-26 Study. J Clin Oncol. 2014;32(17):1769–75.
34. Dunleavy K, Pittaluga S, Maeda LS, et al. Dose-adjusted EPOCH-rituximab therapy in primary mediastinal B-cell lymphoma. N Engl J Med. 2013;368(15):1408–16.
35. Savage KJ, Yenson PR, Shenkier T, Klasa R, Villa D, Goktepe O et al. The outcome of primary mediastinal large B-cell lymphoma (PMBCL) in the R-CHOP treatment era. In: Proceedings from the 54th annual American Society of Hematology conference, Atlanta, GA. 2012.
36. Allen-Auerbach M, Weber WA. Measuring response with FDG-PET: methodological aspects. Oncologist. 2009;14:369–77.
37. National Comprehensive Cancer Network. B-cell lymphomas (Version 1.2018). https://www.nccn.org/professionals/physician_gls/pdf/b-cell.pdf. Accessed 1 Feb 2018.
38. Melani C, Advani RH, Roschewski M, et al. End-of-treatment CT and serial FDG-PET imaging to assess residual disease in primary mediastinal B-cell lymphoma. In: Proceedings from the 59th American Society of Hematology annual meeting, Atlanta, GA. 2017. https://ash.confex.com/ash/2017/webprogram/Paper108834.html.
39. Kuruvilla J, Pintillie M, Tsang R, et al. Salvage chemotherapy and autologous stem cell transplantation are inferior for relapsed or refractory primary mediastinal large B-cell lymphoma compared with diffuse large B-cell lymphoma. Leuk Lymphoma. 2008;49(7):1329–36.
40. Aoki T, Shimada K, Suzuki R, et al. High-dose chemotherapy followed by autologous stem cell transplantation for relapsed/refractory primary mediastinal large B-cell lymphoma. Blood Cancer J. 2015;e372:1–5.

41. Avivi I, Boumendil A, Finel H, et al. Autologous stem cell transplantation for primary mediastinal B-cell lymphoma: long-term outcome and role of post-transplant radiotherapy. A report of the European Society for Blood and Marrow Transplantation. Bone Marrow Transplant. 2018;53:1001–9.. Epub ahead of print.
42. Crump M, Neelapu SS, Farooq U, et al. Outcomes in refractory diffuse large B-cell lymphoma: results from the international SCHOLAR-1 study. Blood. 2017;130(16):1800–8.
43. Khouri IF, Saliba RM, Xu-Monette ZY, et al. Outcomes following allogeneic stem cell transplantation (AlloSCT) in patients with primary mediastinal (PMBL), germinal center B (GCB) and non-GCB cell-like diffuse large B cell lymphomas (DLBCL). In: Proceedings from the 56th American Society of Hematology annual meeting, San Francisco, CA. 2014. http://www.bloodjournal.org/content/124/21/2563?sso-checked=true.
44. Giulino-Roth L, O'Donohue T, Chen Z, et al. Outcomes of adults and children with primary mediastinal B-cell lymphoma treated with dose-adjusted EPOCH-R. Br J Haematol. 2017;179(5):739–47.
45. Shah NN, Szabo A, Huntington SF, et al. R-CHOP versus dose-adjusted R-EPOCH in frontline management of primary mediastinal B-cell lymphoma: a multi-centre analysis. Br J Haematol. 2018;180(4):534–44.
46. Gharwan H, Lai C, Grant C, Dunleavy K, Steinberg SM, Shovlin M, Fojo T, Wilson WH. Female fertility following dose-adjusted EPOCH-R chemotherapy in primary mediastinal B-cell lymphomas. Leuk Lymphoma. 2016;57(7):1616–24.
47. Brudno JN, Kochenderfer JN. Chimeric antigen receptor T-cell therapies for lymphoma. Nat Rev Clin Oncol. 2018;15(1):31–46.
48. Neelapu SS, Locke FL, Barlett NL, et al. Axicabtagene ciloleucel CAR T-cell therapy in refractory large B-cell lymphoma. N Engl J Med. 2017;377(26):2531–44.
49. Gravelle P, Burroni B, Pericart S, et al. Mechanisms of PD-1/PD-L1 expression and prognostic relevance in non-Hodgkin lymphoma: a summary of immunohistochemical studies. Oncotarget. 2017;4(27):44960–75.
50. Zinzani PL, Ribrag V, Moskowitz CH, et al. Safety and tolerability of pembrolizumab in patients with relapsed/refractory primary mediastinal large B-cell lymphoma. Blood. 2017;130(3):267–70.
51. Zinzani PL, Pellegrini C, Chiappella A, et al. Brentuximab vedotin in relapsed primary mediastinal large B-cell lymphoma: results from a phase 2 clinical trial. Blood. 2017;129(16):2328–30.
52. Jacobsen ED, Sharman JP, Oki Y, et al. Brentuximab vedotin demonstrates objective responses in a phase 2 study of relapsed/refractory DLBCL with variable CD30 expression. Blood. 2015;125(9):1394–402.
53. Higgins JP, Warnke RA. CD30 expression is common in mediastinal large B-cell lymphoma. Am J Clin Pathol. 1999;112(2):241–7.
54. Hutchinson CB, Wang E. Primary mediastinal (thymic) large B-cell lymphoma: a short review with brief discussion of mediastinal gray zone lymphoma. Arch Pathol Lab Med. 2011;135(3):394–8.
55. Cherkassky L, Morello A, Villena-Vargas J, et al. Human CAR T cells with cell-intrinsic PD-1 checkpoint blockade resistant tumor-mediated inhibition. J Clin Invest. 2016;126(8):3130–44.
56. Hao Y, Chapuy B, Monti S, et al. Selective JAK2 inhibition specifically decreases Hodgkin lymphoma and mediastinal large B-cell lymphoma growth in vitro and in vivo. Clin Cancer Res. 2014;20(10):2674–83.
57. Philip T, Guglielmi C, Hagenbeek A, et al. Autologous bone marrow transplantation as compared with salvage chemotherapy in relapses of chemotherapy-sensitive non-Hodgkin's lymphoma. N Engl J Med. 1995;333(23):1540–5.

Chapter 7
Plasmablastic Lymphoma and Primary Effusion Lymphoma

Thomas A. Guerrero-Garcia and Jorge J. Castillo

Plasmablastic Lymphoma

Introduction

Despite its original description almost 20 years ago [1], plasmablastic lymphoma (PBL) remains a clinical and pathological challenge to the hematologist, oncologist, and pathologist providing care for these complicated patients. PBL is a rare CD20-negative lymphoma with morphological, immunophenotypical, and genomic features intermediate between aggressive diffuse large B-cell lymphoma (DLBCL) and plasma cell neoplasms [2]. The tumor cells express CD138, CD38, and IRF4/MUM1 – plasma cell markers – and lack expression of typical B-cell markers such as CD19, CD20, or PAX5. Key molecular players in the pathogenesis of PBL are *MYC* gene rearrangements and EBV-encoded RNA (EBER) [3]. Historically, this tumor was reported in association with HIV infection. More recently, it has become evident that PBL can also arise in immunocompetent patients. As in other high-grade B-cell lymphomas, PBL has a MYC rearrangement in about 50% of cases. Although, it is not completely understood how EBV plays a role in the pathogenesis of PBL, in most cases tumor cells are infected with EBV, usually a latency type 1. EBV-encoded RNA (EBER) has been reported as high as 80% and 50% in HIV-positive and HIV-negative PBL, respectively [4]. Despite improvements in the understanding of the biology of the disease by clinicians and pathologists, PBL

T. A. Guerrero-Garcia
Division of Hematologic Malignancies, Dana-Farber Cancer Institute, Harvard Medical School, Boston, MA, USA
e-mail: ThomasA_GuerreroGarcia@DFCI.Harvad.edu

J. J. Castillo (✉)
Bing Center for Waldenström Macroglobulinemia, Dana-Farber Cancer Institute, Harvard Medical School, Boston, MA, USA
e-mail: JorgeJ_Castillo@DFCI.Harvard.edu

C. Dittus (ed.), *Novel Therapeutics for Rare Lymphomas*,
https://doi.org/10.1007/978-3-030-25610-4_7

carries a poor outcome and prognosis. In this chapter our efforts are to focus on the latest research in the treatment of PBL and provide a comprehensive novel therapeutic approach.

An accurate incidence of PBL is yet to be determined by large epidemiological studies. Previous studies have reported an incidence of 2–10% of HIV-associated lymphoma cases and in less than 1% of all diffuse large B-cell lymphoma (DLBCL) cases [5–8]. PBL has also been identified in other immunosuppressive states such as posttransplantation, in immunocompetent individuals, in the elderly, and in the context of other lymphoproliferative disorders, plasma cell dyscrasias, or autoimmune disorders [3, 9, 10].

Although the median age at diagnosis is in the fifth or sixth decade of life, PBL cases have been described in pediatric and elderly patients [11–13]. HIV-associated PBL occurs predominantly in younger men (male-to-female ratio of 7:1) with advanced stage and predilection for the oral cavity [14]. HIV-negative PBL cases were older at presentation (57 years) with a male-to-female ratio of 1.7:1 and a lower frequency of advanced stage [9, 15]. This is consistent with other case series on HIV-negative PBL [16, 17].

Based on the initial seminal report, PBL affects mainly young men with HIV infection and involves the oral cavity. Several recent case series show that the oral cavity remains a common area of involvement in HIV-associated PBL. Most patients however present with extranodal involvement, regardless of their HIV status [15]. The gastrointestinal tract is the second most common site of involvement by PBL. In addition, there are multiple case reports in which PBL has been reported in the central nervous system (CNS), skin, paranasal sinus, soft tissue, mediastinum, lungs, heart, liver, breast, and testes. Bone marrow involvement has been reported in 10–30% of patients with PBL [10, 17–23]. B-symptoms have been reported in 40–60% of patients with PBL [8, 15]. In 50% of cases in multiple cohorts, both HIV-negative and HIV-positive PBL patients had presented with advanced stage (i.e., stage III or IV) [8, 10, 17, 18, 22].

Diagnosis and Evaluation

PBL is morphologically characterized by a monomorphic proliferation of round- to oval-shaped cells with plasmacytoid features. A perinuclear hof is frequently seen. The background infiltrate contains small mature lymphocytes and may include apoptotic bodies, mitotic figures, and tingible body macrophages, imparting a "starry-sky" appearance [2]. Immunophenotypically, PBL demonstrates little to no expression of leukocyte common antigen (CD45) or the B-cell markers CD20, CD79a, and PAX5. However, the plasma cell markers CD38, IRF4, BLIMP-1, and CD138 seem to be almost universally expressed [2, 24]. The proliferation marker Ki-67 is almost always expressed in neoplastic cells.

EBV infection has been associated with the development of PBL [3], and EBV-encoded RNA (EBER) is frequently detected in patients with PBL. Its detection by means of fluorescent or chromogenic in situ hybridization (ISH) has become the standard for evaluating the presence of EBV genome within tumor cells. Several studies have showed detection rates of EBER at 50% or higher in PBL [10, 14, 23, 25]. Molecular testing of MYC in PBL is of importance, as MYC rearrangement or amplification can be detected in a substantial number of patients with PBL [18, 26, 27]. The most common translocation gene occurring within MYC, at about 50–60% prevalence, is the immunoglobulin heavy chain gene, c-MYC/IGH fusion, t(8;14).

PBL should be differentiated from other CD20-negative DLBCL variants, specifically extracavitary PEL and ALK-positive DLBCL. MYC rearrangement could be helpful in distinguishing PBL from ALK-positive DLBCL, as the latter lacks MYC translocation. Also, PBL lacks rearrangements in BCL2 and BCL6, commonly seen in ALK-positive DLBCL. ALK-positive DLBCL is rarely associated with HIV, EBV, or HHV8 infections. Extracavitary forms of PEL can be difficult to differentiate from PBL. The identification of HHV8 genome in the malignant cells should suggest PEL rather than PBL in these cases. Differential features of PBL, PEL, and ALK-positive DLBCL are shown in Table 7.1. A representative case of PBL is shown in Fig. 7.1.

The diagnosis of PBL should be established by obtaining adequate tissue for pathological evaluation. Although the staging of patients with PBL should mimic DLBCL, the data on the use of PET/CT scans are scarce. Extrapolating from other aggressive lymphomas, it follows that a PET/CT scan would be valuable at choosing a desired biopsy location, for staging and also for assessing response to therapy. For staging, current NCCN guidelines recommend PET/CT scans, bone marrow aspirate and biopsy, and a lumbar puncture [28].

Unfortunately, the prognosis of PBL continues being poor with most case series and population-based studies reporting median survival times ranging between 12 and 18 months [7, 8, 10, 18, 21, 22, 28]. Not surprisingly, patients with early stages (i.e., stage I or II) exhibit better outcomes. In addition, studies have found that patients with low or low-intermediate international prognosis index (IPI) scores had longer survival than patients with high or high-intermediate IPI scores [8, 18]. The IPI score, therefore, should be used for risk stratification and prognostic estimates in PBL patients. HIV-positive PBL patients who received antiretroviral therapy (ART) fared better when compared with patients in whom ART was not instituted or continued

Table 7.1 Differential diagnosis of PBL

	PBL	PEL	ALK+ DLBCL
Disease location	Extranodal	Extranodal	Nodal
HIV infection	++	+++	–
EBV infection	++	+++	–
HHV8 infection	–	+++	–
Pathogenesis	EBV, MYC	HHV8, EBV	ALK
Positive markers	CD38,IRF4,MYC,CD30+/–	CD38,IRF4,CD30+/–	CD45, CD38, ALK
Negative markers	CD20, PAX5	CD20, PAX5	CD20, CD30, MYC
Proliferation rate	>90%	>90%	>90%

ALK anaplastic lymphoma kinase, *FISH* fluorescence in situ hybridization, *GR* gene rearrangement, *IRF-4/MUM-1* interferon regulatory factor 4/multiple myeloma 1, *PBL* plasmablastic lymphoma, *PEL* primary effusion lymphoma

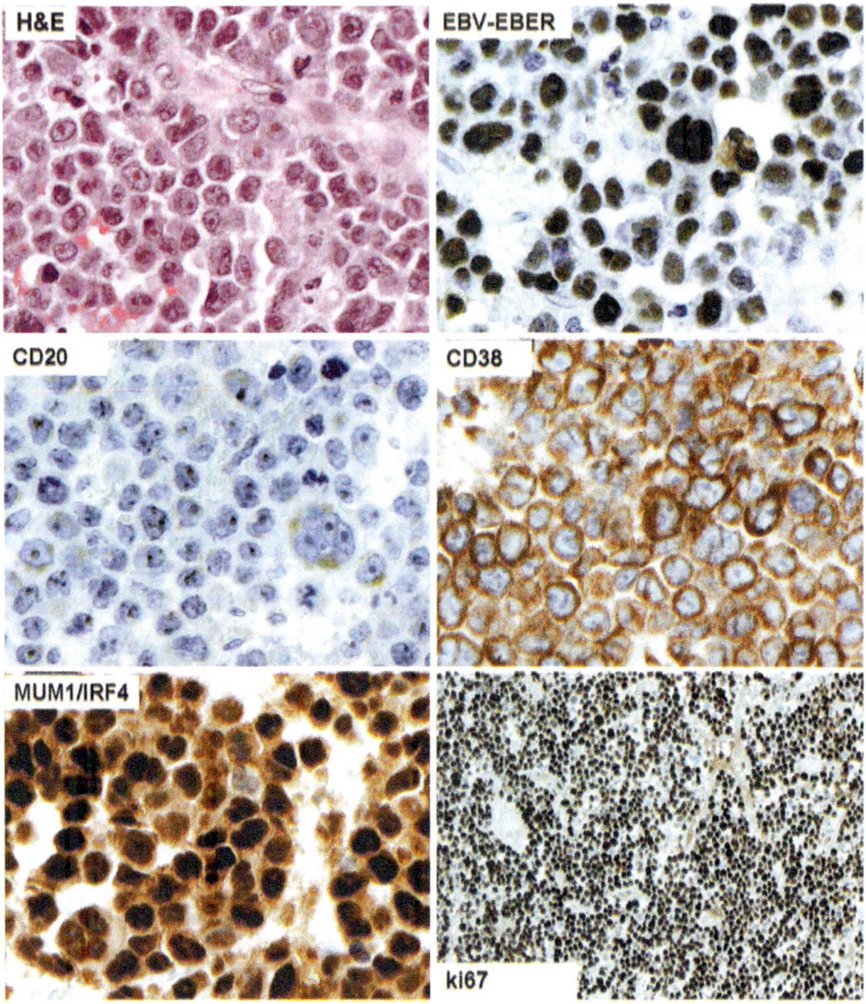

Fig. 7.1 Immunophenotype of PBL. Immunohistochemistry with hematoxylin counterstain shows lack of expression of CD20 and CD10 and positive expression of IRF4/MUM1, Ki67, and MYC (magnification, ×400). Detection of EBER by in situ hybridization shows that neoplastic cells are positive; nuclear reactivity (×400)

[17]. This has been replicated in a smaller Italian study [29]. It is possible that the induction of a virological and/or immunological response positively impacts the response and survival in HIV-infected patients. HIV-negative patients might have a worse outcome than HIV-infected individuals. This idea has been supported by case series as well as a large US population-based study [8, 15, 17]. The prognostic role of EBER expression is unclear. EBER expression was significantly associated with better OS in some studies, while no relation between EBER expression and survival was observed in others [10, 14, 15, 17, 22, 30]. The presence of MYC gene rearrangement appears consistently associated with a worse outcome in PBL [10, 18, 27].

Traditional Treatment Approach

There is not a standard treatment for PBL, and current treatment recommendations are mostly based on small case series, case reports, and experts' opinion. Current NCCN guidelines emphasize that standard CHOP is inadequate therapy for PBL. Regimens with higher intensity such as EPOCH, CODOX-M/IVAC, and Hyper-CVAD are suggested with the use of autologous hematopoietic stem cell transplant for those with high risk and CR in first remission. However, two studies of patients with PBL treated with chemotherapy regimens more intensive than CHOP did not identify a survival benefit [18, 31]. In a large European study, higher-intensity regimens, like DA-EPOCH, ACVBP, and COPADM, did not show significantly higher CR rates compared with patients receiving CHOP therapy [17]. A recent pooled analysis suggested that infusional EPOCH might be more effective than standard CHOP [32]. In HIV-infected patients, initiation or optimization of HAART is highly recommended and should be directed by an infectious disease specialist. For these patients, appropriate antibiotic prophylaxis should be considered, especially with low CD4+ cell counts. For the small portion of PBL cases that express CD20, rituximab should be considered in addition to chemotherapy given better outcomes seen in CD20-positive HIV-positive lymphomas treated with rituximab [33]. The use of G-CSF should be strongly considered in all patients with PBL undergoing chemotherapy. The use of CNS prophylaxis is debatable and should probably mimic recommendations for DLBCL. Radiotherapy should be used as consolidation in patients with early stage disease, similar to DLBCL, and can be considered in the palliative setting. NCCN recommends autologous SCT after achieving a first CR in a case-by-case basis. However, these recommendations come from a limited data source. After the introduction of ART, autologous SCT in HIV-positive patients with NHL has shown to be feasible [34, 35]. A small group of PBL patients was included in a recent prospective phase II multicenter trial conducted by the BMT CTN in collaboration with the AIDS Malignancy Consortium. The authors concluded that the outcomes between HIV-infected patients and controls were not significantly different, and HIV-infected patients should be considered candidates for autologous SCT if they met standard transplant criteria [36]. Both the European and American groups found in different analyses that autologous SCT might be beneficial both in the salvage setting and for consolidation after first responses [37, 38]. However, both analyses have limitations with the retrospective design, small study populations, and lack of consensus about pretransplant regimens used.

Novel Agents

Given the poor outcomes and survival of patients with PBL, novel agents have been evaluated in the treatment of PBL; however these strategies are in the context of small case reports and series. Given the plasmacytic differentiation of PBL cells, one of the agents evaluated was the proteasome inhibitor bortezomib. Bortezomib has been shown to be effective in patients with non-germinal center DLBCL, inducing higher responses and survival rates when used in combination with anthracycline-containing regimens [39]. Bortezomib alone and in combination with chemotherapy has been used with limited efficacy in HIV-positive and HIV-negative patients with relapsed PBL [40–45]. However, a case series of three previously untreated patients with PBL, two of them HIV-positive, showed efficacy with the combination of bortezomib and dose-adjusted EPOCH [46]. The experience was recently extended to two larger case series of 16 and 8 patients, respectively, in which high response rates and longer survival than expected were observed [47, 48]. In the study by Castillo and colleagues, a 5-year overall survival of 52% was reported. Likewise, a Spanish group reported three cases in which upfront bortezomib was added to CHOP [49]. Here, all three patients underwent autologous SCT at first CR. At the time of the report, two out of the three patients remained alive, one with a maximum follow-up of 22 months [50]. Moreover, in a systematic review of the use of upfront bortezomib-containing regimens in 19 patients with PBL, the study suggested an ORR of 74% as well as 3-year OS rate of approximately 60% [51].

The other novel agent of interest is the immunomodulator lenalidomide, which is largely used in the treatment of plasma cell neoplasms. The cell of origin in PBL is thought to be the plasmablast, an activated B-cell that has undergone somatic hypermutation and class switching recombination and is in the process of becoming a plasma cell. The pathogenesis of PBL is poorly understood, but inhibition of the NF-kB pathway seems to be important. This pathway might also play an important role in PBL as plasmablasts are closely related to activated B-cells, which often show NF-kB activation. Immunomodulating agents have multiple mechanisms of action, which include inhibition of angiogenesis and NF-kB downregulation, among others. Clinically, lenalidomide alone or in combination with chemotherapy has shown to induce responses in patients with PBL [40, 52–55].

Studies have shown that approximately 30% of PBL cases express the activation marker CD30 [19, 27, 56], and a recent report showed a rapid, but very short, response to brentuximab vedotin in a patient with CD30-positive relapsed PBL. Unfortunately, the patient developed complications and could not get further treatment and eventually passed away [57]. Recently, another case report showed a fast response to brentuximab vedotin in combination with lenalidomide in the fourth line setting, but the patient unfortunately passed away shortly after treatment was started [58].

Given the poor response in the frontline setting, PBL patients in the relapsed setting have very poor outcomes, short survival, and very limited options. Lenalidomide, bortezomib, and brentuximab vedotin have been used in the relapsed setting with limited success. Interestingly, one HIV-positive patient underwent autologous SCT after salvage therapy with daratumumab in combination with ifosfamide, carboplatin, and etoposide [47, 51]. That patient was alive after 2 years of follow-up.

Immune checkpoint inhibitors are of great interest in PBL. In the tumor microenvironment, PD-1 and its ligand PD-L1 perform a vital role in tumor progression and survival by escaping tumor neutralizing immune surveillance. A recent study found that PBL expresses PD-1/PD-L1 in the microenvironment and the malignant cells, particularly in EBV-positive PBL [59]. PD-L1 expression was positive in tumor cells in 22.5% of PBL cases showing a high PD-L1 score in 77% of cases compared to PD-1 which was expressed in tumor cells in 5% of PBL cases. These findings represent an important step to support further implementation of newer strategies with immunotherapy for patients with PBL who have very limited therapeutic options. Currently, a randomized phase 2 study of CDX-1127 (varlilumab) in combination with nivolumab in patients with relapsed and/or refractory aggressive B-cell lymphomas, including PBL, is ongoing (**NCT03038672**).

Several clinical trials that will include PBL are ongoing. DA-EPOCH-R regimen is being evaluated prospectively in untreated BL and c-MYC high-risk DLBCL patients, in which PBL is included (**NCT01092182**). A sequential phase I/II trial of vorinostat and chemotherapy with rituximab in HIV-related lymphoma including PBL is ongoing (**NCT01193842**). In the phase II portion of the trial, patients will be randomized to vorinostat plus R-DA-EPOCH or R-DA-EPOCH. In the phase I, the response rate in high-risk patients treated with vorinostat plus R-DA-EPOCH was 100% (complete 83% and partial 17%) with a 1-year event-free survival of 83% [60].

Gene therapy is another strategy being studied in HIV-associated lymphomas after frontline chemotherapy. Researchers are using peripheral blood stem cells treated with a lentivirus vector-encoding multiple anti-HIV RNAs targeted to the HIV-1 TAT/REV (SHL)-trans-active response element-chemokine cysteine-cysteine receptor 5 ribozyme-treated hematopoietic stem progenitor cells and then transferring this via SCT to patients with HIV-associated lymphoma (**NCT01961063**). Patients with PBL can be included in this study. The NCI group is using the same approach but with frontline R-EPOCH (**NCT02337985**).

An ongoing study is evaluating the therapeutic value of autologous EBV-specific CAR T-cells with CD30 as the main target (**NCT01192464**). Potentially, CAR T-cells can be directed against EBV antigens in patients with EBV-associated lymphomas including PBL, especially if they express CD30.

A group of reader proteins named bromodomain and extra-terminal (BET) domain has gained popularity as emerging anticancer strategy. In PBL, however it would make sense to target MYC given that >50% of patients with PBL would have MYC gene rearrangements. Yet, targeting MYC is cumbersome as it lacks a ligand-binding domain. Therefore, through epigenetics perhaps the transcriptional function of MYC can be modified. The BET family members (BRD2, BRD3, BRD4, and BRDT) comprise a class of epigenetic reader proteins, which bind acetylated lysine residues on histones to facilitate the recruitment of transcriptional elongation complexes [61]. MYC transcription depends on the assembly of these proteins. Therefore, small-molecule BET inhibitors have been proposed as a MYC pathway-targeted therapeutic. JQ1 is a small molecule inhibitor of BET, with the highest affinity for BRD4. BRD4 is a scaffolding factor that associates with acetylated chromatin to facilitate active transcription. JQ1 competitively interacts with BRD4, thus preventing BRD4 from binding to chromatin [62]. A study in DLBCL cells hypothesized that JQ1 treatment would result in decreased cell proliferation and viability in a MYC-dependent manner. The study showed that JQ1 efficiently inhibited proliferation of human DLBCL cells in a dose-dependent manner regardless of their molecular subtypes. The expression of MYC was suppressed by JQ1. Furthermore, JQ1 treatment significantly suppressed growth of DLBCL cells engrafted in mice and improved survival of engrafted mice [63]. Combining anti-PD-1 antibodies and JQ1 caused synergistic responses in mice bearing MYC-driven lymphomas [64]. Lastly, the BET inhibitor BAY 1238097 has shown strong antitumor efficacy in vivo as a single agent in two DLBCL models [65]. When DLBCL cells were treated with BAY 1238097, downregulation of EZH2 was observed. Interestingly, this led to a synergism between pharmacological inhibition of BET and EZH2, suggesting that this combination of epigenetic drugs is worth further preclinical and clinical investigation. Interestingly, BAY 1238097 decreased MYC signaling and downregulated target genes of MYC, NOTCH, and E2F, as well as members of the NF-kB/MYD88 and mTOR/AKT signaling pathways.

Recommended Treatment Approach

Our recommendation for first-line treatment of PBL is six cycles of infusional dose-adjusted EPOCH in combination with bortezomib and consideration of consolidative autologous SCT in first remission for appropriate candidates. In HIV-positive patients, ART should be started or optimized under the supervision of an infectious disease specialist with experience in the potential interactions between anticancer agents and ART. For the relapsed patient, treatment remains a challenge. Treatment with proteasome inhibitors, immunomodulators, and anti-CD30, anti-CD38, or anti-PD-1 monoclonal antibodies can be considered alone or in combination with chemotherapy. If a response is obtained, selected patients should be considered for autologous SCT.

Primary Effusion Lymphoma

Introduction

Primary effusion lymphoma (PEL) was first reported in 1989 [66]. In the initial report, a patient with a history of AIDS was diagnosed with a body cavity lymphoma of B-cell lineage that was lacking typical B-cell markers, such as CD20. In 1995, a larger case series showed seven HIV-infected individuals who presented with a malignant pleural effusion and in some cases concomitant Kaposi sarcoma (KS) [67]. DNA analysis found HHV-8 and EBV genome sequences in the neoplastic cells.

PEL is now considered a CD20-negative aggressive B-cell lymphoma and comprises 2–4% of all HIV-associated lymphomas and 0.5% of all DLBCL cases in the USA [8]. Besides association with HIV infection, PEL has also been reported in the setting of solid organ transplantation and elderly individuals. Patients with PEL can present with concurrent KS and multicentric Castleman disease. The median age at presentation is in the mid-50s [8]. However, HIV-negative cases tend to present at a later age. There is a male predominance, especially in HIV-infected individuals. There is also a higher proportion of Blacks and Hispanics among patients with PEL, when compared to DLBCL patients.

PEL typically manifests as a malignant pleural, pericardial, or peritoneal effusion without evidence of lymphadenopathy, masses, or tumors [68]. By definition, PEL is a stage IV disease. Due to the presence of effusions, patients can present with chest pain, shortness of breath, dyspnea of exertion, or abdominal distention. Constitutional symptoms are reported in about half of the patients at diagnosis. Pleural is the most commonly affected body cavity, followed by peritoneum and pericardium. Rarely, the scrotum can be affected [69]. Furthermore, there can be extracavitary PEL variants [70]. Extracavitary PEL is morphologically and genetically identical to classical PEL. The gastrointestinal tract is the commonly affected, but there have been cases of extracavitary PEL involving the skin, lungs, lymph nodes, and central nervous system.

Diagnosis and Evaluation

The diagnosis of PEL is made by demonstrating the presence of malignant lymphocytes in the affected tissue and confirming HHV-8 infection [68]. Fluid should be obtained from the effusion, which can then be prepared as cell block or cytospin. PEL cells are typically large with variable nuclear size and prominent nucleoli, and in some cases, they can resemble plasmablasts or immunoblasts. Immunophenotypic studies reveal a null lymphocyte phenotype with positive expression of CD45 but negative expression of typical B-cell markers (i.e., CD19, CD20, CD79a) or T-cell makers (i.e., CD3, CD4, CD8). PEL cells can express lymphocyte activation markers (i.e., CD30, CD71) as well as markers of plasmacytic differentiation (i.e., CD38, CD138, IRF4). The Ki67 index is typically high. In addition, concomitant HHV-8 and EBV infection is demonstrated by positive expression of HHV-8 latent nuclear antigen and EBV-encoded RNA, respectively. A representative case of PEL is shown on Fig. 7.2.

Pleural, peritoneal, and/or pericardial effusions are typically suspected by physical examination and confirmed by x-rays, computed tomography (CT) scans, or echocardiogram. It is important to evaluate all body cavities, as the number of body cavities involved might have prognostic implications [71]. Also, patients with peritoneal involvement or extracavitary PEL seem to have a worse prognosis than patients with pleural involvement [8, 71]. The prognosis of PEL remains poor. A recent US population-based study reported a median overall survival of 5 months [8]. Other case series have reported median OS ranging between 4 and 9 months. HIV, HBV, and HCV testing should be performed in all cases with PEL, and appropriate treatment for active viral infections should be started, as antiretroviral therapy (ART) seems to improve the survival of HIV-infected patients with PEL. HIV-infected PEL patients appear to have a better prognosis than HIV-negative patients [8].

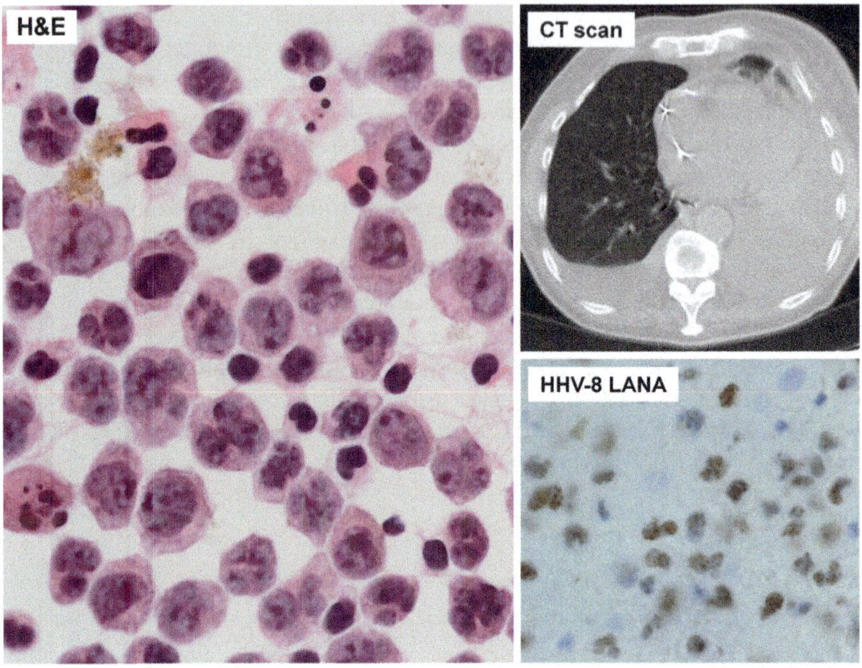

Fig. 7.2 Representative case of primary effusion lymphoma. H&E (×400) staining from a pleural effusion cytoprep in a typical case of PEL is shown here. CT scan shows a left-sided pleural effusion. HHV-8 infection can be demonstrated by the expression of LANA (×400) in these cases

Traditional Treatment Approach

The treatment for PEL is not standardized. Response rates to standard CHOP are approximately 40% with a median OS of 6 months. Other more intensive regimens such as ACVBP and dose-adjusted EPOCH have been reported in patients with PEL, but it is unclear if these regimens are associated with higher rates of response and/or survival than CHOP. Based on a recent patient-level meta-analysis showing survival benefits of EPOCH over CHOP in HIV-infected individuals with aggressive lymphoma [32], it is common practice to use EPOCH in patients with PEL. This is supported by current NCCN guidelines. To further support the use of chemotherapy in PEL, a population-based study from the USA showed that the median OS of HIV-positive PEL patients who receive chemotherapy is longer than in HIV-positive PEL patients who do not receive chemotherapy (0.7 vs. 0.4 years, respectively) [7]. However, the same study showed that only 60% of HIV-positive PEL patients actually receive chemotherapy when compared to 80–90% in HIV-positive patients with DLBCL or Burkitt lymphoma. G-CSF support should be provided to all patients with PEL. As there is negative expression of CD20, rituximab is typically not indicated; however, it can be considered in rare cases of CD20-positive PEL. ART should be instituted in HIV-infected individuals, and complete remissions have rarely been seen in PEL patients with ART alone [72, 73]. Autologous and allogeneic hematopoietic stem cell transplantation can be considered in the young and/or fit patient with relapsed and/or refractory PEL.

Novel Agents

Responses have been seen to antiviral therapy such as cidofovir, ganciclovir, or valganciclovir. Cidofovir was tested in vitro against two HHV8-positive PEL cell lines (i.e., BCBL-1 and HBL-6) [74]. Cidofovir inhibited dose-dependent cell proliferation and viability and induced apoptosis in both cell lines. Based on these results, intracavitary infusions of cidofovir were administered to three elderly patients with HHV8-positive, HIV-negative PEL. All patients tolerated cidofovir well and responded with resolution of the effusion as confirmed by x-rays or CT scans. Relapse, however, was observed in two patients. Another patient who failed two lines of chemotherapy had a durable response to intracavitary cidofovir lasting for 15 months [50]. Initial preclinical studies evaluating the role of the tumor microenvironment in PEL showed no effect of ganciclovir on cell growth in culture or in a xenograft model [75]. However, another study suggested that the combination of ganciclovir and valproate would promote lytic replication of HHV8 promoting tumor cell apoptosis without increasing viral load [76]. One case reported on the use of ganciclovir in a 31-year-old HIV-infected man with HHV8 and EBV-positive PEL [77]. Therapy consisted of ganciclovir and CHOP and induced a remission that was ongoing at 48 months after therapy. A randomized, double-blind placebo-controlled study evaluated the role of valganciclovir on suppression of HHV-8 replication and showed that valganciclovir administered daily reduced the frequency and quantity of HHV-8 replication [78]. The use of valganciclovir has also been reported in PEL patients with limited success [79], although it was successful at achieving a radiological response with clearance of HHV8 DNA after failure of bortezomib-containing therapy [80].

Preclinical data support a constitutive activation of the NF-kB pathway in PEL cells [81], suggesting that proteasome inhibitors such as bortezomib can be effective in PEL patients. Specifically, PEL cells treated with an inhibitor of IkB-alpha downregulated IL6, inducing apoptosis of PEL cells. Furthermore, a direct xenograft murine PEL model was developed, and exposure to bortezomib induced remission of PEL and prolonged the survival of NOD/SCID mice bearing PEL [82]. Transcriptome analysis revealed that bortezomib downregulated DNA replication and MYC target genes. However, the preclinical activity of bortezomib has not translated into clinical efficacy [83].

As the cell of origin on PEL is theorized to be a B-cell with plasmacytic differentiation, anti-myeloma agents such as immunomodulatory drugs (IMIDs) have been studied preclinically with evidence of efficacy against PEL cell lines [84]. In this study, clinically achievable levels of IMIDs induced an antiproliferative effect against a majority of PEL cell lines exposed and suggested that the anti-PEL effect of IMIDs involved cereblon-dependent suppression of IRF4. Clinically, there have been a few case reports suggesting activity of lenalidomide in patients with PEL. A 77-year-old man, who was felt not to be a good candidate for chemotherapy, was treated with lenalidomide 25 mg/day and experienced a decrease in his pleural effusion and tolerated lenalidomide for 18 months until the time of the report [85]. Another 80-year-old male patient obtained a complete radiologic response within 6 months of therapy with lenalidomide at a dose of 15 mg/day [86].

CD30 is frequently expressed in PEL cells [71, 87]. Targeting of PEL cells with the anti-CD30 conjugated monoclonal antibody brentuximab vedotin improved the survival of a xenograft mouse model by inhibiting proliferation and causing arrest in the G2/M cell cycle phase [88]. Similarly, CD38 is almost universally expressed in PEL [71]. However, the role of CD38 expression or inhibition in PEL cells has not been evaluated in PEL either preclinically or clinically. Targeting CD38 is of interest given the number of anti-CD38 monoclonal antibodies under development, specifically daratumumab, which is already approved by the FDA for the treatment of patients with multiple myeloma.

PEL cells have a deregulated MYC protein likely due to the activity of HHV-8-encoded latent proteins. Although MYC is considered "untargetable," genes associated with regulation of MYC can be targeted. Specifically, bromodomain and extra-terminal (BET) bromodomain inhibitors have shown activity against PEL cells [89]. Treatment of PEL cells with BET inhibitors suppressed expression of MYC and dysregulated MYC-dependent genes inhibiting cell growth and inducing cell cycle arrest, apoptosis, and cellular senescence. In a xenograft murine model, the BET inhibitor JQ1 reduced tumor burden and improved survival of PEL-bearing mice. Furthermore, the combination of BET inhibitors and IMIDs might be synergistic against PEL cells, and the combination of JQ1 and lenalidomide increased the survival of PEL-bearing NOD/SCID mice when compared with either agent alone [84].

Several other pathways have been evaluated in preclinical cell and/or animal models. Increased PD-L1 expression was found in HHV8-associated PEL cells and also in tumor-infiltrating macrophages [90]. These findings suggest that immunotherapeutic agents with activity against the PD-1/PD-L1 pathway, such as nivolumab, pembrolizumab, or atezolizumab, can be of interest for clinical development in PEL. HSP90 inhibitors have shown preclinically to be active against PEL cells [91]. Specifically, HSP90 inhibition leads to the degradation of vFLIP and IKK-gamma, as well as NF-kB downregulation, which promotes apoptosis and autophagy. Interestingly, there was synergy when a BCL2 inhibitor was added to the HSP90 inhibitor. These findings suggest the potential clinical application of HSP90 inhibitors such as tanespimycin in combination with BCL2 inhibitors such as venetoclax in PEL. IRAK1 mutations were present in virtually 100% of the cases evaluated in a preclinical study and were associated with cell survival [92]. IRAK1, along with MYD88, mediates toll-like receptor signaling. IRAK1 inhibitors are undergoing clinical development for B-cell lymphomas and could be effective in PEL. Another study reported that the hepatocyte growth factor/c-MET pathway was highly activated by HHV8. A c-MET inhibitor was able to induce cell cycle arrest and cause

DNA damage, which resulted in PEL cell apoptosis and suppressed tumor progression in a xenograft murine model [93]. Targeting of the glycolytic phenotype of PEL cells by PI3K, Akt, and mTOR inhibitors showed increased cytotoxicity against PEL cells [94]. Inhibitors of the PI3K/Akt/mTOR pathway reduce lactate production and could shift cell metabolism from aerobic glycolysis toward oxidative respiration. Cytotoxic synergy was observed when combining PI3K/Akt/mTOR inhibitors with a glycolysis inhibitor. A recent study identified MALT1 as one of the main mediators of NF-kB activation in PEL cells [95]. MALT1 inhibition induced a switch from latent to lytic stages of viral infection and impacted growth and survival of PEL cells in a xenograft model.

Recommended Treatment Approach

In patients with PEL and HIV infection, we initiate or modify ART as spontaneous remission has rarely been seen with ART alone. We also recommend draining any effusions for symptomatic comfort as frequently as needed. With regard to therapy, our typical frontline approach for PEL is to use infusional EPOCH. Given the encouraging results with the addition of bortezomib to infusional EPOCH in PBL, we feel that V-EPOCH is reasonable in PEL patients as well. Daratumumab or lenalidomide in combination with chemotherapy followed by autologous SCT can be considered in selected relapsed patients.

References

1. Delecluse HJ, Anagnostopoulos I, Dallenbach F, et al. Plasmablastic lymphomas of the oral cavity: a new entity associated with the human immunodeficiency virus infection. Blood. 1997;89(4):1413–20.
2. Stein H, Harris N, Campo E. Plasmablastic lymphoma. In: Swerdlow S, et al., editors. WHO classification of tumours of the haematopoietic and lymphoid tissues. Lyon: IARC; 2008. p. 256–7.
3. Castillo JJ, Bibas M, Miranda RN. The biology and treatment of plasmablastic lymphoma. Blood. 2015;125(15):2323–30.
4. Castillo JJ, Chavez JC, Hernandez-Ilizaliturri FJ, Montes-Moreno S. CD20-negative diffuse large B-cell lymphomas: biology and emerging therapeutic options. Expert Rev Hematol. 2015;8(3):343–54.
5. Carbone A. AIDS-related non-Hodgkin's lymphomas: from pathology and molecular pathogenesis to treatment. Hum Pathol. 2002;33(4):392–404.
6. Engels EA, Biggar RJ, Hall HI, et al. Cancer risk in people infected with human immunodeficiency virus in the United States. Int J Cancer. 2008;123(1):187–94.
7. Olszewski AJ, Fallah J, Castillo JJ. Human immunodeficiency virus-associated lymphomas in the antiretroviral therapy era: analysis of the National Cancer Data Base. Cancer. 2016;122(17):2689–97.
8. Qunaj L, Castillo JJ, Olszewski AJ. Survival of patients with CD20-negative variants of large B-cell lymphoma: an analysis of the National Cancer Data Base. Leuk Lymphoma. 2017;59:1–9.

9. Castillo JJ, Winer ES, Stachurski D, et al. HIV-negative plasmablastic lymphoma: not in the mouth. Clin Lymphoma Myeloma Leuk. 2011;11(2):185–9.
10. Morscio J, Dierickx D, Nijs J, et al. Clinicopathologic comparison of plasmablastic lymphoma in HIV-positive, immunocompetent, and posttransplant patients: single-center series of 25 cases and meta-analysis of 277 reported cases. Am J Surg Pathol. 2014;38(7):875–86.
11. Pather S, MacKinnon D, Padayachee RS. Plasmablastic lymphoma in pediatric patients: clinicopathologic study of three cases. Ann Diagn Pathol. 2013;17(1):80–4.
12. Vaubell JI, Sing Y, Ramburan A, et al. Pediatric plasmablastic lymphoma: a clinicopathologic study. Int J Surg Pathol. 2014;22(7):607–16.
13. Liu F, Asano N, Tatematsu A, et al. Plasmablastic lymphoma of the elderly: a clinicopathological comparison with age-related Epstein-Barr virus-associated B cell lymphoproliferative disorder. Histopathology. 2012;61(6):1183–97.
14. Castillo J, Pantanowitz L, Dezube BJ. HIV-associated plasmablastic lymphoma: lessons learned from 112 published cases. Am J Hematol. 2008;83(10):804–9.
15. Castillo JJ, Winer ES, Stachurski D, et al. Clinical and pathological differences between human immunodeficiency virus-positive and human immunodeficiency virus-negative patients with plasmablastic lymphoma. Leuk Lymphoma. 2010;51(11):2047–53.
16. Liu M, Liu B, Liu B, et al. Human immunodeficiency virus-negative plasmablastic lymphoma: a comprehensive analysis of 114 cases. Oncol Rep. 2015;33(4):1615–20.
17. Tchernonog E, Faurie P, Coppo P, et al. Clinical characteristics and prognostic factors of plasmablastic lymphoma patients: analysis of 135 patients from the LYSA group. Ann Oncol. 2017;28(4):843–8.
18. Castillo JJ, Furman M, Beltran BE, et al. Human immunodeficiency virus-associated plasmablastic lymphoma: poor prognosis in the era of highly active antiretroviral therapy. Cancer. 2012;118(21):5270–7.
19. Colomo L, Loong F, Rives S, et al. Diffuse large B-cell lymphomas with plasmablastic differentiation represent a heterogeneous group of disease entities. Am J Surg Pathol. 2004;28(6):736–47.
20. Liu JJ, Zhang L, Ayala E, et al. Human immunodeficiency virus (HIV)-negative plasmablastic lymphoma: a single institutional experience and literature review. Leuk Res. 2011;35(12):1571–7.
21. Montes-Moreno S, Gonzalez-Medina AR, Rodriguez-Pinilla SM, et al. Aggressive large B-cell lymphoma with plasma cell differentiation: immunohistochemical characterization of plasmablastic lymphoma and diffuse large B-cell lymphoma with partial plasmablastic phenotype. Haematologica. 2010;95(8):1342–9.
22. Schommers P, Wyen C, Hentrich M, et al. Poor outcome of HIV-infected patients with plasmablastic lymphoma: results from the German AIDS-related lymphoma cohort study. AIDS. 2013;27(5):842–5.
23. Teruya-Feldstein J, Chiao E, Filippa DA, et al. CD20-negative large-cell lymphoma with plasmablastic features: a clinically heterogenous spectrum in both HIV-positive and -negative patients. Ann Oncol. 2004;15(11):1673–9.
24. Vega F, Chang CC, Medeiros LJ, et al. Plasmablastic lymphomas and plasmablastic plasma cell myelomas have nearly identical immunophenotypic profiles. Mod Pathol. 2005;18(6):806–15.
25. Kim JE, Kim YA, Kim WY, et al. Human immunodeficiency virus-negative plasmablastic lymphoma in Korea. Leuk Lymphoma. 2009;50(4):582–7.
26. Bogusz AM, Seegmiller AC, Garcia R, et al. Plasmablastic lymphomas with MYC/IgH rearrangement: report of three cases and review of the literature. Am J Clin Pathol. 2009;132(4):597–605.
27. Valera A, Balague O, Colomo L, et al. IG/MYC rearrangements are the main cytogenetic alteration in plasmablastic lymphomas. Am J Surg Pathol. 2010;34(11):1686–94.
28. NCCN Guidelines Version 1.2018. AIDS-related B-cell lymphomas. AIDS-2. Available at http://www.nccn.org/professionals/physician_gls/pdf/nhl.pdf. Accessed 2 Feb 2018.

29. Cattaneo C, Re A, Ungari M, et al. Plasmablastic lymphoma among human immunodeficiency virus-positive patients: results of a single center's experience. Leuk Lymphoma. 2015;56(1):267–9.
30. Loghavi S, Alayed K, Aladily TN, et al. Stage, age, and EBV status impact outcomes of plasmablastic lymphoma patients: a clinicopathologic analysis of 61 patients. J Hematol Oncol. 2015;8:65.
31. Castillo JJ, Winer ES, Stachurski D, et al. Prognostic factors in chemotherapy-treated patients with HIV-associated plasmablastic lymphoma. Oncologist. 2010;15(3):293–9.
32. Barta SK, Lee JY, Kaplan LD, Noy A, Sparano JA. Pooled analysis of AIDS malignancy consortium trials evaluating rituximab plus CHOP or infusional EPOCH chemotherapy in HIV-associated non-Hodgkin lymphoma. Cancer. 2012;118(16):3977–83.
33. Barta SK, Xue X, Wang D, et al. Treatment factors affecting outcomes in HIV-associated non-Hodgkin lymphomas: a pooled analysis of 1546 patients. Blood. 2013;122(19):3251–62.
34. Krishnan A, Molina A, Zaia J, et al. Autologous stem cell transplantation for HIV-associated lymphoma. Blood. 2001;98(13):3857–9.
35. Re A, Cattaneo C, Michieli M, et al. High-dose therapy and autologous peripheral-blood stem-cell transplantation as salvage treatment for HIV-associated lymphoma in patients receiving highly active antiretroviral therapy. J Clin Oncol. 2003;21(23):4423–7.
36. Alvarnas JC, Le Rademacher J, Wang Y, et al. Autologous hematopoietic cell transplantation for HIV-related lymphoma: results of the BMT CTN 0803/AMC 071 trial. Blood. 2016;128(8):1050–8.
37. Al-Malki MM, Castillo JJ, Sloan JM, Re A. Hematopoietic cell transplantation for plasmablastic lymphoma: a review. Biol Blood Marrow Transplant. 2014;20(12):1877–84.
38. Cattaneo C, Finel H, McQuaker G, et al. Autologous hematopoietic stem cell transplantation for plasmablastic lymphoma: the European Society for Blood and Marrow Transplantation experience. Biol Blood Marrow Transplant. 2015;21(6):1146–7.
39. Dunleavy K, Pittaluga S, Czuczman MS, et al. Differential efficacy of bortezomib plus chemotherapy within molecular subtypes of diffuse large B-cell lymphoma. Blood. 2009;113(24):6069–76.
40. Bibas M, Grisetti S, Alba L, et al. Patient with HIV-associated plasmablastic lymphoma responding to bortezomib alone and in combination with dexamethasone, gemcitabine, oxaliplatin, cytarabine, and pegfilgrastim chemotherapy and lenalidomide alone. J Clin Oncol. 2010;28(34):e704–8.
41. Bose P, Thompson C, Gandhi D, Ghabach B, Ozer H. AIDS-related plasmablastic lymphoma with dramatic, early response to bortezomib. Eur J Haematol. 2009;82(6):490–2.
42. Dasanu CA, Bauer F, Codreanu I, Padmanabhan P, Rampurwala M. Plasmablastic haemato-lymphoid neoplasm with a complex genetic signature of Burkitt lymphoma responding to bortezomib. Hematol Oncol. 2013;31(3):164–6.
43. Hirosawa M, Morimoto H, Shibuya R, Shimajiri S, Tsukada J. A striking response of plasmablastic lymphoma of the oral cavity to bortezomib: a case report. Biomark Res. 2015;3:28.
44. Saba NS, Dang D, Saba J, et al. Bortezomib in plasmablastic lymphoma: a case report and review of the literature. Onkologie. 2013;36(5):287–91.
45. Yan M, Dong Z, Zhao F, et al. CD20-positive plasmablastic lymphoma with excellent response to bortezomib combined with rituximab. Eur J Haematol. 2014;93(1):77–80.
46. Castillo JJ, Reagan JL, Sikov WM, Winer ES. Bortezomib in combination with infusional dose-adjusted EPOCH for the treatment of plasmablastic lymphoma. Br J Haematol. 2015;169(3):352–5.
47. Castillo JJ, Guerrero-Garcia T, Baldini F, et al. Bortezomib plus EPOCH is effective as front-line treatment in patients with plasmablastic lymphoma. Br J Haematol. 2018;59:1730–3.
48. Dittus C, Grover N, Ellsworth S, Tan X, Park SI. Bortezomib in combination with dose-adjusted EPOCH (etoposide, prednisone, vincristine, cyclophosphamide, and doxorubicin) induces long-term survival in patients with plasmablastic lymphoma: a retrospective analysis. Leuk Lymphoma. 2018;59:1–7.

49. Fernandez-Alvarez R, Gonzalez-Rodriguez AP, Rubio-Castro A, et al. Bortezomib plus CHOP for the treatment of HIV-associated plasmablastic lymphoma: clinical experience in three patients. Leuk Lymphoma. 2016;57(2):463–6.
50. Halfdanarson TR, Markovic SN, Kalokhe U, Luppi M. A non-chemotherapy treatment of a primary effusion lymphoma: durable remission after intracavitary cidofovir in HIV negative PEL refractory to chemotherapy. Ann Oncol. 2006;17(12):1849–50.
51. Guerrero-Garcia TA, Mogollon RJ, Castillo JJ. Bortezomib in plasmablastic lymphoma: a glimpse of hope for a hard-to-treat disease. Leuk Res. 2017;62:12–6.
52. Carras S, Regny C, Peoc'h M, et al. Dramatic efficacy of low dose lenalidomide as single agent in a patient with refractory gastric non-human immunodeficiency virus-associated plasmablastic lymphoma. Leuk Lymphoma. 2015;56(10):2986–8.
53. Schmit JM, DeLaune J, Norkin M, Grosbach A. A case of plasmablastic lymphoma achieving complete response and durable remission after lenalidomide-based therapy. Oncol Res Treat. 2017;40(1–2):46–8.
54. Sher T, Miller KC, Lee K, Chanan-Khan A. Remission induction with lenalidomide alone in a patient with previously untreated plasmablastic myeloma: a case report. Clin Lymphoma Myeloma. 2009;9(4):328–30.
55. Yanamandra U, Sahu KK, Jain N, et al. Plasmablastic lymphoma: successful management with CHOP and lenalidomide in resource constraint settings. Ann Hematol. 2016;95(10):1715–7.
56. Folk GS, Abbondanzo SL, Childers EL, Foss RD. Plasmablastic lymphoma: a clinicopathologic correlation. Ann Diagn Pathol. 2006;10(1):8–12.
57. Holderness BM, Malhotra S, Levy NB, Danilov AV. Brentuximab vedotin demonstrates activity in a patient with plasmablastic lymphoma arising from a background of chronic lymphocytic leukemia. J Clin Oncol. 2013;31(12):e197–9.
58. Pretscher D, Kalisch A, Wilhelm M, Birkmann J. Refractory plasmablastic lymphoma-a review of treatment options beyond standard therapy. Ann Hematol. 2017;96(6):967–70.
59. Laurent C, Fabiani B, Do C, et al. Immune-checkpoint expression in Epstein-Barr virus positive and negative plasmablastic lymphoma: a clinical and pathological study in 82 patients. Haematologica. 2016;101(8):976–84.
60. Ramos JC, Sparano JA, Rudek MA, et al. Safety and preliminary efficacy of vorinostat with R-EPOCH in high-risk HIV-associated non-Hodgkin's lymphoma (AMC-075). Clin Lymphoma Myeloma Leuk. 2018;18(3):180–190 e2.
61. Hogg SJ, Newbold A, Vervoort SJ, et al. BET inhibition induces apoptosis in aggressive B-cell lymphoma via epigenetic regulation of BCL-2 family members. Mol Cancer Ther. 2016;15(9):2030–41.
62. Filippakopoulos P, Qi J, Picaud S, et al. Selective inhibition of BET bromodomains. Nature. 2010;468(7327):1067–73.
63. Trabucco SE, Gerstein RM, Evens AM, et al. Inhibition of bromodomain proteins for the treatment of human diffuse large B-cell lymphoma. Clin Cancer Res. 2015;21(1):113–22.
64. Hogg SJ, Vervoort SJ, Deswal S, et al. BET-bromodomain inhibitors engage the host immune system and regulate expression of the immune checkpoint ligand PD-L1. Cell Rep. 2017;18(9):2162–74.
65. Bernasconi E, Gaudio E, Lejeune P, et al. Preclinical evaluation of the BET bromodomain inhibitor BAY 1238097 for the treatment of lymphoma. Br J Haematol. 2017;178(6):936–48.
66. Knowles DM, Inghirami G, Ubriaco A, Dalla-Favera R. Molecular genetic analysis of three AIDS-associated neoplasms of uncertain lineage demonstrates their B-cell derivation and the possible pathogenetic role of the Epstein-Barr virus. Blood. 1989;73(3):792–9.
67. Cesarman E, Chang Y, Moore PS, Said JW, Knowles DM. Kaposi's sarcoma-associated herpesvirus-like DNA sequences in AIDS-related body-cavity-based lymphomas. N Engl J Med. 1995;332(18):1186–91.
68. Said J, Cesarman E. Primary effusion lymphoma. In: Swerdlow S, et al., editors. WHO classification of tumours of haematopoietic and lymphoid tissues. Lyon: IARC; 2008. p. 260–1.

69. Nakamura Y, Tajima F, Omura H, et al. Primary effusion lymphoma of the left scrotum. Intern Med. 2003;42(4):351–3.
70. Pan ZG, Zhang QY, Lu ZB, et al. Extracavitary KSHV-associated large B-cell lymphoma: a distinct entity or a subtype of primary effusion lymphoma? Study of 9 cases and review of an additional 43 cases. Am J Surg Pathol. 2012;36(8):1129–40.
71. Castillo JJ, Shum H, Lahijani M, Winer ES, Butera JN. Prognosis in primary effusion lymphoma is associated with the number of body cavities involved. Leuk Lymphoma. 2012;53(12):2378–82.
72. Bower M, Newsom-Davis T, Naresh K, et al. Clinical features and outcome in HIV-associated multicentric Castleman's disease. J Clin Oncol. 2011;29(18):2481–6.
73. Ripamonti D, Marini B, Rambaldi A, Suter F. Treatment of primary effusion lymphoma with highly active antiviral therapy in the setting of HIV infection. AIDS. 2008;22(10):1236–7.
74. Luppi M, Trovato R, Barozzi P, et al. Treatment of herpesvirus associated primary effusion lymphoma with intracavity cidofovir. Leukemia. 2005;19(3):473–6.
75. Staudt MR, Kanan Y, Jeong JH, et al. The tumor microenvironment controls primary effusion lymphoma growth in vivo. Cancer Res. 2004;64(14):4790–9.
76. Klass CM, Krug LT, Pozharskaya VP, Offermann MK. The targeting of primary effusion lymphoma cells for apoptosis by inducing lytic replication of human herpesvirus 8 while blocking virus production. Blood. 2005;105(10):4028–34.
77. Pereira R, Carvalho J, Patricio C, Farinha P. Sustained complete remission of primary effusion lymphoma with adjunctive ganciclovir treatment in an HIV-positive patient. BMJ Case Rep. 2014;2014:pii: bcr2014204533.
78. Casper C, Krantz EM, Corey L, et al. Valganciclovir for suppression of human herpesvirus-8 replication: a randomized, double-blind, placebo-controlled, crossover trial. J Infect Dis. 2008;198(1):23–30.
79. Ozbalak M, Tokatli I, Ozdemirli M, et al. Is valganciclovir really effective in primary effusion lymphoma: case report of an HIV(−) EBV(−) HHV8(+) patient. Eur J Haematol. 2013;91(5):467–9.
80. Marquet J, Velazquez-Kennedy K, Lopez S, et al. Case report of a primary effusion lymphoma successfully treated with oral valganciclovir after failing chemotherapy. Hematol Oncol. 2018;36(1):316–9.
81. Keller SA, Schattner EJ, Cesarman E. Inhibition of NF-kappaB induces apoptosis of KSHV-infected primary effusion lymphoma cells. Blood. 2000;96(7):2537–42.
82. Sarosiek KA, Cavallin LE, Bhatt S, et al. Efficacy of bortezomib in a direct xenograft model of primary effusion lymphoma. Proc Natl Acad Sci U S A. 2010;107(29):13069–74.
83. Boulanger E, Meignin V, Oksenhendler E. Bortezomib (PS-341) in patients with human herpesvirus 8-associated primary effusion lymphoma. Br J Haematol. 2008;141(4):559–61.
84. Gopalakrishnan R, Matta H, Tolani B, Triche T Jr, Chaudhary PM. Immunomodulatory drugs target IKZF1-IRF4-MYC axis in primary effusion lymphoma in a cereblon-dependent manner and display synergistic cytotoxicity with BRD4 inhibitors. Oncogene. 2016;35(14):1797–810.
85. Antar A, El Hajj H, Jabbour M, et al. Primary effusion lymphoma in an elderly patient effectively treated by lenalidomide: case report and review of literature. Blood Cancer J. 2014;4:e190.
86. Chan TSY, Mak V, Kwong YL. Complete radiologic and molecular response of HIV-negative primary effusion lymphoma with short-course lenalidomide. Ann Hematol. 2017;96(7):1211–3.
87. Michai M, Goto H, Hattori S, et al. Soluble CD30: a possible serum tumor marker for primary effusion lymphoma. Asian Pac J Cancer Prev. 2012;13(10):4939–41.
88. Bhatt S, Ashlock BM, Natkunam Y, et al. CD30 targeting with brentuximab vedotin: a novel therapeutic approach to primary effusion lymphoma. Blood. 2013;122(7):1233–42.
89. Tolani B, Gopalakrishnan R, Punj V, Matta H, Chaudhary PM. Targeting Myc in KSHV-associated primary effusion lymphoma with BET bromodomain inhibitors. Oncogene. 2014;33(22):2928–37.

90. Chen BJ, Chapuy B, Ouyang J, et al. PD-L1 expression is characteristic of a subset of aggressive B-cell lymphomas and virus-associated malignancies. Clin Cancer Res. 2013;19(13):3462–73.
91. Nayar U, Lu P, Goldstein RL, et al. Targeting the Hsp90-associated viral oncoproteome in gammaherpesvirus-associated malignancies. Blood. 2013;122(16):2837–47.
92. Yang D, Chen W, Xiong J, et al. Interleukin 1 receptor-associated kinase 1 (IRAK1) mutation is a common, essential driver for Kaposi sarcoma herpesvirus lymphoma. Proc Natl Acad Sci U S A. 2014;111(44):E4762–8.
93. Dai L, Trillo-Tinoco J, Cao Y, et al. Targeting HGF/c-MET induces cell cycle arrest, DNA damage, and apoptosis for primary effusion lymphoma. Blood. 2015;126(26):2821–31.
94. Mediani L, Gibellini F, Bertacchini J, et al. Reversal of the glycolytic phenotype of primary effusion lymphoma cells by combined targeting of cellular metabolism and PI3K/Akt/ mTOR signaling. Oncotarget. 2016;7(5):5521–37.
95. Bonsignore L, Passelli K, Pelzer C, et al. A role for MALT1 activity in Kaposi's sarcoma-associated herpes virus latency and growth of primary effusion lymphoma. Leukemia. 2017;31(3):614–24.

Chapter 8
Novel Agents in Primary Central Nervous System Lymphoma

Raghuveer Ranganathan and Natalie Sophia Grover

Introduction

Primary central nervous system lymphoma (PCNSL) is an uncommon subclass of extranodal non-Hodgkin lymphoma (NHL) that can occur in the brain, cerebrospinal fluid (CSF), spinal column, or eyes, in the absence of systemic disease. It has an archetypally aggressive clinical phenotype but is chemo- and radiosensitive. However, it tends to have inferior survival compared to systemic lymphomas, with relapsed and refractory disease having especially abysmal long-term outcomes. Though there are several widely used therapeutic regimens, there is no accepted standard for PCNSL treatment, and the disease continues to be a challenge clinically. However, there has been progress in the utilization of novel agents and cellular immunotherapies, which show clinical promise. After a brief review of the most current treatment regimens, this chapter will explore the ongoing studies with novel therapeutic modalities addressing PCNSL.

Epidemiology

PCNSL accounts for approximately 3% of newly diagnosed CNS tumors and 5% of extranodal lymphomas, with about 1200 new cases per year arising in the United States [1, 2]. It is an AIDS-defining illness, and its overall incidence increased during the AIDS epidemic from the mid-1980s to the mid-1990s but has since decreased [2]. Since the year 2000, the demographics of PCNSL have changed, and incidence in

R. Ranganathan · N. S. Grover (✉)
Department of Medicine, Division of Hematology and Oncology,
University of North Carolina at Chapel Hill, Chapel Hill, NC, USA
e-mail: raghuveer.ranganathan@unchealth.unc.edu; natalie_grover@med.unc.edu

C. Dittus (ed.), *Novel Therapeutics for Rare Lymphomas*,
https://doi.org/10.1007/978-3-030-25610-4_8

patients aged 65 and older has increased, particularly in those patients older than 75 years of age [2]. Median age at diagnosis is between 61 and 65.

Clinical Presentation

PCNSL patients can present with a constellation of neurologic symptoms. Focal neurologic deficits (~70%), neuropsychiatric changes (~43%), and nausea, headaches, and vomiting associated with increased intracranial pressure (33%) are the primary presenting symptoms [3]. Neuropsychiatric changes can present as behavioral or mental status changes. Seizures are a somewhat infrequent manifestation, occurring less than 15% of the time. Twenty percent of PCNSL develop in, or eventually involve, the eyes, with primary complaints being vision changes, vitreous floaters, or even complete blindness [4]. Seven to forty-two percent of PCNSL patients have morphological CSF involvement, while primary meningeal involvement without concurrent parenchymal evidence of disease is very rare (7% of cases) [5–7].

Diagnosis and Workup

Neuroimaging with magnetic resonance imaging (MRI) is the accepted gold standard imaging modality [8, 9]. MRI with and without contrast of the brain, ophthalmologic evaluation, and CSF examination by lumbar puncture are the standard elements of the initial workup [9]. MRI of the spine can be completed if spinal involvement is suspected. Nearly 70% of immunocompetent PCNSL patients present with a solitary, homogenously enhancing brain lesion on T1-weighted MRI imaging, while 30% have multiple lesions; both presentations are usually accompanied by varying degrees of surrounding vasogenic edema [10]. Up to a quarter of PCNSL tumors are associated with separate, non-enhancing lesions that are hyperintense on T2 fluid-attenuated inversion recovery (FLAIR)-weighted imaging, which points to promulgation of the lymphoma [11, 12]. Due to their high cellularity, PCNSL also display hyperintensity on diffusion-weighted imaging and hypointensity on apparent diffusion coefficient valuations [13]. On retrospective analysis, close to 90% of PCNSL tumors are found in a supratentorial location, with the most common lesion sites being the frontal lobe, parietal lobe, temporal lobe, basal ganglia, corpus callosum, and cerebellum [3].

Histopathological confirmation is compulsory and usually requires a sample of the affected brain tissue. A stereotactic biopsy is the procedure of choice. Steroid pretreatment is often given to alleviate symptoms from the tumor but should be delayed, if possible, until after the biopsy has been collected, as it can lead to decreased sensitivity and specificity of biopsy results. However, in the setting of unstable neurologic status, steroid use is sometimes unavoidable and should be implemented to reduce the risk of neurologic complications and sequelae.

In addition to pathological confirmation, 5–10 mL of CSF by lumbar puncture should be collected either 1 week before or after surgical biopsy to reduce risk of false-positive results. The CSF should be examined for cytology, flow cytometry, cell count, and protein. In some cases, if CSF is diagnostic of PCNSL, brain biopsy may be deferred.

Between 4% and 8% of patients initially thought to have PCNSL end up having systemic occult disease, so a PET CT or CT with contrast should be done to rule out systemic lymphoma [14]. Ophthalmologic evaluation usually includes fundoscopy and slit lamp examination. Testicular exam as part of the overall physical exam is also warranted to rule out testicular lymphoma as the primary cause for CNS disease. All patients' HIV status should be confirmed, and antiretroviral therapy should be initiated in HIV patients not already on therapy.

Pathology

The majority of PCNSL are of the diffuse large B cell lymphoma (DLBCL) subtype [15]. However, there are occasional cases of T-cell lymphoma [16], Hodgkin lymphoma [17], and low-grade lymphomas [18]. This chapter will focus on the DLBCL subtype.

Prognosis

Two scoring systems are used to stratify the prognosis of PCNSL: the International Extranodal Lymphoma Study Group (IELSG) and the Memorial Sloan Kettering Cancer Center (MSKCC) prognostic scores. The IELSG score is based on five risk factors: age above 60 years, Eastern Cooperative Oncology Group performance status above 1, elevated LDH, elevated CSF protein, and whether the tumor arises within the deep regions of the brain (periventricular regions, basal ganglia, brainstem, and/or cerebellum) [19]. The 2-year overall survival (OS) rates were 80%, 48%, and 15% for patients having zero to one, two to three, and four to five of the risk factors, respectively. The MSKCC score has two characteristics: age and Karnofsky Performance Score (KPS). Patients are divided into three prognostic groups: age ≤ 50 plus KPS ≥ 70, age > 50 plus KPS ≥ 70, and age > 50 plus KPS < 70. These groups correspond to median OS of 5.2, 2.1, and 0.9 years, respectively.

Conventional Treatment

A major problem with the treatment of PCNSL is that no unanimity on the ideal therapeutic approach exists. This is primarily due to the lack of randomized studies comparing different regimens because of the rarity of the disease. Additionally, there is difficulty enrolling patients with PCNSL on clinical trials, due to their frequent poor performance status at diagnosis. However, over the past two decades, certain requisite elements have been identified and form the basis for modern PCNSL therapy.

Historically, treatment of PCNSL was solely dependent on whole-brain radiation (WBRT) with doses of 45–51 Gy; while the overall response rates (ORR) were high, the ensuing median OS was only 1–1.5 years with a 5-year survival of 25% [20–23]. The high doses of WBRT also resulted in debilitating neurotoxicity, especially in patients older than 60 years of age. Targeted radiation to just the tumor involved areas of the brain demonstrated increased relapse rates in the regions that were not radiated [22, 23]. Traditional chemotherapy regimens used for systemic DLBCL, when combined with WBRT, did not show adequate efficacy for PCNSL due to low penetration of the blood-brain barrier (BBB) [23–25].

High-dose methotrexate (HD-MTX) (at doses >1.0 g/m^2) has been used to treat other hematologic malignancies at high risk of CNS involvement or relapse, such as acute lymphoblastic leukemia [26–28]. While doses >1.0 g/m^2 yield therapeutic levels in the brain parenchyma, MTX doses >3.0 g/m^2 produce tumoricidal concentrations in the cerebrospinal fluid as well as brain parenchyma [29]. As a result, the majority of PCNSL chemotherapy regimens incorporate a HD-MTX dose >3.0 g/m^2 and up to 8 g/m^2 [5]. When combined with WBRT for PCNSL treatment, there was an improved OS rate compared to WBRT alone. In single-arm, phase II trials, HD-MTX plus WBRT showed similar ORR of 88–95% compared to historical controls of WBRT alone but with improved median OS of 33–42 months [30–32]. A seminal, randomized phase II trial by Ferreri and colleagues illustrated HD-MTX with cytarabine followed by WBRT showed better ORR and PFS than HD-MTX alone plus WBRT [33]. This finding led to additional polychemotherapy regimens being examined with WBRT or modifying consolidation strategies in lieu of WBRT due to concerns over long-term neurocognitive toxicity with radiation. Since rituximab greatly enhances efficacy in systemic, non-CNS DLBCL, it was included in many PCNSL treatment regimens. The Cancer and Leukemia Group B (CALGB) 50202 single-arm study treated newly diagnosed PCNSL patients with an induction regimen of rituximab, HD-MTX, and the alkylating agent temozolomide (R-MT) followed by consolidation with cytarabine plus etoposide and omitting WBRT altogether. The ORR was 77%, with a CR rate of 66% and 2-year PFS and time to progression (TTP) of 57% and 59%, respectively; those patients who completed consolidation had a 2-year TTP of 77% and estimated 4-year OS of 65% [34]. The Radiation Therapy Oncology Group (RTOG) 0227 phase I/II study also looked at induction therapy with R-MT but added consolidation with WBRT and maintenance temozolomide following radiation. The induction alone resulted in ORR 84% with CR rate of 51%; after completion of induction and consolidation, 2-year PFS and OS were 64% and 81%, respectively, with an estimated median PFS and OS of 5.4 years and 7.5 years, respectively [35].

Concerns with the neurocognitive toxicity from WBRT-containing treatment regimens, which became more apparent with the improving survival of PCNSL patients, prompted trials investigating decreasing the radiation doses or possibly circumventing the need for it completely. The aforementioned CALGB 50,202 study included consolidation with chemotherapy alone and excluded WBRT. A multicenter phase II study evaluated the effectiveness of combining induction rituximab, HD-MTX, procarbazine, and vincristine (R-MPV) with reduced WBRT consolidation with a dose of 23.4 Gy. Induction therapy alone resulted in an ORR of 97% and CR of 47% (increased to 79% after patients with a PR were given two additional R-MPV cycles); 2-year PFS was 77% and 5-year OS was 80% [36]. The median PFS for all patients was 7.7 years, with the median PFS in patients ≤60 years of age not being reached. The median OS was not reached for patients regardless of age category. Importantly, with the reduced WBRT dose, there was less neurocognitive decline or deterioration among the evaluable patients.

One of the largest randomized trials comparing different induction and consolidation regimens was a phase II study by the IELSG32 group, which randomized the combination of the alkylating agent thiotepa with rituximab, HD-MTX, and cytarabine (MATRix) against HD-MTX plus cytarabine with or without rituximab for induction [37]. There was an additional randomization arm for investigating autologous stem cell transplant (auto-SCT) versus WBRT as consolidation. The MATRix regimen showed ORR of 87%, with CR of 49% compared to CR rates of 23% and 30% with the HD-MTX plus cytarabine with and without rituximab arms, respectively. The 2-year PFS and OS for MATRix was 61% and 69%, respectively. The second randomization arm for consolidation demonstrated no significant differences in outcomes; the 2-year PFS was 76% for WBRT and 75% for auto-SCT, with a 4-year OS of 85% versus 83% for WBRT and auto-SCT, respectively [38]. A phase II study examining auto-SCT following R-MPV induction showed both a 2-year PFS and OS of 81% post-transplant [39]. Subsequent studies with auto-SCT suggest that a standard conditioning regimen like BEAM (BCNU, etoposide, cytarabine, melphalan) does not have good efficacy due to decreased penetration of the BBB [40, 41]. Two thiotepa-containing regimens, thiotepa plus busulfan and cyclophosphamide as well as thiotepa with BCNU, show excellent efficacy due to their CNS bioavailability with the BCNU-thiotepa regimen showing lower toxicities, better tolerance, and less patient mortality compared to thiotepa-busulfan-cyclophosphamide (TBC) [40, 42–45].

Though there is no accepted standard regimen for PCNSL therapy, the results from these trials strongly suggest that PCNSL treatment should consist of an induction phase followed by consolidative therapy. The induction backbone should comprise HD-MTX (>3 g/m^2), alkylating agents, and likely rituximab for a polychemotherapeutic approach. Consolidation could consist of either WBRT and chemotherapy or auto-SCT. The induction treatment regimens exhibiting efficacy with minimal neurotoxicities or patient morbidity/mortality are R-MPV and MATRix. Induction should be followed by consolidation with either reduced-dose WBRT or auto-SCT with BCNU-thiotepa conditioning appearing to be better tolerated than TBC.

Relapsed/Refractory PCNSL

Although the prognosis of PCNSL has improved with the incorporation of HD-MTX-based regimens and consolidation therapy, there is still a substantial proportion of patients with relapsed or refractory disease. Unfortunately, treatment options for patients with recurrent or progressive disease are limited. Patients who did not get radiation up front may be treated with WBRT at time of relapse. Patients with a response duration greater than 1 year may be retreated with HD-MTX [8, 46]. Patients are also considered for other systemic chemotherapy options including temozolomide [47], high-dose cytarabine [48], topotecan [49], and pemetrexed [50], which have modest efficacy and brief duration of response. Novel therapeutic agents are urgently needed for this disease.

Basis for Novel Agents

Pathophysiologic findings and gene-expression profiles reveal unique features for the possible pathogenesis of PCNSL (Fig. 8.1). Immunophenotypically, PCNSL is predominantly of the activated B cell (ABC) classification, based on the expression of MUM-1 and BCL-6 [51]. NFκB, a protein complex involved with controlling DNA transcription and promoting cell survival and proliferation, has been shown to be constitutively active and required for blocking apoptosis in ABC-DLBCL subtypes [52]. Mutations affecting proteins which regulate NFκB also result in increased activation of NFκB [53]. MYD88, an intracellular adapter protein, is a commonly mutated target in PCNSL, affecting more than half of PCNSL cases. It actuates NFκB through interleukin-1 receptor-associated kinases (IRAKs). Activating mutations in MYD88 result in upregulation of IRAK activity and, consequently, NFκB. CD79B, a B cell receptor (BCR)-associated protein, is a second frequently mutated target in PCNSL. Other proteins that are implicated in the dysregulation of NFκB activation include CARD11 and TNFAIP3 (an inhibitory mediator of NFκB) [54]. Critically, chronic BCR signaling through BCR clustering and utilization of BCR-related kinases such as SYK or Bruton's tyrosine kinase (BTK) can also promote survival of PCNSL [55]. Additional pro-survival circuits harnessed by PCNSL are the PI3K/mTOR and JAK/STAT pathways and increased copy number gains of the chromosomal locus 9p24.1, which correlates with increased PDL1 expression. This preponderance of mutational and dysregulatory aberrations has been a primary reason for the study of new immunotherapeutic and immunomodulatory agents in PCNSL.

Ibrutinib

Due to the high incidence of BCR pathway aberrations, ibrutinib has become an attractive novel agent to investigate in PCNSL. It is an oral inhibitor of BTK that has gained significant attention as a therapeutic modality in NHL. The ABC subtype of DLBCL shows a dependence upon BTK for survival, and blocking the kinase can

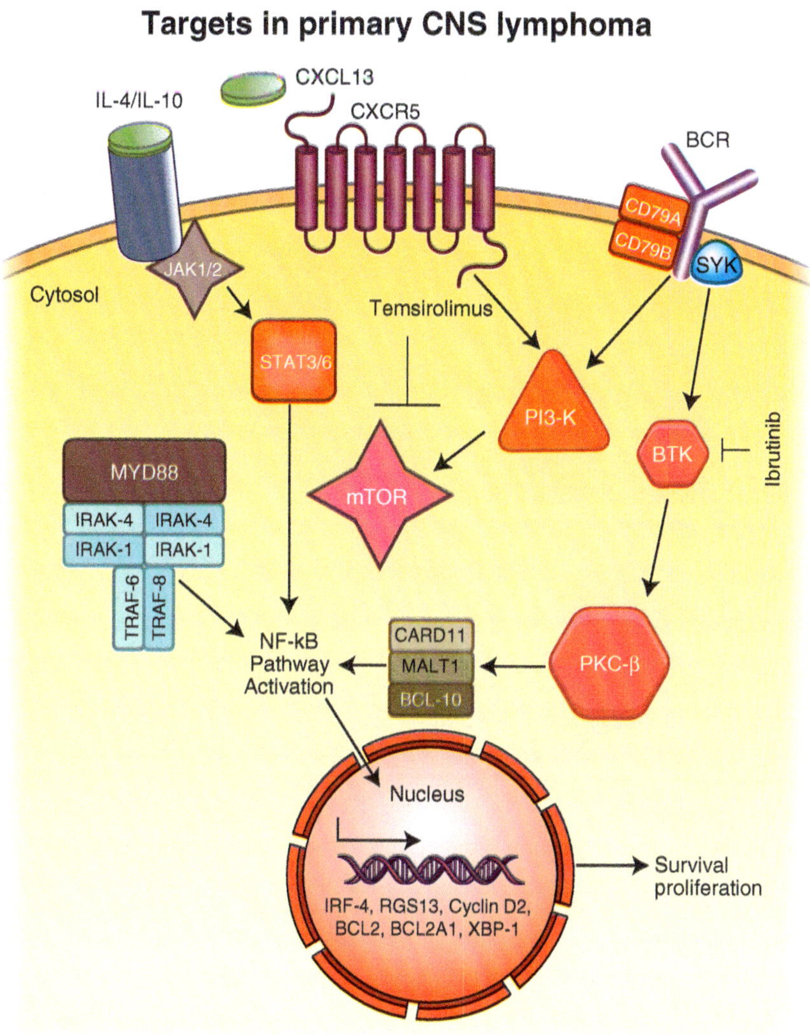

Fig. 8.1 Targets in primary CNS lymphoma. The activation of NF-κB allows for survival and proliferation of PCNSL tumor cells and is controlled by a myriad of signalling pathways. Some novel agents target these pathways. Blocking Bruton's tyrosine kinase (BTK), which acts downstream from the B cell receptor (BCR), is the primary mode of action for ibrutinib. Close to 60% of PCNSL cases harbor the L265P mutation in MYD88, resulting in constitutive activity of IRAK kinases and subsequent NF-κB-dependent transcription of pro-survival genes such as BCL-2, IRF-4, etc. Temsirolimus inhibits the mTOR pathway, which is another pro-survival pathway

instigate apoptosis [55, 56]. A phase I/II clinical trial in 80 patients with relapsed/refractory DLBCL receiving ibrutinib showed an ORR of 25% with CR of 10%, with a relatively short PFS and OS of 1.64 and 6.41 months, respectively [56]. However, in the subset of patients with ABC-DLBCL, there was a notable increased response with ORR of 37% and CR of 16%, with a PFS and OS of 2.02 and 10.35 months, respectively. The ABC-DLBCLs that had BCR mutations in CD79B with concurrent MYD88 mutations exhibited favorable responses of 55%; interestingly, the highest rate of response occurred in ABC patients who had wild-type BCR, suggesting non-genetic processes can be the driving force for oncogenesis. A small case series involving three mantle cell lymphoma patients having relapsed disease in the CNS showed two CRs and one PR at 6–12-month follow-up, with confirmation of CNS penetration by ibrutinib through CSF analysis of the patients [57].

One of the first PCNSL studies with ibrutinib was a non-randomized, single-center phase I trial with 20 relapsed/refractory CNS lymphoma patients [58]. Thirteen had PCNSL, while seven had secondary CNS involvement from systemic DLBCL (SCNSL); all of them had received HD-MTX-based chemotherapy prior to enrollment. Of the 13 PCNSL patients, 10 patients or 77% showed a clinical response, with a CR in 5 patients (38%). The three patients who had malignant cells detected in the CSF had no lymphoma cells detected during follow-up evaluations. After a median follow-up of 15.5 months, the median PFS and OS were 4.6 and 15 months, respectively. Sixty percent of patients who had been receiving steroids for symptomatic relief prior to ibrutinib were able to be tapered off the steroids once therapy was initiated. Overall, ibrutinib was well tolerated with the most commonly observed adverse effects being grade 1–2: hyperglycemia (80%), anemia and/or thrombocytopenia (60–65%), hypercholesterolemia and/or hypertriglyceridemia (60–65%), and hypoalbuminemia or AST elevation (40–50%). Grade 3–4 toxicities involved neutropenia in 15%, with febrile neutropenia occurring in 5%. These abnormalities resolved with the drug being held temporarily. One patient, however, had to be permanently taken off ibrutinib due to pulmonary aspergillosis. Among the tumors that had genomic analyses, mutations in CARD11 appeared to be a harbinger of partial or complete resistance to ibrutinib. Unexpectedly, none of the PCNSL patients with concomitant MYD88 and CD79B mutations showed a CR, which is contradictory to reported responses in systemic ABC-DLBCL.

A prospective, multicenter, open-label phase II trial enrolled 52 patients with either relapsed/refractory PCNSL or primary vitreoretinal lymphoma (PVRL), who were administered ibrutinib monotherapy at 560 mg until disease progression or adverse toxicity [59]. Concurrent steroid use was allowed during the initial 4 weeks for symptomatic cerebral edema. All the patients had exposure to HD-MTX-based chemotherapy prior to the trial, with four patients having auto-SCT as consolidation. An interim analysis after 2 months of treatment revealed an ORR of 55.6%, with CR of 16.7%. One patient developed pulmonary aspergillosis but recovered, and no treatment-related mortality overall was reported up to the time of interim analysis.

Since ibrutinib monotherapy showed modest PFS results, approaches incorporating it with chemotherapy were examined in a phase Ib study. In this trial, ibrutinib monotherapy was initiated for 2 weeks, followed by a polychemotherapy-ibrutinib combination with temozolomide, etoposide, liposomal doxorubicin, dexamethasone, rituximab, and ibrutinib (TEDDi-R) [60]. Liposomal doxorubicin was incorporated into the regimen because non-liposomal doxorubicin does not penetrate the blood-brain barrier (BBB). Using in vitro assays with ABC-DLBCL cell lines, the investigators noted anti-folate agents such as HD-MTX showed antagonism when implemented concurrently with ibrutinib, while the chemotherapy agents included in the final TEDDi-R regimen showed high synergistic action with ibrutinib. Eighteen patients with PCNSL were enrolled in the study; thirteen of whom were relapsed/refractory and five were newly diagnosed. All patients were treated at ibrutinib dose levels of 560, 700, or 800 mg for 2 weeks. Two patients developed grade 5 pulmonary/CNS aspergillosis during the ibrutinib lead-in period, while the remaining 16 patients proceeded to receive TEDDi-R chemotherapy. There was an ORR of 94% (17/18) on ibrutinib monotherapy alone, with two relapsed/refractory patients eventually achieving CR. Twenty-two percent of patients with CSF involvement became negative by flow cytometry on monotherapy. There was an 86% CR rate in the patients who received TEDDi-R, with median PFS of 15.5 months and median OS that was not reached. However, 39% of patients contracted invasive pulmonary/CNS aspergillosis infections during the trial. Two patients died from aspergillosis during the ibrutinib monotherapy phase, while five cases of aspergillosis infections occurred during the TEDDi-R treatment. A patient also died from neutropenic sepsis while receiving TEDDi-R. In contrast, PCNSL treatment-related mortality with conventional chemotherapy and consolidation modalities is quite low at 1–8% [61]. In addition, 56% developed grade 4 thrombocytopenia and 94% had grade 4 neutropenia. The authors cited their preclinical studies showing more susceptibility to *Aspergillus fumigatus* exposure in mice lacking BTK compared to those with wild-type BTK. Their findings suggested that BTK plays a role as part of macrophage and neutrophil response mechanisms to control aspergillosis infections and initiate adaptive immunity. Corticosteroid use with dexamethasone as part of the regimen with ibrutinib was also mentioned as a possible contributory factor. However, previous trials with ibrutinib monotherapy had patients taking concurrent steroids with ibrutinib and reported a much lower occurrence of aspergillosis infection [58, 59]. Nevertheless, if ibrutinib continues to show promise as a therapeutic adjunct for PCNSL treatment, fungal prophylaxis may need to be incorporated with ibrutinib treatment.

Future directions of ibrutinib in PCNSL involve designing combinations that can lead to more durable responses while maintaining a good safety profile. An ongoing clinical trial is investigating the combination of ibrutinib with HD-MTX and rituximab in patients with relapsed or refractory PCNSL and SCNSL (NCT02315326) (Table 8.1). In this trial, to avoid interactions, ibrutinib is stopped on the day of HD-MTX infusion and only restarted 5 days after HD-MTX or at time of clearance. Preliminary results suggest that this combination is tolerable but enrollment is ongoing [62]. Another clinical trial is evaluating the role of ibrutinib as maintenance in elderly patients with PCNSL after induction with a polychemotherapy regimen of rituximab, methotrexate, and another agent (NCT02623010) (Table 8.1).

Table 8.1 Active clinical trials for primary CNS lymphoma

Clinicaltrials.gov identifier	Drug	Design/concept
NCT02315326	Ibrutinib	Phase 1/2 trial in relapsed/refractory primary and secondary CNS lymphoma
		One arm investigating combination of high-dose methotrexate and ibrutinib
NCT02623010	Ibrutinib	Studying maintenance ibrutinib in elderly (age 60–85) patients with primary CNS lymphoma
		Patients initially receive induction with rituximab and high-dose methotrexate protocol and patients with response will receive maintenance ibrutinib until relapse or disease progression
NCT02857426	Nivolumab	Phase 2 trial of nivolumab in relapsed/refractory primary CNS lymphoma or primary testicular lymphoma
NCT02779101	Pembrolizumab	Phase 2 trial of pembrolizumab in relapsed/refractory primary CNS lymphoma
NCT03255018	Pembrolizumab	Phase 2 trial of pembrolizumab in relapsed/refractory gray-zone lymphoma, primary CNS lymphoma, and other extranodal DLBCL
NCT03212807	Durvalumab and lenalidomide	Phase 2 trial of durvalumab and lenalidomide in relapsed/refractor primary CNS lymphoma and other types of DLBCL
NCT02669511	PQR309	Phase 2 trial of PQR309, PI3K, and mTOR inhibitor, in patients with relapsed/refractory primary CNS lymphoma
NCT02498951	Obinutuzumab	Randomized trial studying maintenance obinutuzumab in patients who achieved complete response to first-line treatment with high-dose methotrexate-based chemotherapy
		Patients are randomized to obinutuzumab every 60 days for 2 years or until progression or observation

Ibrutinib appears to have high response rates but suboptimal duration of response as a single agent in PCNSL. We await results of combination studies that may improve the efficacy of ibrutinib, as well as further clarify the toxicity profile.

Checkpoint Inhibitors

PD-1 is an inhibitory receptor expressed by activated T cells on the cell surface. Its ligands, PD-L1 and PD-L2, are upregulated in expression in many cancers. Evidence of increased expression of the PD-1/PD-L1 signaling pathway in PCNSL has spawned interest in checkpoint inhibition as an investigative modality. PD-L1 over-expression, while a relatively uncommon feature in NHL, happens in subsets of

ABC-DLBCL [63], which is the most frequently seen subtype in PCNSL. PD-1 checkpoint inhibitors have shown efficacy in heavily pretreated DLBCL in a phase I trial [64]. PCNSL has been noted to have increased PD-L1 expression secondary to chromosomal gains at the 9p24.1 genetic locus, which contains the PD-L1/PD-L2 genes [54, 65]. The presence of reactive, perivascular T cell infiltrates at PCNSL tumor sites has been shown to correlate with a survival benefit [65]. This suggests that PD-1/PD-L1 checkpoint inhibition could augment this survival advantage by thwarting the immunosuppression imparted by the PD-1/PD-L1 axis upon the reactive T cells.

Nivolumab and pembrolizumab are both anti-PD-1, humanized IgG4 antibodies which have FDA approval for use in many solid malignancies such as melanoma, renal cell, and non-small cell lung cancers. Both immunotherapies are also being actively studied in hematologic malignancies that show PD-L1 overexpression and have been FDA approved for the treatment of Hodgkin lymphoma. While investigation with these medications in PCNSL is in the nascent stages, PD-1 inhibition shows potential for clinical use. In a small pilot study of five patients, four with relapsed/refractory PCNSL and one with CNS relapse of primary testicular lymphoma (PTL), PD-1 blockade with nivolumab induced clinical responses in all five patients [66]. Among the four PCNSL patients, all achieved a CR, with two patients relapsing after 14 and 17 months, respectively. The remaining two patients were disease-free at the time of study publication (13 and 17 months, respectively). Nivolumab was relatively well-tolerated by the patients overall. The only significant complication involved one patient with a history of chronic renal insufficiency who developed renal failure requiring hemodialysis, which was not thought to be due to nivolumab. Currently there is an ongoing multicenter, phase II, single-arm study investigating nivolumab in relapsed/refractory PCNSL or PTL (NCT02857426). Additionally, there are two ongoing studies evaluating the use of pembrolizumab in PCNSLs. One is an ongoing, single-center, open-label, single-arm phase II study examining pembrolizumab use in recurrent PCNSL (NCT02779101); the other is a study investigating the use of pembrolizumab in extranodal lymphomas including PCNSL (NCT03255018) (Table 8.1). Although preliminary data on checkpoint inhibitors in PCNSL is very promising, we await further data to better clarify their role in the treatment of PCNSL.

Pomalidomide and Lenalidomide

Immunomodulatory imide drugs (IMiDs) such as pomalidomide and lenalidomide display particularly heightened cytotoxicity toward ABC-DLCBL tumor cells [67]. This is partly explained by their cereblon-mediated degradation of the MUM1/IRF4 transcription factor, a protein highly expressed in PCNSL [68]. IMiDs also synergistically boost the NK cell-driven antibody-dependent cellular cytotoxicity of rituximab [69]. The combination of lenalidomide with rituximab demonstrated efficacy in DLBCL in phase II trials [70, 71]. The same combination was tried in

PCNSL patients as a phase I trial, with the addition of lenalidomide maintenance following initial treatment. The rituximab was administered both intravenously and intraventricularly. Thirteen relapsed/refractory patients, eight with PCNSL and five with SCNSL, were recruited onto the study in total and given either 10, 20, or 30 mg dose levels. Preliminary results show 8 out of 13 patients achieving PR or better, with 4 CRs in patients with either parenchymal or intraocular disease [72]. At a median follow-up of >18 months, five patients had maintained remissions for >2 years. Ventricular CSF analysis also demonstrated CNS penetration by lenalidomide. The final results of the study are still pending with regards to PFS, OS, and adverse events.

A multicenter, phase II study, also looking at lenalidomide-rituximab, enrolled 50 patients with relapsed/refractory PCNSL or PVRL, all with prior exposure to HD-MTX therapies [73]. There was an induction phase of lenalidomide-rituximab, followed by lenalidomide maintenance. Interim analysis showed an ORR of 39% with a CR rate of 30% at the end of the induction phase. After a median follow-up of 9 months during the maintenance lenalidomide period, median PFS and OS were 8.1 and 15.3 months, respectively. Completed results of this investigation are forthcoming.

A phase I study combined pomalidomide, a second-generation IMiD, with dexamethasone in 25 relapsed/refractory PCNSL or PVRL patients [74]. Treatment consisted of pomalidomide at four-dose escalation levels for 21 out of 28 days with dexamethasone daily for two cycles, followed by pomalidomide alone for subsequent cycles until progression or toxicity. Interim analysis showed an ORR of 43% with CR of 24%. Grade 3/4 hematologic toxicities with either neutropenia, anemia, or thrombocytopenia occurred in 38% of patients, while non-hematologic toxicities of either fatigue, sepsis, rash, or respiratory issues happened in 33%.

With the molecular pathogenetic mechanisms of PCNSL bearing similarity to ABC-DLBCL and IMiDs showing viability as an effective second-line therapy, further studies are in progress to validate pomalidomide and lenalidomide use in PCNSL and PVRL. There is also an ongoing study investigating the combination of durvalumab (a PD-L1 inhibitor) with lenalidomide in relapsed or refractory PCNSL [NCT03212807] (Table 8.1).

Temsirolimus

The PI-3/AKT/mTOR signaling axis can be an additional pathway to promote anti-apoptotic behavior in PCNSL. Temsirolimus had previously been found to possess CNS penetrance at high concentrations within tumor specimens of malignant glioma patients [75]. A phase II study tested temsirolimus monotherapy in 37 relapsed/refractory PCNSL patients [76]. It exhibited an ORR of 56% with a CR rate of 21.5% and a median PFS of 2.1 months. However, a high degree of toxicity was observed, with an associated 13.5% treatment-associated mortality mostly from sepsis. There was also a question of whether cases of pneumonia were instead cases of pneumonitis, which is a well-known side effect of the drug. While temsirolimus does show activity against PCNSL, its high rate of treatment-related mortality would likely make it a less desirable therapeutic option.

Chimeric Antigen Receptor T Cells

Chimeric antigen receptor T (CAR-T) cells genetically engineered to target CD19, an antigen found on most B cells, have shown significant promise in B cell malignancies including DLBCL and have recently been FDA approved for the treatment of relapsed or refractory DLBCL [77, 78]. However, studies of CAR-T cells have generally excluded patients with CNS involvement although it is known that CAR-T cells can cross the BBB and are found in patients' CSF [79, 80]. There was a recent case report published of a patient with refractory DLBCL with CNS relapse involving the brain parenchyma who was treated with CD19-directed CAR-T cells and achieved a CR which was durable with ongoing remission at 12 months [81]. Of course, more data is needed to make any conclusions, but this is encouraging and hopefully future studies will include some patients with CNSL.

Conclusion

While there has been recent incremental progress in PCNSL, especially in the front-line setting, there is still a poor prognosis in relapsed/refractory patients. It remains a difficult disease to study not only due to its rarity and, often, serious clinical presentation but also because many trials exclude patients with CNS involvement. However, novel agents offer promise for forthcoming treatments, especially in the relapsed/refractory setting. Though the studies are small, they offer potential avenues for improvement in PCNSL treatment. Future directions should focus on combining different novel immunotherapies with or without standard chemotherapy regimens that are currently used for PCNSL.

References

1. Hoffman SPJ, McCarthy BJ. Temporal trends in incidence of primary brain tumors in the United States, 1985–1999. Neuro-Oncology. 2006;8(1):27–37.
2. Villano JLKM, Shaikh H, Dolecek TA, McCarthy BJ. Age, gender, and racial differences in incidence and survival in primary CNS lymphoma. Br J Cancer. 2011;105(9):1414–8.
3. Bataille BDV, Menet E, et al. Primary intracerebral malignant lymphoma: report of 248 cases. Neurosurgery. 2000;92(2):261–6.
4. Chan CC, Rubenstein J, Coupland SE, Davis JL, et al. Primary vitreoretinal lymphoma: a report from an International Primary Central Nervous System Lymphoma Collaborative Group symposium. Oncologist. 2011;16(11):1589–99.

5. Batchelor T, Carson K, O'Neill A, Grossman SA, et al. Treatment of primary CNS lymphoma with methotrexate and deferred radiotherapy: a report of NABTT 96-07. J Clin Oncol. 2003;21(6):1044–9.
6. Jahnke K, Korfel A, Martus P, et al. High-dose methotrexate toxicity in elderly patients with primary central nervous system lymphoma. Ann Oncol. 2005;16(3):445–9.
7. Taylor JW, Flanagan E, O'Neill BP, Siegal T, et al. Primary leptomeningeal lymphoma: International Primary CNS Lymphoma Collaborative Group report. Neurology. 2013;81(19):1690–6.
8. Network NCC. Central nervous system cancers 2018. 2018. Available from: https://www.nccn.org/professionals/physician_gls/pdf/cns.pdf.
9. Abrey LE, Batchelor T, Ferreri AJ, International Primary CNS Lymphoma Collaborative Group, et al. Report of an international workshop to standardize baseline evaluation and response criteria for primary CNS lymphoma. J Clin Oncol. 2005;23(22):5034–43.
10. Bühring U, Herrlinger U, Krings T, Thiex R, et al. MRI features of primary central nervous system lymphomas at presentation. Neurology. 2001;57(3):393–6.
11. Rubenstein JL. Biology of CNS lymphoma and the potential of novel agents. Hematol Am Soc Hematol Educ Program. 2017;1:556–64.
12. Tabouret E, Houillier C, Martin-Duverneuil N, et al. Patterns of response and relapse in primary CNS lymphomas after first-line chemotherapy: imaging analysis of the ANOCEF-GOELAMS prospective randomized trial. Neuro-Oncology. 2017;19(3):422–9.
13. Haldorsen IS, Espeland A, Larsson EM. Central nervous system lymphoma: characteristic findings on traditional and advanced imaging. Am J Neuroradiol. 2010;32(6):984–92.
14. O'Neill BP, Dinapoli R, Kurtin PJ, et al. Occult systemic non-Hodgkin's lymphoma in patients initially diagnosed as primary central nervous system lymphoma: how much staging is enough? J Neuro-Oncol. 1995;25(1):67–71.
15. Miller DC, Hochberg FH, Harris NL, Gruber ML, Louis DN, Cohen H. Pathology with clinical correlations of primary central nervous system non-Hodgkin's lymphoma. The Massachusetts General Hospital experience 1958–1989. Cancer. 1994;74(4):1383–97.
16. Gijtenbeek JM, Rosenblum MK, DeAngelis LM. Primary central nervous system T-cell lymphoma. Neurology. 2001;57(4):716–8.
17. de Castro AF, Junior AS, de Lins e Horta H, Neuenschwander LC, Fonseca RP, Lima SS, et al. Primary intracerebral Hodgkin lymphoma. Br J Haematol. 2007;138(5):562.
18. Jahnke K, Korfel A, O'Neill BP, Blay JY, Abrey LE, Martus P, et al. International study on low-grade primary central nervous system lymphoma. Ann Neurol. 2006;59(5):755–62.
19. Ferreri AJ, Blay J, Reni M, Pasini F, et al. Prognostic scoring system for primary CNS lymphomas: The International Extranodal Lymphoma Study Group experience. J Clin Oncol. 2003;21(2):266–72.
20. Shibamoto Y, Ogino H, Hasegawa M, Suzuki K, et al. Results of radiation monotherapy for primary central nervous system lymphoma in the 1990s. Int J Radiat Oncol Biol Phys. 2005;62(3):809–13.
21. Nelson DF, Martz K, Bonner H, Nelson JS, et al. Non-Hodgkin's lymphoma of the brain: can high dose, large volume radiation therapy improve survival? Report on a prospective trial by the Radiation Therapy Oncology Group (RTOG): RTOG 8315. Int J Radiat Oncol Biol Phys. 1992;23(1):9–17.
22. Shibamoto Y, Hayabuchi N, Hiratsuka J, et al. Is whole-brain irradiation necessary for primary central nervous system lymphoma? Patterns of recurrence after partial-brain irradiation. Cancer. 2003;97(1):128–33.
23. Grommes C, DeAngelis L. Primary CNS lymphoma. J Clin Oncol. 2017;35(21):2410–8.
24. Schultz C, Scott C, Sherman W, et al. Preirradiation chemotherapy with cyclophosphamide, doxorubicin, vincristine, and dexamethasone for primary CNS lymphomas: initial report of radiation therapy oncology group protocol 88-06. J Clin Oncol. 1996;14(2):556–64.
25. Mead GM, Bleehen N, Gregor A, Bullimore J, et al. A medical research council randomized trial in patients with primary cerebral non-Hodgkin lymphoma: cerebral radiotherapy with and

without cyclophosphamide, doxorubicin, vincristine, and prednisone chemotherapy. Cancer. 2000;89(6):1359–70.
26. Surapaneni UR, Cortes J, Thomas D, O'Brien S, et al. Central nervous system relapse in adults with acute lymphoblastic leukemia. Cancer. 2002;94(3):773–9.
27. Kantarjian HM, O'Brien S, Smith TL, Cortes J, et al. Results of treatment with hyper-CVAD, a dose-intensive regimen, in adult acute lymphocytic leukemia. J Clin Oncol. 2000;18(3):547–61.
28. Sancho JM, Ribera J, Oriol A, Hernandez-Rivas JM, et al. Central nervous system recurrence in adult patients with acute lymphoblastic leukemia: frequency and prognosis in 467 patients without cranial irradiation for prophylaxis. Cancer. 2006;106(12):2540–6.
29. Lippens RJ, Winograd B. Methotrexate concentration levels in the cerebrospinal fluid during high-dose methotrexate infusions: an unreliable prediction. Pediatr Hematol Oncol. 1988;5(2):115–24.
30. DeAngelis LM, Yahalom J, Thaler HT, Kher U, et al. Combined modality therapy for primary CNS lymphoma. J Clin Oncol. 1992;10(4):635–43.
31. O'Brien P, Roos D, Pratt G, Liew K, et al. Phase II multicenter study of brief single-agent methotrexate followed by irradiation in primary CNS lymphoma. J Clin Oncol. 2000;18(3):519–26.
32. Glass J, Gruber M, Cher L, Hochberg FH. Preirradiation methotrexate chemotherapy of primary central nervous system lymphoma: long-term outcome. J Neurosurg. 1994;81(2):188–95.
33. Ferreri AJ, Reni M, Foppoli M, Martelli M, et al. High-dose cytarabine plus high-dose methotrexate versus high-dose methotrexate alone in patients with primary CNS lymphoma: a randomised phase 2 trial. Lancet Oncol. 2009;374(9700):1512–20.
34. Rubenstein JL, Hsi E, Johnson JL, Jung SH, et al. Intensive chemotherapy and immunotherapy in patients with newly diagnosed primary CNS lymphoma: CALGB 50202 (Alliance 50202). J Clin Oncol. 2013;31(25):3061–8.
35. Glass J, Won M, Schultz CJ, Brat D, et al. Phase I and II study of induction chemotherapy with methotrexate, rituximab, and temozolomide, followed by whole-brain radiotherapy and postirradiation temozolomide for primary CNS lymphoma: NRG oncology RTOG 0227. J Clin Oncol. 2016;34(14):1620–5.
36. Morris PG, Correa D, Yahalom J, Raizer JJ, et al. Rituximab, methotrexate, procarbazine, and vincristine followed by consolidation reduced-dose whole-brain radiotherapy and cytarabine in newly diagnosed primary CNS lymphoma: final results and long-term outcome. J Clin Oncol. 2013;31(31):3971–9.
37. Ferreri AJ, Cwynarski K, Pulczynski E, Ponzoni M, et al. Chemoimmunotherapy with methotrexate, cytarabine, thiotepa, and rituximab (MATRix regimen) in patients with primary CNS lymphoma: results of the first randomisation of the International Extranodal Lymphoma Study Group-32 (IELSG32) phase 2 trial. Lancet Haematol. 2016;3(5):217–27.
38. Ferreri AJM, Cwynarski K, Pulczynski E, Fox CP, et al. Whole-brain radiotherapy or autologous stem-cell transplantation as consolidation strategies after high-dose methotrexate-based chemoimmunotherapy in patients with primary CNS lymphoma: results of the second randomisation of the International Extranodal Lymphoma Study Group-32 phase 2 trial. Lancet Haematol. 2017;4(11):510–23.
39. Omuro A, Correa D, DeAngelis LM, Moskowitz CH, et al. R-MPV followed by high-dose chemotherapy with TBC and autologous stem-cell transplant for newly diagnosed primary CNS lymphoma. Blood. 2015;125(9):1403–10.
40. Ferreri AJ, Illerhaus G. The role of autologous stem cell transplantation in primary central nervous system lymphoma. Blood. 2016;127(13):1642–9.
41. Wiebe VJ, Smith B, DeGregorio MW, Rappeport JM. Pharmacology of agents used in bone marrow transplant conditioning regimens. Crit Rev Oncol Hematol. 1992;13(3):241–70.
42. Cote GM, Hochberg E, Muzikansky A, Hochberg FH, et al. Autologous stem cell transplantation with thiotepa, busulfan, and cyclophosphamide (TBC) conditioning in patients with CNS involvement by non-Hodgkin lymphoma. Biol Blood Marrow Transplant. 2012;18(1):76–83.
43. Cheng T, Forsyth P, Chaudhry A, Morris D, et al. High-dose thiotepa, busulfan, cyclophosphamide and ASCT without whole-brain radiotherapy for poor prognosis primary CNS lymphoma. Bone Marrow Transplant. 2003;31(8):679–85.

44. Illerhaus G, Müller F, Feuerhake F, Schäfer AO, et al. High-dose chemotherapy and autologous stem-cell transplantation without consolidating radiotherapy as first-line treatment for primary lymphoma of the central nervous system. Haematologica. 2008;93(1):147–8.
45. Bojic M, Berghoff A, Troch M, Agis H, et al. Haematopoietic stem cell transplantation for treatment of primary CNS lymphoma: single-centre experience and literature review. Eur J Haematol. 2015;95(1):75–82.
46. Network NCC. Central nervous system cancers: National Comprehensive Cancer Network. 2018. Available from: https://www.nccn.org/professionals/physician_gls/pdf/cns.pdf.
47. Enting RH, Demopoulos A, DeAngelis LM, Abrey LE. Salvage therapy for primary CNS lymphoma with a combination of rituximab and temozolomide. Neurology. 2004;63(5):901–3.
48. Chamberlain MC. High-dose cytarabine salvage therapy for recurrent primary CNS lymphoma. J Neuro-Oncol. 2016;126(3):545–50.
49. Fischer L, Thiel E, Klasen HA, Birkmann J, Jahnke K, Martus P, et al. Prospective trial on topotecan salvage therapy in primary CNS lymphoma. Ann Oncol. 2006;17(7):1141–5.
50. Raizer JJ, Rademaker A, Evens AM, Rice L, Schwartz M, Chandler JP, et al. Pemetrexed in the treatment of relapsed/refractory primary central nervous system lymphoma. Cancer. 2012;118(15):3743–8.
51. Camilleri-Broët S, Crinière E, Broët P, Delwail V, et al. A uniform activated B-cell-like immunophenotype might explain the poor prognosis of primary central nervous system lymphomas: analysis of 83 cases. Blood. 2006;107(1):190–6.
52. Davis RE, Brown K, Siebenlist U, Staudt LM. Constitutive nuclear factor kappaB activity is required for survival of activated B cell-like diffuse large B cell lymphoma cells. J Exp Med. 2001;194(12):1861–74.
53. Vlahopoulos SA. Aberrant control of NF-κB in cancer permits transcriptional and phenotypic plasticity, to curtail dependence on host tissue: molecular mode. Cancer Biol Med. 2017;14(3):254–70.
54. Chapuy B, Roemer M, Stewart C, et al. Targetable genetic features of primary testicular and primary central nervous system lymphomas. Blood. 2016;127(7):869–81.
55. Davis RE, Ngo V, Lenz G, Tolar P, et al. Chronic active B-cell-receptor signalling in diffuse large B-cell lymphoma. Nature. 2010;463(7277):88–92.
56. Wilson WH, Young R, Schmitz R, Yang Y, et al. Targeting B cell receptor signaling with ibrutinib in diffuse large B cell lymphoma. Nat Med. 2015;21(8):922–6.
57. Bernard S, Goldwirt L, Amorim S, Brice P, et al. Activity of ibrutinib in mantle cell lymphoma patients with central nervous system relapse. Blood. 2015;126(14):1695–8.
58. Grommes C, Pastore A, Palaskas N, Tang SS, et al. Ibrutinib unmasks critical role of Bruton tyrosine kinase in primary CNS lymphoma. Cancer Discov. 2017;7(9):1018–29.
59. Choquet S, Houillier C, Bijou F, Houot R, et al. Ibrutinib monotherapy in relapse or refractory Primary CNS Lymphoma (PCNSL) and Primary Vitreo-Retinal Lymphoma (PVRL). Result of the Interim Analysis of the iLOC Phase II Study from the Lysa and the French LOC Network. Blood. 2016;128(22):784.
60. Lionakis MS, Dunleavy K, Roschewski M, Widemann BC, et al. Inhibition of B cell receptor signaling by ibrutinib in primary CNS lymphoma. Cancer Cell. 2017;31(6):833–43.
61. Grommes C, Younes A. Ibrutinib in PCNSL: the curious cases of clinical responses and aspergillosis. Cancer Cell. 2017;31(6):731–3.
62. Grommes C, Stone J, Nolan C, Tsyvkin E, Wolfe J, Mellinghoff IK, et al. Phase 1B of ibrutinib and high-dose methotrexate for recurrent/refractory CNS lymphoma. J Clin Oncol. 2017;35(15_suppl):7533.
63. Andorsky DJ, Yamada R, Said J, Pinkus GS, et al. Programmed death ligand 1 is expressed by non-Hodgkin lymphomas and inhibits the activity of tumor-associated T cells. Clin Cancer Res. 2011;17(13):4232–44.
64. Lesokhin AM, Ansell S, Armand P, Scott EC, et al. Nivolumab in patients with relapsed or refractory hematologic malignancy: preliminary results of a phase Ib study. J Clin Oncol. 2016;34(23):2698–704.

65. Rubenstein JL, Fridlyand J, Shen A, Aldape K, et al. Gene expression and angiotropism in primary CNS lymphoma. Blood. 2006;107(9):3716–23.
66. Nayak L, Iwamoto F, LaCasce A, Mukundan S, et al. PD-1 blockade with nivolumab in relapsed/refractory primary central nervous system and testicular lymphoma. Blood. 2017;129(23):3071–3.
67. Hernandez-Ilizaliturri FJ, Deeb G, Zinzani PL, Pileri SA, et al. Higher response to lenalidomide in relapsed/refractory diffuse large B-cell lymphoma in nongerminal center B-cell-like than in germinal center B-cell-like phenotype. Cancer. 2011;117(22):5058–66.
68. Yang Y, Shaffer AI, Emre NC, Ceribelli M, et al. Exploiting synthetic lethality for the therapy of ABC diffuse large B cell lymphoma. Cancer Cell. 2012;21(6):723–37.
69. Wu L, Adams M, Carter T, Chen R, et al. Lenalidomide enhances natural killer cell and monocyte-mediated antibody-dependent cellular cytotoxicity of rituximab-treated CD20+ tumor cells. Clin Cancer Res. 2008;14(14):4650–7.
70. Wang M, Fowler N, Wagner-Bartak N, Feng L, et al. Oral lenalidomide with rituximab in relapsed or refractory diffuse large cell, follicular and transformed lymphoma: a phase II clinical trial. Leukemia. 2013;27(9):1902–9.
71. Zinzani PL, Pellegrini C, Gandolfi L, Stefoni V, et al. Combination of lenalidomide and rituximab in elderly patients with relapsed or refractory diffuse large B-cell lymphoma: a phase 2 trial. Clin Lymphoma Myeloma Leuk. 2011;11(6):462–6.
72. Rubenstein JL, Fraser E, Formaker P, Lee JCC, et al. Phase I investigation of lenalidomide plus rituximab and outcomes of lenalidomide maintenance in recurrent CNS lymphoma. J Clin Oncol. 2016;34(15 Suppl):7502.
73. Ghesquieres H, Houillier C, Chinot O, Choquet S, et al. Rituximab-Lenalidomide (REVRI) in relapse or refractory Primary Central Nervous System (PCNSL) or Vitreo Retinal Lymphoma (PVRL): results of a "Proof of Concept" phase II study of the French LOC Network. Blood. 2016;128(22):785.
74. Tun HW, Johnston P, Grommes C, Reeder CB, et al. Phase I clinical trial on pomalidomide and dexamethasone in treating patients with relapsed/refractory primary central nervous system lymphoma (PCNSL) or primary vitreoretinal lymphoma (PVRL). J Clin Oncol. 2017;35(15 Suppl):7516.
75. Kuhn JG, Chang S, Wen PY, et al. Pharmacokinetic and tumor distribution characteristics of temsirolimus in patients with recurrent malignant glioma. Clin Cancer Res. 2007;13(24):7401–6.
76. Korfel A, Schlegel U, Herrlinger U, Dreyling M, et al. Phase II trial of temsirolimus for relapsed/refractory primary CNS lymphoma. J Clin Oncol. 2016;34(15):1757–63.
77. Schuster SJ, Svoboda J, Chong EA, Nasta SD, et al. Chimeric antigen receptor T cells in refractory B-cell lymphomas. N Engl J Med. 2017;377(26):2545–54.
78. Neelapu SS, Locke F, Bartlett NL, Lekakis LJ, et al. Axicabtagene ciloleucel CAR T-cell therapy in refractory large B-cell lymphoma. N Engl J Med. 2017;377(26):2531–44.
79. Kochenderfer JN, Dudley M, Kassim SH, Somerville RP, et al. Chemotherapy-refractory diffuse large B-cell lymphoma and indolent B-cell malignancies can be effectively treated with autologous T cells expressing an anti-CD19 chimeric antigen receptor. J Clin Oncol. 2015;33(6):540–9.
80. Grupp SA, Kalos M, Barrett D, Aplenc R, et al. Chimeric antigen receptor–modified T cells for acute lymphoid leukemia. N Engl J Med. 2013;368(16):1509–18.
81. Abramson JS, McGree B, Noyes S, Plummer S, et al. Anti-CD19 CAR T cells in CNS diffuse large-B-cell lymphoma. N Engl J Med. 2017;377(8):783–4.

Chapter 9
Adult T-Cell Leukemia/Lymphoma

Luis Malpica Castillo and Christopher Dittus

Introduction

Adult T-cell leukemia/lymphoma (ATLL) is a mature peripheral T-cell neoplasm caused by human T-cell leukemia virus type 1 (HTLV-1). The clinical entity was proposed by Takatsuki et al. in 1977 [1], with HTLV-1 discovered as the causative virus in 1980 by Poiesz et al. [2]. Beyond ATLL, HTLV-1 is associated with several entities, including HTLV-1-associated myelopathy/tropical spastic paraparesis (HAM/TSP), infective dermatitis, and severe forms of parasitic infections (disseminated strongyloidiasis, crusted scabies) [3, 4]. ATLL carries a dismal prognosis and is essentially incurable by conventional drugs. The largest updated retrospective Japanese study published by Katsuya et al. included 1594 patients treated with modern aggressive therapies, with reported median survival (MS) of 8.3 and 10.6 months for acute and lymphomatous types, respectively [5]. Only allogeneic hematopoietic stem cell transplantation (HSCT) appeared to be curative in a group of patients who are eligible for this approach [6–8]. This chapter will review the epidemiology, clinical manifestations, diagnostic considerations, and conventional and novel treatment approaches, including ongoing clinical trials and preclinical agents.

L. Malpica Castillo
Division of Hematology and Oncology, University of North Carolina at Chapel Hill, Chapel Hill, NC, USA
e-mail: luis.malpicacastillo@unchealth.unc.edu

C. Dittus (✉)
Department of Medicine, Division of Hematology and Oncology, University of North Carolina at Chapel Hill, Chapel Hill, NC, USA
e-mail: chris_dittus@med.unc.edu

C. Dittus (ed.), *Novel Therapeutics for Rare Lymphomas*,
https://doi.org/10.1007/978-3-030-25610-4_9

Epidemiology

ATLL geographic distribution is primarily driven by HTLV-1 epidemiology. HTLV-1 prevalence has been estimated at ten million individuals worldwide and is most endemic in southwestern Japan, the Caribbean Basin, Central and South America, and western Africa (Fig. 9.1) [3, 9, 10]. In the western world, the highest prevalence of HTLV-1 infection is found in Haiti, Jamaica, Dominican Republic, northeastern Brazil, and Peru [3]. In the United States, cases of HTLV-1 and ATLL are seen as an effect of migration, particularly from West Africa and the Caribbean (Fig. 9.1). South Florida is the continental region most proximal to the Caribbean; therefore HTLV-1-associated diseases are commonly encountered in Miami [11–13]. Large metropolitan regions along the Eastern Seaboard also have significant populations with HTLV-1, particularly Boston and New York [11, 14]. Boston, in particular, has a large population of Cape Verdean immigrants, who are likely at risk for HTLV-1 infection, but few data exist. HTLV-1 has rarely been described in the US-born population [13].

The virus is primarily transmitted via breastfeeding. The risk of infection in children of seropositive mothers correlates with the viral load in breast milk, the concordance of HLA class I type between mother and child, and the duration of breastfeeding [15, 16]. In Japan, screening of pregnant women and avoiding breastfeeding in those infected has reduced transmission by 80% [17, 18]. Other modes of transmission include blood transfusion, sharing of needles, and sexual intercourse [3, 11]. Most people infected with HTLV-1 remain asymptomatic throughout life, and it is difficult to determine which individuals will develop symptomatic HTLV-1-associated disease [19, 20]. Among HTLV-1 carriers, the general lifetime risk of developing any HTLV-1-associated disease, including ATLL, HAM/TSP, uveitis, polymyositis, and arthropathy, may be close to 10% [21–24].

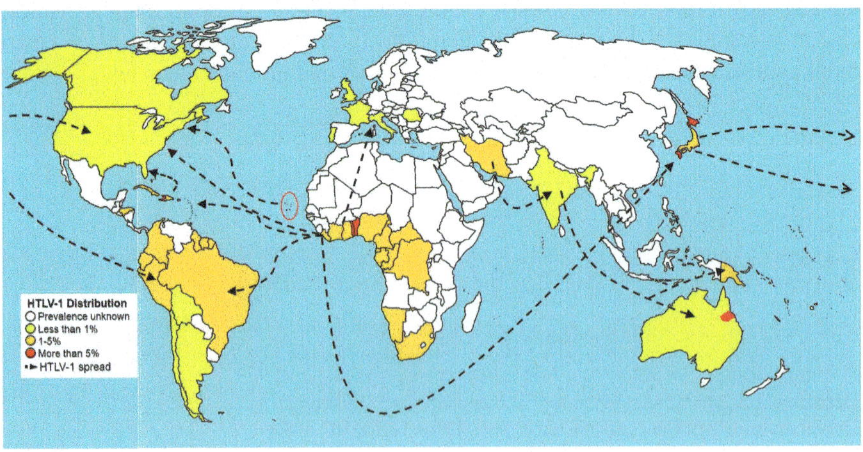

Fig. 9.1 Geographic distribution and spread of HTLV-1

ATLL is associated with some intriguing characteristics. First, ATLL seems to be hyperendemic in southwestern Japan, particularly the Kyushu region [25]. Second, HTLV-1 establishes a lifelong latent infection in human CD4+ T-cells. ATLL, in particular, has a very long latency period, and only patients infected with HTLV-1 early in life (via breastfeeding) are generally at risk. Those individuals infected later in life via blood transfusions, intravenous drug use, or sexual contact are more at risk for HAM/TSP and other HTLV-1-associated illnesses [26]. Malignant transformation leading to ATLL develops in HTLV-1-infected individuals with a cumulative lifetime risk of 4–7% [27]. Third, ATLL occurs predominantly in adults between the sixth and seventh decades in Japan [27, 28] and fourth to fifth decades in the Caribbean Basin and Central and South America [25, 29, 30]. Unfortunately, there is no clear evidence on why this regional discrepancy exists.

The viral oncogenic protein Tax is responsible for transforming the CD4+ T-cell into a cancerous ATLL cell [26, 31]. Infection of T lymphocytes with HTLV-1 results in an increase in proviral loads, with a more pronounced effect for HTLV-1 proviral DNA load. An antibody response against Gag and Env (viral proteins) and Tax-specific cytotoxic T-cell responses induces killing of infected cells. HTLV-1 can evade the immune response by reducing Tax and stimulating HBZ (basic leucine zipper factor) expression. HBZ would subsequently promote the establishment of a chronic infection by inhibiting Tax-dependent viral transcription, stimulating its own expression, and inducing T-cell proliferation [31]. Tax protein expression is undetectable in circulating ATLL cells; HBZ is the only viral protein consistently expressed in ATLL [26, 31].

Clinical Features

Clinically, ATLL is classified into four subtypes, namely, acute, lymphomatous, chronic, and smoldering, as defined by the Shimoyama criteria [32]. The acute and lymphomatous forms are by far the most common subtypes and are often grouped as "aggressive ATLL." The acute subtype presents with a leukemic phase consisting of circulating atypical lymphocytes (ATLL cells) known as "flower cells" (Fig. 9.2), profoundly increased calcium level, and high serum lactate dehydrogenase (LDH). Additionally, the acute type will often present with diffuse lymphadenopathy (LAD) and organ infiltration. The lymphomatous subtype presents with extensive (often bulky) lymphadenopathy, markedly elevated LDH, organ infiltration, and, by definition, an absence of circulating ATLL cells in the peripheral blood (<1%). The smoldering and chronic forms present with circulating ATLL cells (absolute lymphocyte count $<4 \times 10^3$ cells/μL or $\geq 4 \times 10^3$ cells/μL, respectively), normal or mildly elevated LDH (<1.5 or <2 times the upper limit of normal, ULN, respectively), and involvement of the lung, skin, or liver (in chronic only), but no other extranodal sites, and no hypercalcemia. The chronic subtype is further divided into unfavorable and favorable, based on the presence or absence of risk factors such as elevated LDH level greater than the ULN, serum blood urea nitrogen level greater than the ULN,

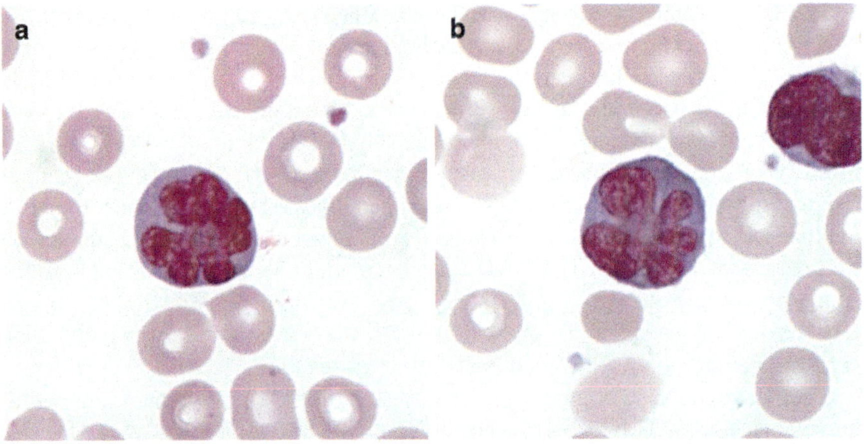

Fig. 9.2 (**a**, **b**) Flower cells (atypical lymphocytes). (Photos courtesy of UNC Hematopathology)

and serum albumin level lower than the normal lower limit [32]. In summary, the smoldering, chronic, and acute subtypes of ATLL can be viewed on a continuum of leukemic involvement, with the smoldering subtype representing the mildest form of the disease. The acute and lymphomatous subtypes represent the most aggressive forms of the disease, with risk for tumor lysis syndrome (TLS) and central nervous system (CNS) involvement. All subtypes of ATLL have variable dermatologic manifestations.

Comorbid opportunistic infections are often seen in ATLL patients as a result of immunosuppression caused by dysfunctional HTLV-1-infected T-cells. Parasitic (especially strongyloidiasis), fungal, and viral infections are frequently associated with all forms of ATLL [3, 30, 33, 34]. Because of the risk of severe infection in patients with ATLL, prophylaxis against these infectious complications is paramount.

Diagnosis and Pertinent Workup

The diagnosis of ATLL involves a comprehensive history which will include epidemiologic, clinical, and laboratory/pathologic data. Although almost all patients diagnosed with ATLL were born in HTLV-1 endemic areas, there are rare cases where the patient was born in a non-endemic region [13]. Clinically, hypercalcemia is an important marker; it occurs in up to 70% of patients with ATLL during the entire course of their disease and is often accompanied by lytic lesions [35]. Hypercalcemia is most associated with the acute-type ATLL; the indolent subtypes would only develop hypercalcemia on progression to an aggressive type. A parathyroid hormone-related peptide is frequently increased in ATLL patients [35, 36].

Severe eosinophilia has been described in ATLL patients [37]; however, most recent data relate this finding to dysregulation of an appropriate Th2 response against opportunistic pathogens. Conversely, patients with disseminated strongyloidiasis may present with eosinopenia [3, 38, 39]. In the leukemic phase, the white blood cell count may increase into the hundreds of thousands, and the peripheral blood smear may have "flower cells" which are pathognomonic for ATLL. Any suspicion must still be confirmed by HTLV-1 testing. Confirmation of infection is generally performed by enzyme-linked immunosorbent assay (ELISA) and should always be confirmed by Western blot and/or polymerase chain reaction (PCR) [25–27, 32]. Although a positive test does not confirm ATLL, a negative test does rule out ATLL.

The predominant immunological phenotype of neoplastic cells is that of a CD4+ helper T-cell: CD3+, CD4+, CD7−, CD8−, and CD25+ [40]. CD30 expression is variable in ATLL, with a lower percentage of CD30+ cells in the acute than in the lymphomatous ATLL subtype (positive in 28% and 47%, respectively) [41]. Lymphomatous presentations depend on an excisional lymph node biopsy for diagnosis, which should have flow cytometry and immunohistochemical (IHC) testing. Additional IHC tests include anaplastic lymphoma kinase (ALK), paired box 5 (PAX5), and terminal deoxynucleotidyl transferase (TdT) which are all negative in ATLL. The Ki-67 proliferation index is very high in aggressive ATLL [40]. Bone marrow aspiration and biopsy may be performed to obtain a diagnosis or to complete staging and have prognostic relevance [42].

In clinical practice, evaluation of ATLL patients should always include a complete cell blood count with differential and peripheral blood smear; additionally, all patients with ATLL should have an LDH, a TLS panel, including uric acid, phosphate, calcium, potassium, and creatinine levels, and a soluble interleukin 2 (IL-2) receptor test. Glucose-6-phosphate dehydrogenase (G6PD) testing should also be sent with the initial work-up in order to evaluate for the presence of a hereditary deficiency that would preclude the use of the recombinant urate oxidase enzyme rasburicase. Patients should be evaluated for coinfections, including human immunodeficiency virus, hepatitis B virus, and hepatitis C virus. Additionally, all patients with aggressive ATLL that are potentially curable candidates for allogeneic stem cell transplant should have a human leukocyte antigen (HLA) typing of their siblings immediately after diagnosis [43], since this process can take time and remissions after chemotherapy are often transient.

All aggressive ATLL patients should have imaging to evaluate the extent of lymphadenopathy (LAD), splenomegaly, organ infiltration, and skeletal involvement. Ann Arbor clinical staging is used in both acute and lymphomatous ATLL subtypes. When circulating ATLL cells are visualized in peripheral blood, the patient has stage IV disease but still requires imaging at baseline. Imaging with either computed tomography (CT) with intravenous contrast or positron-emission tomography-computed tomography (PET-CT) is adequate; however, given the rapid progression of this disease, treatment should not be delayed to obtain PET imaging unless it is readily available. Aggressive ATLL often invades the CNS; therefore, all newly diagnosed patients with either the acute or lymphomatous ATLL subtypes should have brain imaging (CT or MRI), along with a lumbar puncture (LP) sent for cytology and flow cytometry [42]. Intrathecal chemotherapy should be given at the time of the initial LP [44].

Lastly, the histopathological patterns of ATLL vary and mimic different types of T-cell lymphoma. The differential diagnosis of ATLL includes mature T-cell neoplasms such as peripheral T-cell lymphoma not otherwise specified (PTCL-NOS), anaplastic large cell lymphoma (ALCL), angioimmunoblastic T-cell lymphoma (AITL), and even Hodgkin lymphoma (HL). Because of frequent dermatologic manifestations and a leukemic component, ATLL can also be confused with cutaneous T-cell lymphomas (CTCL). Importantly, though, in the World Health Organization's classification, the pathologists can only diagnose this disease if they are aware of the HTLV-1 status [45, 46].

Prognosis

ATLL carries a dismal prognosis and is essentially incurable by conventional drugs. Since its initial description in the 1970s until Shimoyama published his review in 1991, patients with acute and lymphomatous ATLL subtypes had a median survival (MS) time of just 6 and 10 months, respectively [32]. The largest updated retrospective Japanese study published by Katsuya et al. [47] included 1594 patients treated with modern aggressive therapies and reported MS times of 8.3 and 10.6 months for acute and lymphomatous types, respectively. The MS times for the chronic and smoldering types were 31.5 months and 55 months, respectively. The 4-year overall survival (OS) rates for acute, lymphomatous, chronic, and smoldering subtypes were 11%, 16%, 36%, and 52%, respectively [47]. Although there is some improvement in the 4-year OS when comparing both studies (except for smoldering subtype that had a lower than expected OS), the long-term prognosis of ATLL remains poor, thus urging the development of novel therapeutic strategies for this disease.

Factors that have been associated with a poor prognosis in aggressive ATLL include high expression of the Ki67 antigen [40], high serum levels of calcium, parathyroid hormone-related protein, lactate dehydrogenase, thymidine kinase, soluble interleukin-2 receptor (sIL-2R), β2-microglobulin, and neuron-specific enolase. These have been particularly associated with the acute ATLL subtype [48–51]. Based on these data, researchers have developed prognostic scores. The most recent study by Katsuya et al. included 807 patients with newly diagnosed aggressive ATLL (acute and lymphomatous subtypes) [52]. The Ann Arbor stage (stage III/IV, 2 points), performance status (ECOG score 2–4, 1 point), and three continuous variables (age greater than 70, serum albumin level less than 3.5 g/dL, and sIL-2R level greater than 20,000 U/mL; each 1 point) were identified as independent poor prognostic factors. A low score (0–2 points) correlated with a median OS of 16.2 months, an intermediate score (3–4 points) correlated with a median OS of 7 months, and a high score (5–6 points) correlated with a median OS of 4.6 months [52].

Additionally, several studies have identified other poor prognostic factors in aggressive ATLL such as bone marrow involvement, skin involvement, and monocytosis [53]. Eosinophilia [54], high levels of serum LDH and serum urea, and low levels of serum albumin were associated with poor prognosis in chronic ATLL subtype (also known as "chronic ATLL with unfavorable features") [48]. CD30 positivity has been associated with poor prognosis in the acute and chronic with unfavorable feature subtypes (MS time in the CD30+ and CD30− groups were 10.1 weeks vs. 33.7 weeks, respectively) [55], but not in the lymphomatous ATLL subtype. Expression of c-Rel and interferon regulatory factor-4 (IRF-4 also known as MUM-1 or multiple myeloma oncogene-1) has also been associated with antiviral resistance and poor prognosis [55]. Lastly, CC chemokine receptor 4 (CCR4) expression has been associated with skin involvement and shorter overall survival (OS; median 9.5 months) compared with CCR4-negative (20.6 months) patients [56].

Conventional Treatment Approach

Antiretroviral Therapy

The treatment of ATLL remains challenging and is based on the clinical subtype. In several countries, including Japan, patients with aggressive ATLL (acute, lymphomatous, and chronic with unfavorable feature subtypes) often receive chemotherapy as first-line treatment; in contrast, in the United States, Europe, and some South American countries (e.g., Brazil and Peru), zidovudine (AZT) and interferon-α (IFN) are considered the first-line treatment for non-lymphomatous subtypes, and it is recommended under the National Comprehensive Cancer Network treatment guidelines [48, 57]. Patients with smoldering and favorable chronic subtypes are either observed or started on AZT-IFN [51]. In these groups, narrowband ultraviolet B (NB-UVB) phototherapy can be used to treat symptomatic, superficial skin lesions, and PUVA (psoralen and ultraviolet A) can treat symptomatic, infiltrated skin lesions [58, 59]. One study showed improved survival in those with smoldering ATLL treated with phototherapy combined with oral etoposide (25–75 mg/day for 2–4 weeks with a 1-week interval or on alternate weeks) [60]. Notably, treating smoldering and favorable chronic ATLL with frontline chemotherapy has shown worse survival [51].

The use of AZT-IFN was proposed in 1995 by Gill PS et al. as an attempt to improve mortality in ATLL patients given the short survival despite the use of cytotoxic chemotherapy [61]. The study showed a good response even in patients in whom prior cytotoxic chemotherapy failed. Subsequent studies have supported this finding. The only prospective study to evaluate the efficacy of AZT-IFN in ATLL was a small phase II trial that included 13 frontline patients and 6 relapsed patients [67]. The study only included the aggressive ATLL subtypes (15 acute and 4 lymphomatous). For the 17 patients with evaluable tumor, 13 responses were obtained with 9 complete remissions (CR) and 4 partial remissions (PR). The overall response rate (ORR) was 92% for patients who received AZT-IFN as first-line therapy (58% CR and 33% PR). The median event-free survival (EFS) was 7 months (10 months with AZT-IFN as first-line and 2 months when used after chemotherapy). Median overall survival (OS) was 11 months, with a 28-month survival for patients who entered CR [62]. Despite impressive responses, most of the patients ultimately relapsed and required further treatment. A meta-analysis by Bazarbachi et al. evaluated the effect of AZT-IFN in 254 patients from four Western countries [63]. Patients with chronic and smoldering ATLL that were initially treated with AZT-IFN had a 5-year OS of 100% and those with acute ATLL who achieved a complete response (CR) while on AZT-IFN had a 5-year survival of 82%. In June 2013, the "16th International Conference on HTLV-1" held in Montreal summarized these findings and concluded that AZT-IFN was effective in the leukemic forms of ATLL and should be considered the first-line therapy in this setting; chemotherapy was only recommended if there was no response to AZT-IFN [64]. Another study has evaluated the role of concurrent chemotherapy and AZT-IFN, which has shown some advantage in aggressive ATLL [65]. Arsenic trioxide may induce cell-cycle arrest and apoptosis in leukemic ATLL cells and has been studied in combination with IFN [66] and with AZT-IFN [67]. The latter study showed an overall response rate (ORR) of 100% in chronic ATLL [67]. Although promising, more prospective data are required to better assess these results.

Chemotherapy

Several combinations of chemotherapeutic agents have been evaluated among ATLL patients. The most commonly used chemotherapy regimens are CHOP (cyclophosphamide, doxorubicin, vincristine, and prednisone), CHOEP (cyclophosphamide, doxorubicin, etoposide, vincristine and prednisone), VCAP-AMP-VECP (vincristine, cyclophosphamide, doxorubicin, prednisone-doxorubicin, ranimustine, and prednisone-vindesine, etoposide, carboplatin, prednisone), ATL-G-CSF (vincristine, vindesine, doxorubicin, mitoxantrone, cyclophosphamide, etoposide, ranimustine, and prednisolone with prophylactic support by granulocyte colony-stimulating factor), and modified EPOCH (etoposide, prednisolone, vincristine, carboplatin, and doxorubicin; carboplatin is substituted for cyclophosphamide). Despite intensive therapy, MS only ranges between 6 and 8.5 months [40, 42, 47, 48, 68, 69]. The Japanese Clinical Oncology Group (JCOG) has conducted several clinical trials assessing different chemotherapy regimens. A representative study from this group was published by Tsukasaki K et al. in 2007 and showed good results with the VCAP-AMP-VECP regimen (also known as LSG-15), when compared to bi-weekly CHOP for aggressive ATLL subtypes; a complete response rate of 40% vs. 25% and a MS of 13 vs. 11 months were observed [64]. This regimen is currently the standard of care for aggressive ATLL in Japan, although with significant toxicity (including three treatment-related deaths). As some of these drugs are not available in the United States, regimens like dose-adjusted EPOCH, CHOP, CHOEP, and hyper-CVAD (cyclophosphamide, vincristine, doxorubicin, and dexamethasone-methotrexate, cytarabine) are acceptable alternatives [57, 70]. Because of frequent CNS involvement in aggressive ATLL subtypes (ranging from 10% to 25%), intrathecal chemotherapy prophylaxis is recommended [44, 57].

Novel Agents

Conventional approaches for the treatment of ATLL have failed to achieve long-term survival. Because of this, there has been a shift to evaluate agents with a novel mechanism of action. Several of these agents have been studied for the treatment of ATLL, but none are currently approved by the Food and Drug Administration (FDA). For the remainder of this chapter, we will focus on the research behind these novel agents. Table 9.1 compares various treatments for frontline and relapsed ATLL. Table 9.2 lists ongoing clinical trials in the United States with various novel agents.

Monoclonal Antibody Therapy

Brentuximab Vedotin

Brentuximab vedotin (BV) is an antibody-drug conjugate that combines an anti-CD30 monoclonal antibody with the microtubule disrupting agent, monomethyl auristatin E (MMAE) [71]. BV is an effective treatment option for Hodgkin lymphoma (HL), anaplastic large cell lymphoma (ALCL), CD30+ peripheral T-cell lymphoma (PTCL), CD30+ cutaneous T-cell lymphoma (CTCL), and CD30+ diffuse large B-cell lymphoma (DLBCL) [71–76]. However, the impact of BV in ATLL has not been established. As previously discussed, a study published by Campuzano-Zuluaga et al. in 2013 showed a variable CD30 expression in ATLL specimens [55] with 22.1% of ATLL cases positive for CD30. Importantly, the cutoff for CD30 expression in this study was high at 30%. BV has been shown to be effective in cases

Table 9.1 Treatment regimens used in frontline and relapsed setting

Treatment regimen	*N*	Study	ORR (%)	CR (%)	PFS	OS
AZT-IFN	19	Phase II	76.5	53	10 months	11 months
CHOP-14	61	Randomized phase II	66	21	5.4	11
LSG15	57	Randomized phase II	72	40	7	13
Lenalidomide	26	Phase II	42	19	3.8	20.3
BV-CHP	2	Phase I	100	100	18.5	NR
Mogamulizumab	27	Phase II	50	31	5.2	13.7
Mogamulizumab-LSG15	29	Randomized phase II	86	52	8.5	NR

AZT-IFN zidovudine-interferon-alpha; *BV-CHEP* brentuximab vedotin with cyclophosphamide, doxorubicin, etoposide, prednisone; *CHOP-14* cyclophosphamide, doxorubicin, vincristine, and prednisone as a 14-day cycle; *CR* complete response; *LSG-15* VCAP-AMP-VECP (vincristine, cyclophosphamide, doxorubicin, prednisone-doxorubicin, ranimustine, and prednisone-vindesine, etoposide, carboplatin, prednisone); *N* number of patients, *ORR* overall response rate; *OS* overall survival, *PFS* progression-free survival

Table 9.2 Ongoing clinical trials available for ATLL patients in the United States

Status	Study title	Conditions	Interventions	Location
Recruiting	BV-CHEP chemotherapy for frontline treatment of adult T-cell leukemia or lymphoma	ATLL	Drug: BV-CHEP	Chapel Hill, North Carolina (UNC Hospital and Clinics) and other centers in Boston and NYC
Recruiting	Belinostat therapy with zidovudine for frontline treatment of adult T-cell leukemia-lymphoma	ATLL	Drugs: belinostat, AZT-IFN, pegylated-IFN	Miami, FL (University of Miami)
Recruiting	Subcutaneous recombinant human IL-15 (s.c. rhIL-15) and alemtuzumab for people with refractory or relapsed chronic and acute adult T-cell leukemia (ATL)	ATLL	Biological: IL-15 plus alemtuzumab	Bethesda, Maryland (NIH)
Recruiting	Ruxolitinib for adult T-cell leukemia	ATLL	Drug: ruxolitinib	Bethesda, Maryland (NIH)

ATLL adult T-cell leukemia/lymphoma, *AZT* zidovudine, *BV-CHEP* brentuximab vedotin with cyclophosphamide, doxorubicin, etoposide, prednisone, *IFN* interferon-alpha, *IL-15* interleukin 15, *NIH* National Institutes of Health

of CTCL with levels of CD30 expression lower than 10% [75]. In 2014, Fanale et al., as part of a Phase I multicenter clinical trial that evaluated the safety and efficacy of BV in CD30-positive PTCL [77], two patients with ATLL were treated with BV-CHP (cyclophosphamide, doxorubicin, and prednisone) and achieved a complete response (one patient was stage IV with an International Prognostic Index [IPI] score of 3% and 25% of CD30 expression with a progression-free survival [PFS] of 7.1 months, and one patient was stage IV with an IPI score of 5% and 98% CD30 expression with a PFS of 22.8 months) [77]. Updated results from this study were recently published, and one ATLL patient remained in remission with a PFS of 56.7+ months and an OS of 64.1+ months [78]. At present, a Phase III trial (ECHELON-2 trial) comparing BV-CHP with CHOP in the initial treatment of CD30-positive mature T-cell lymphomas is not recruiting patients as of July 2017, but data analysis is ongoing [79, 80]. Two promising Phase II clinical trials are currently recruiting patients. One trial, based on the west coast, is assessing BV and combination chemotherapy in the treatment of patients with CD30-positive PTCL that will include ATLL patients [81]. The other trial will target the ATLL population specifically and is focused where the majority of ATLL patients are located in the United States, on the Eastern Seaboard [84]. This trial is based at the University of North Carolina at Chapel Hill and will collaborate with Rare Lymphoma Working Group (RLWG) sites in Boston to capture more cases of ATLL. This study will evaluate four to six cycles of the regimen BV-CHEP (brentuximab vedotin, cyclophosphamide, doxorubicin, etoposide, and prednisone) in ATLL patients. Patients who are eligible for allogeneic transplant will be consolidated with this modality in the first complete response (CR1). Patients who are not eligible for transplant but are CD30-positive will continue maintenance BV after they complete six cycles of BV-CHEP. CD30-negative patients who are not transplant eligible will complete six cycles of BV-CHEP and then enter a follow-up period.

Mogamulizumab

Mogamulizumab is a humanized monoclonal antibody targeting CC chemokine receptor 4 (CCR4), which was found to be overexpressed in 99 (88.3%) out of 103 patients with ATLL and was associated with a poor prognosis [82]. Mogamulizumab was approved in Japan in 2012 based on a Phase II trial for the treatment of relapsed or refractory ATLL [83, 84]. The study included 27 CCR4-positive patients with aggressive, relapsed ATLL, and mogamulizumab was given at a dose of 1.0 mg/kg intravenous weekly for 8 weeks. The median PFS was 5.2 months and a median OS of 13.7 months. Common adverse events were cytopenias, fever, rash, chills, and one case of erythema multiforme. In 2015, Ishida et al. conducted a Phase II randomized trial comparing mogamulizumab in combination with LSG-15 regimen versus LSG-15 alone in newly diagnosed patients with aggressive ATLL [85]. The study showed a complete response (CR) rate of 52% vs. 33% and a median PFS of 8.5 months vs. 6.3 months, in the combination arm vs. the LSG15-alone arm, respectively. Median OS was not reached in either arm after 413 and 502 days of follow-up, respectively [85]. In October 2016, a retrospective study evaluated 82 ATLL patients who underwent allogeneic stem cell transplant who received mogamulizumab-based regimen as first-line therapy, found a significant association between mogamulizumab, and increased risk of grade 3–4 acute graft-versus-host disease (GVHD; relative risk, 1.80; $p < 0.01$), nonrelapse mortality ($p < 0.01$), and decreased overall survival ($p < 0.01$) [89]. Based on these findings, mogamulizumab should be used cautiously in transplant-eligible patients. In October 2017, an updated follow-up analysis of the Phase I and Phase II mogamulizumab studies was published [86]. The analysis reported a 3-year OS of 31% and 23%, in the Phase I and Phase II studies, respectively. An interesting conclusion from this study was that patients who developed a grade 2 or greater skin rash as an immune-related adverse event had a better PFS and OS (1-year PFS of 0% vs. 50% and 3-year OS of 8% vs. 36%, in patients with grade 1 vs. ≥ grade 2 skin rash, respectively) [86].

Alemtuzumab

Alemtuzumab is a monoclonal antibody that binds to CD52, an antigen present on normal and pathologic B- and T-cells. It has shown activity in chronic lymphocytic leukemia (CLL), cutaneous T-cell lymphoma (CTCL), and PTCL [87]. ATLL cells frequently express CD52 as compared to other PTCLs [88]. The combination of alemtuzumab with a standard-dose CHOP regimen as a first-line treatment was studied in 24 patients with PTCL and showed a CR rate in 17 (71%) patients, with an overall median duration of response of 11 months; however, it was associated with CMV reactivation [89]. In the United States, a phase II study conducted by the National Institute of Health treated 29 patients with chronic, acute, or lymphomatous-type ATLL with alemtuzumab as frontline therapy [90]. Alemtuzumab induced responses in patients with acute HTLV-1-associated ATLL (15 of 29 patients); however, duration of responses, progression-free survival, and overall survival were short (median response duration 1.4 months, PFS 2.0 months, OS 5.9 months). Although alemtuzumab has shown activity in ATLL, the modest survival rates and risk of CMV infection limit its effectiveness in treating ATLL.

Daclizumab

Because CD25 (interleukin-2 receptor alpha chain) is universally expressed in ATLL, it is an obvious target for monoclonal antibody therapy. An anti-CD25 agent, daclizumab, which is used to prevent rejection in organ transplantation, was evaluated in two different ATLL clinical trials. One study evaluated daclizumab alone (8 mg/kg) in 34 patients and found no response in the 18 patients with aggressive ATLL [91], and the second study, a Phase II trial, evaluated 15 patients with ATLL treated with a lower dose of daclizumab (1 mg/kg) in combination with standard CHOP chemotherapy and showed median OS of 10 months, with CR and PR of 33% and 20%, respectively [92]. Taken together, the response to daclizumab was not as robust as was hoped; therefore use of this agent has not been widely adopted.

Immunomodulatory Therapy

Lenalidomide is an immunomodulatory agent currently used in multiple hematologic malignancies. Its role in ATLL has been evaluated in Phase I and Phase II trials in the relapsed/recurrent ATLL setting, demonstrating clinically meaningful antitumor activity [93–95]. An updated follow-up analysis from the Phase II trial (ATLL-002) by Ishida et al. was published in December 2016 [95]. Twenty-six ATLL patients (median age 68.5 years) with aggressive ATLL ($n = 22$) and chronic unfavorable ($n = 4$) subtypes, which had relapsed after at least one prior therapy, were included in this study and received lenalidomide 25 mg oral daily continuously until disease progression or unacceptable toxicity. The median PFS and OS were 3.8 and 20.3 months, respectively. The CR and OR rates were 15% and 42%, respectively. Responses according to disease subtype were 33% (5 of 15) for acute, 57% (4 of 7) for lymphoma, and 50% (2 of 4) for unfavorable chronic ATLL. Responses according to disease site were 31% for target (nodal and extranodal) lesions, 75% for skin, and 60% for peripheral blood. Responses were also analyzed according to prior mogamulizumab treatment and were 18% in patients who had previously received mogamulizumab and 60% in mogamulizumab-naïve patients [95]. Based on these results, further investigations of lenalidomide in ATLL are warranted.

PD-1/PD-L1 Pathway

Programmed cell death protein 1 (PD-1) and programmed cell death ligand 1 (PD-L1) are expressed on both tumor and tumor-infiltrating nonmalignant cells in lymphoid malignancies [96, 97]. Increasing data have shown that PD-1 is expressed at a higher level in T-cells from tumor patients [98]. The presence of high levels of plasma-soluble PD-L1 and PD-L1 expression on lymphoma cells is associated with poor overall survival (OS) and is considered an important biomarker in diffuse large B-cell lymphoma (DLBCL) [99, 100]; additionally, blockade therapy of the PD-1/PD-L1 pathway showed a remarkable effect for Hodgkin lymphoma (HL) [101]. These results suggest that the PD-1/PD-L1 pathway might support tumor cell survival and that blockade of this pathway could be an effective therapeutic method in lymphoid malignancies other than DLBCL and HL. Studies performed on ATLL cells have shown increased PD-1 expression on both CD4+CD25+ and CD4+CD25− T-cells, but not in CD8+T cells [102, 103]. Similarly, higher expression of PD-L1 has been found in the majority of different hematological malignant cells, including ATLL cells [103, 104]. A study published in September 2016 by Miyoshi et al. performed PD-L1 immunostaining in 135 ATLL biopsy samples (51%, 48%, and 1% were acute, lymphomatous, and smoldering subtypes, respectively) [104]. They observed that PD-L1 (+) ATLL had inferior OS compared with PD-L1 (−) ATLL (MS times 7.5 vs. 14.5 months, respectively; $p = 0.0085$). This is the first report describing the clinicopathological features and outcomes of PD-L1 expression in ATLL. In the United States, the National Cancer Institute (NCI) conducted a phase II clinical trial to evaluate nivolumab in the treatment of ATLL patients who had an increased mutational load and overexpression of PD-L1 [105]. After treating the first three patients, they developed worsening leukocytosis, hypercalcemia, renal insufficiency, and increased LDH levels after a single dose of nivolumab [106]. The study was closed due to evidence of rapid disease progression. More studies are needed to elucidate the role of PD-L1 in ATLL.

HDAC Inhibitors

Histone deacetylases (HDACs) are enzymes involved in the remodeling of chromatin and play a key role in the epigenetic regulation of gene expression. Histone deacetylase (HDAC) inhibitors induce the hyperacetylation of nonhistone proteins as well as nucleosomal histones resulting in the expression of repressed genes involved in growth arrest, terminal differentiation, and/or apoptosis among cancer cells. HDAC inhibitors such as vorinostat, romidepsin (depsipeptide), and panobinostat (LBH589) have shown activity in preclinical and clinical studies against T-cell malignancies including ATLL [107, 108]. LBH589 had a significant anti-ATL effect in vitro and in mice. However, a phase II study for CTCL and indolent ATLL in Japan was terminated because of severe infections associated with the shrinkage of skin tumors and formation of ulcers in patients with ATLL [108].

IL-2 Receptor

Denileukin diftitox, an interleukin-2-diphtheria toxin fusion protein targeting IL-2 receptor-expressing malignant T lymphocytes, has also shown efficacy as a single agent [109] or in combination with CHOP with promising results for PTCL [110]. Some ATLL cases successfully treated with this agent have been reported [111].

Anti-Tax Vaccine

Cytotoxic T lymphocyte (CTL) against HTLV-1 Tax has been demonstrated to play a vital role in controlling HTLV-1-infected cells in HTLV-1-carrier patients [112]. Since there is a long latency period between HTLV-1 infection and the onset of ATLL, mechanisms for leukemogenesis in the infected cells present in a multistep fashion; hence, immunization may play a role against it. In Japan, Suehiro et al. developed an anti-ATLL therapeutic vaccine consisting of autologous dendritic cells that is pulsed with Tax peptides (Tax-DC) [112]. The vaccination protocol was completed with three injections at a 2-week interval. This approach was studied in a pilot study of three previously treated ATLL patients (unknown subtypes). All patients had a Tax-specific CTL response, and two patients had a partial response at 8 weeks, which was maintained for at least 19 months. The third patient had stable disease at 8 weeks and then slowly progressed [112]. From this study, investigators have conducted a clinical trial of Tax-DC vaccine combined with anti-CCR4 antibody to enhance the efficacy of the vaccine as next-generation immunotherapy [113]. Results have not been presented yet.

Allogeneic Stem Cell Transplantation

Considering the unsatisfactory results of standard treatments, the role of stem cell transplantation (SCT) in aggressive ATLL has been investigated. Initially, autologous stem cell transplantation (auto-SCT) was attempted, but it did not yield success [114]. In 1996 Borg et al. reported the first successful allogeneic stem cell transplant (allo-SCT) for the treatment of ATLL. This patient remained in a CR with no evidence of disease at 23 months post-transplant [115]. Since that first case, several reports have been published by various Japanese groups mainly in form of retrospective series and Phase I clinical trials. Although the earlier studies were notable for a high incidence of serious infections and other complications, recent experience has been more encouraging. In 2013, The Japan Society for Hematopoietic Cell Transplantation reported that by 2012, more than 1000 ATLL patients had received allo-SCT [116] with an estimate of approximately 120 ATLL patients transplanted a year. This study showed that patients receiving an allogeneic transplant with an HLA-matched donor had a 3-year OS rate of 41% [122]. In another study, researchers found that acute grade I/II GVHD was significantly associated with a longer OS, which was likely from a graft-versus-leukemia effect [117]. Lastly, a study showed no significant difference between myeloablative conditioning (MAC) and reduced-intensity conditioning (RIC) in OS, although there was a mild trend for superior OS with RIC in older patients [118].

Regarding non-Japanese experience, in October 2014, Bazarbachi et al. reported 21 ATLL patients (7 acute, 12 lymphomatous subtypes) that underwent SCT (4 auto-SCT and 17 allo-SCT) [119]. All patients that underwent auto-SCT rapidly died from ATLL. Of 17 patients who underwent allo-SCT (4 myeloablative, 13 reduced intensity), 6 are still alive at the time of this publication (4 were in CR at SCT), and 11 patients died within 2 years (8 from relapse/progression and 3 from transplant toxicity) [119]. The study concluded that, overall, these results indicate that allo-SCT but not auto-SCT may salvage a subset of ATLL patients with relapsed disease, supporting the existence of graft-versus-leukemia/ATLL effect in non-Japanese patients.

Lastly, the largest updated retrospective study published in 2015 by Katsuya et al. reported 214 patients (of age 65 years or younger) with acute and lymphoma subtypes that underwent allo-SCT after first remission (n = 117), in primary refractory ATLL (n = 56), and in the relapsed setting (n = 41) [5]. The MS time after transplant and 4-year OS were 5.9 months and 26%, respectively. The MS times from transplantation showed differences when analyzed by clinical status before transplant. Patients survived 22 months when transplanted in first remission vs. 3 months when the transplant occurred in primary refractory or relapsed disease. Regarding ongoing clinical trials, there is one clinical trial recruiting only ATLL patients at the University Hospital Center of Martinique in the Caribbean; the study will evaluate high-risk adult T-cell leukemia/lymphoma (ATLL-HR) treated with AZT-IFN, AZT-IFN and CHOP, and AZT-DHAP (dexamethasone, cytarabine, and cisplatin) followed by allo-SCT (ATLL-HR-01) [120].

Recommended Treatment Approach in Frontline and Refractory/Relapsed Disease

Treating ATLL represents a challenge because there are few data based on randomized controlled trials due to its rarity. Additionally, several of the abovementioned drugs (e.g., ranimustine, vindesine) are not available in the United States. Figure 9.3 summarizes a treatment strategy in frontline and in refractory/relapsed setting based on available data and the National Comprehensive Cancer Network (NCCN) recommendations.

Frontline

At present, treatment options for ATLL are suboptimal, and all patients diagnosed with ATLL should be evaluated for clinical trials. Regarding current treatment recommendations for ATLL, as previously discussed, it will depend on the clinical

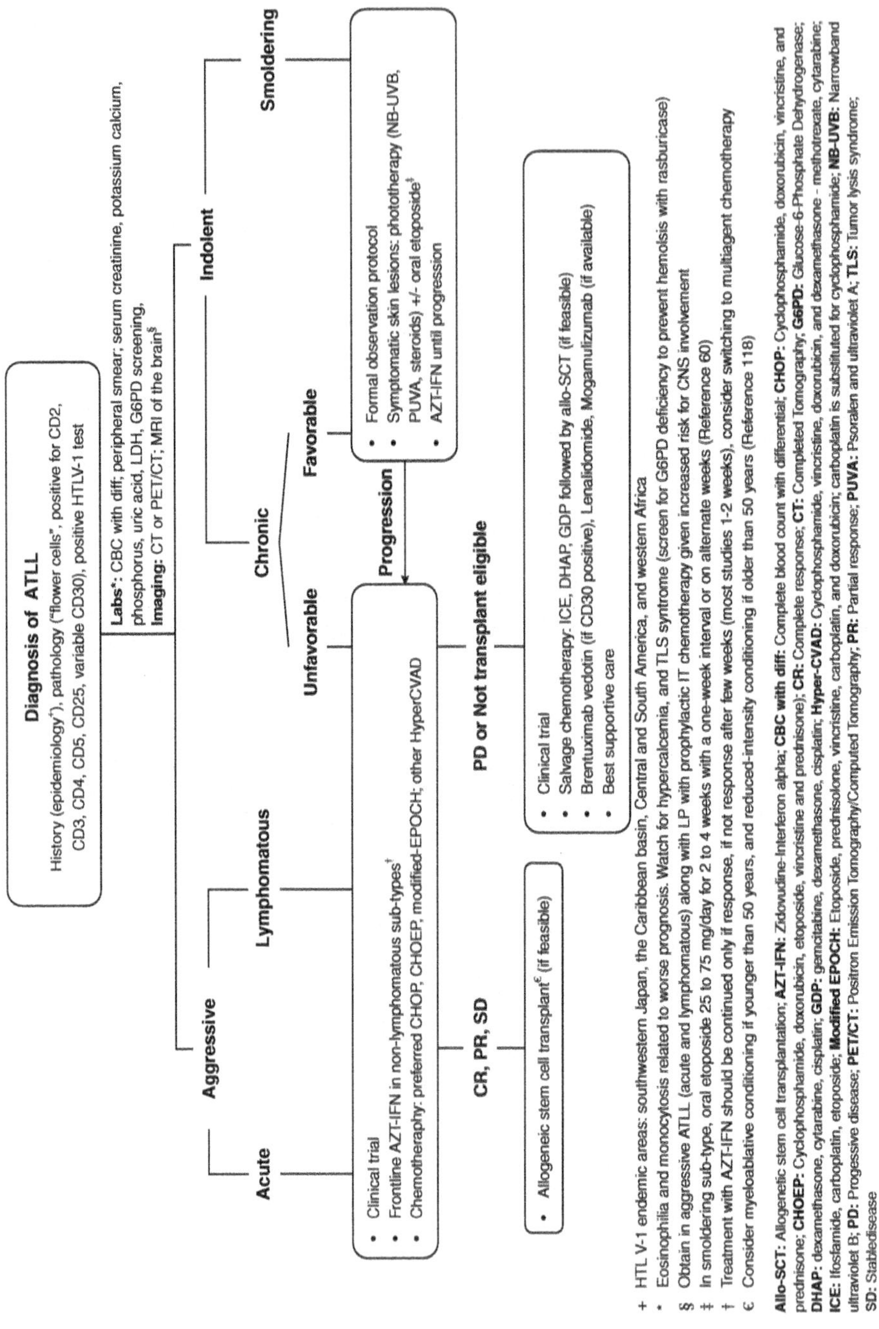

Fig. 9.3 Adapted treatment strategy for ATLL

subtype at diagnosis. Patients with aggressive ATLL should receive immediate treatment with either antiviral therapy with zidovudine and interferon-α (AZT-IFN) (except for those with the lymphomatous subtype) or multiagent chemotherapy [47, 48, 51, 57, 64, 65, 63]. Available chemotherapy regimens recommended by the NCCN are CHOP, CHOEP, modified EPOCH, and hyper-CVAD. Including etoposide in the regimen is reasonable for patients under the age of 60, based on an extrapolation from studies in PTCL [121]. Because of frequent CNS involvement and CNS relapse in aggressive ATLL subtypes, intrathecal chemotherapy prophylaxis is recommended [44, 57]. Any patient achieving a CR (or PR) should be evaluated for an allogeneic stem cell transplantation (allo-SCT), which is particularly effective in young patients with good performance status [47, 118, 119, 122]. In indolent ATLL, AZT-IFN can be initiated at diagnosis or on progression of disease. If surveillance is pursued, patients must be followed very closely for progression. If skin lesions are present, skin-directed therapy with topical steroids, and narrowband ultraviolet B (NB-UVB) phototherapy for superficial lesions, and PUVA (psoralen and ultraviolet A) for more infiltrated lesions are recommended [58, 59].

Refractory/Relapsed Disease

ATLL patients with relapsed or refractory disease should be evaluated for clinical trials. In the aggressive ATLL subtypes, if a patient fails to respond to frontline chemotherapy prior to allo-SCT, the patient should be switched to a salvage regimen (ICE, DHAP, GDP), and if remission/response is achieved, then the patient should be evaluated for allo-SCT. If the patient relapsed after allo-SCT or the patient is not eligible for transplant, CD30 positivity should be evaluated. If positive, patients should receive a trial of brentuximab vedotin. Lenalidomide is another reasonable option in the relapsed setting. Mogamulizumab is an option that should be used in regions where it is available. Other relapsed regimens used in PTCL can also be extrapolated to ATLL, but these will likely have limited effect.

Supportive Care

ATLL is unique in that there are many severe complications that are associated with the disease. Common complications in ATLL include hypercalcemia, tumor lysis syndrome, and severe infections. The hypercalcemia associated with ATLL is often severe, with calcium levels over 20 mg/dL. Treatment should include aggressive hydration and the early administration of a bisphosphonate. Opportunistic infections caused by immunosuppression are common in ATLL. Prophylaxis for *pneumocystis* pneumonia, herpes simplex/zoster virus, fungal infections, and gram negative bacterial infections should be strongly considered for all patients. Patients should be screened for *Strongyloides stercoralis* infection and should receive treatment for any positive screening given the risk for hyperinfection syndrome by *Strongyloides stercoralis* [123–126]. Tuberculosis screening should be considered for patients who are high risk for prior exposure. Tumor lysis syndrome is a known complication in all aggressive hematologic malignancies and can be fatal; hence, early and aggressive intravenous hydration, along with allopurinol administration, and G6PD deficiency screening are recommended. If the patient does not have G6PD deficiency, rasburicase should be considered for severe TLS.

Conclusion

Adult T-cell leukemia/lymphoma (ATLL) is a rare T-cell neoplasm caused by the human T-cell lymphotropic virus type 1 (HTLV-1). ATLL continues to have a poor outcome with currently available therapies. ATLL can be divided into the aggressive (acute, lymphomatous, and chronic with unfavorable features) and indolent (smoldering and chronic with favorable features) subtypes, which influence treatment strategies. AZT-IFN is a reasonable first-line option in patients with the smoldering, chronic, or non-bulky acute subtypes. Chemotherapy remains the preferred choice for lymphomatous or bulky acute ATLL. The current therapeutic approach in the United States is to give a CHOP-like regimen containing etoposide (either CHOEP or dose-adjusted EPOCH), with the intent to achieve remission and proceed to allogeneic transplant. Novel therapeutic approaches include the use of antibody-drug conjugates (brentuximab vedotin), anti-CCR4 therapy, immunomodulatory therapy, and anti-TAX vaccines. The Rare Lymphoma Working Group is focusing future research on multi-institutional clinical trial participation because of the rarity of this disease. We are hopeful that a collaborative effort can help find an effective therapeutic approach to improve survival in ATLL.

References

1. Uchiyama T, Yodoi J, Sagawa K, Takatsuki K, Uchino H. Adult T-cell leukemia: clinical and hematologic features of 16 cases. Blood [Internet]. 1977 [cited 2017 Oct 1];50(3):481–92. Available from: http://www.ncbi.nlm.nih.gov/pubmed/301762.
2. Poiesz BJ, Ruscetti FW, Gazdar AF, Bunn PA, Minna JD, Gallo RC. Detection and isolation of type C retrovirus particles from fresh and cultured lymphocytes of a patient with cutaneous T-cell lymphoma. Proc Natl Acad Sci U S A [Internet]. 1980 [cited 2017 Oct 1];77(12):7415–9. Available from: http://www.ncbi.nlm.nih.gov/pubmed/6261256.
3. Verdonck K, González E, Van Dooren S, Vandamme A-M, Vanham G, Gotuzzo E. Human T-lymphotropic virus 1: recent knowledge about an ancient infection. Lancet Infect Dis [Internet]. 2007 [cited 2015 Mar 9];7(4):266–81. Available from: http://www.ncbi.nlm.nih.gov/pubmed/17376384.

4. Matsuoka M. Human T-cell leukemia virus type I (HTLV-I) infection and the onset of adult T-cell leukemia (ATL). Retrovirology [Internet]. BioMed Central; 2005 [cited 2017 Oct 1];2(1):27. Available from: https://doi.org/10.1186/1742-4690-2-27.
5. Katsuya H, Ishitsuka K, Utsunomiya A, Hanada S, Eto T, Moriuchi Y, et al. Treatment and survival among 1594 patients with ATL. Blood [Internet]. American Society of Hematology; 2015 [cited 2017 Oct 1];126(24):2570–7. Available from: http://www.ncbi.nlm.nih.gov/pubmed/26361794.
6. Ishida T, Hishizawa M, Kato K, Tanosaki R, Fukuda T, Taniguchi S, et al. Allogeneic hematopoietic stem cell transplantation for adult T-cell leukemia-lymphoma with special emphasis on preconditioning regimen: a nationwide retrospective study. Blood [Internet]. American Society of Hematology; 2012 [cited 2017 Oct 1];120(8):1734–41. Available from: http://www.ncbi.nlm.nih.gov/pubmed/9446633.
7. Chihara D, Ito H, Matsuda T, Katanoda K, Shibata A, Taniguchi S, et al. Association between decreasing trend in the mortality of adult T-cell leukemia/lymphoma and allogeneic hematopoietic stem cell transplants in Japan: analysis of Japanese vital statistics and Japan Society for Hematopoietic Cell Transplantation (JSHCT). Blood Cancer J [Internet]. 2013 [cited 2017 Oct 1];3(11):e159. Available from: http://www.ncbi.nlm.nih.gov/pubmed/24241399.
8. Ishitsuka K, Ikeda S, Utsunomiya A, Saburi Y, Uozumi K, Tsukasaki K, et al. Smouldering adult T-cell leukaemia/lymphoma: a follow-up study in Kyushu. Br J Haematol [Internet]. 2008 [cited 2017 Oct 1];143(3):442–4. Available from: http://www.ncbi.nlm.nih.gov/pubmed/18759766.
9. Iwanaga M, Watanabe T, Yamaguchi K. Adult T-cell leukemia: a review of epidemiological evidence. Front Microbiol [Internet]. Frontiers Media SA; 2012 [cited 2017 Nov 13];3:322. Available from: http://www.ncbi.nlm.nih.gov/pubmed/22973265.
10. Gonçalves DU, Proietti FA, Ribas JGR, Araújo MG, Pinheiro SR, Guedes AC, et al. Epidemiology, treatment, and prevention of human T-cell leukemia virus type 1-associated diseases. Clin Microbiol Rev [Internet]. American Society for Microbiology (ASM); 2010 [cited 2017 Nov 13];23(3):577–89. Available from: http://www.ncbi.nlm.nih.gov/pubmed/20610824.
11. Proietti FA, Carneiro-Proietti ABF, Catalan-Soares BC, Murphy EL. Global epidemiology of HTLV-I infection and associated diseases. Oncogene [Internet]. 2005 [cited 2017 Nov 14];24(39):6058–68. Available from: http://www.ncbi.nlm.nih.gov/pubmed/16155612.
12. Harrington WJ, Ucar A, Gill P, Snodgrass S, Sheremata W, Cabral L, et al. Clinical spectrum of HTLV-I in south Florida. J Acquir Immune Defic Syndr Hum Retrovirol [Internet]. 1995 [cited 2017 Nov 14];8(5):466–73. Available from: http://www.ncbi.nlm.nih.gov/pubmed/7697443.
13. Harrington WJ, Miller GA, Kemper RR, Byrne GE, Whitcomb CC, Rabin M. HTLV-I-associated leukemia/lymphoma in south Florida. J Acquir Immune Defic Syndr [Internet]. 1991 [cited 2017 Nov 14];4(3):284–9. Available from: http://www.ncbi.nlm.nih.gov/pubmed/1992105.
14. Moskowitz AJ, Lunning MA, Horwitz SM. Should patients with aggressive peripheral T-cell lymphoma all be treated the same?: no… well yes, …but maybe not for long. Cancer J [Internet]. NIH Public Access; 2012 [cited 2017 Nov 14];18(5):445–9. Available from: http://www.ncbi.nlm.nih.gov/pubmed/23006950.
15. Biggar RJ, Ng J, Kim N, Hisada M, Li H, Cranston B, et al. Human leukocyte antigen concordance and the transmission risk via breast-feeding of human T cell lymphotropic virus type I. J Infect Dis [Internet]. 2006 [cited 2017 Nov 14];193(2):277–82. Available from: http://www.ncbi.nlm.nih.gov/pubmed/16362892.
16. Li H, Biggar RJ, Miley WJ, Maloney EM, Cranston B, Hanchard B, et al. Provirus load in breast milk and risk of mother-to-child transmission of human T lymphotropic virus type I. J Infect Dis [Internet]. 2004 [cited 2017 Nov 14];190(7):1275–8. Available from: http://www.ncbi.nlm.nih.gov/pubmed/15346338.
17. Hino S, Katamine S, Kawase K, Miyamoto T, Doi H, Tsuji Y, et al. Intervention of maternal transmission of HTLV-1 in Nagasaki, Japan. Leukemia [Internet]. 1994 [cited 2017 Nov 14];8 Suppl 1:S68–70. Available from: http://www.ncbi.nlm.nih.gov/pubmed/8152307.

18. Kashiwagi K, Furusyo N, Nakashima H, Kubo N, Kinukawa N, Kashiwagi S, et al. A decrease in mother-to-child transmission of human T lymphotropic virus type I (HTLV-I) in Okinawa, Japan. Am J Trop Med Hyg [Internet]. 2004 [cited 2017 Nov 14];70(2):158–63. Available from: http://www.ncbi.nlm.nih.gov/pubmed/14993627.
19. Hisada M, Stuver SO, Okayama A, Li H, Sawada T, Hanchard B, et al. Persistent paradox of natural history of human T lymphotropic virus type I: parallel analyses of Japanese and Jamaican carriers. J Infect Dis [Internet]. 2004 [cited 2017 Nov 14];190(9):1605–9. Available from: http://www.ncbi.nlm.nih.gov/pubmed/15478065.
20. Maguer-Satta V, Gazzolo L, Dodon M. Human immature thymocytes as target cells of the leukemogenic activity of human T-cell leukemia virus type I. Blood [Internet]. 1995 [cited 2017 Nov 14];86(4):1444–52. Available from: http://www.bloodjournal.org/content/86/4/1444?sso-checked=true.
21. de Thé G, Kazanji M. An HTLV-I/II vaccine: from animal models to clinical trials? J Acquir Immune Defic Syndr Hum Retrovirol [Internet]. 1996 [cited 2017 Nov 14];13 Suppl 1:S191–8. Available from: http://www.ncbi.nlm.nih.gov/pubmed/8797723.
22. Cleghorn FR, Manns A, Falk R, Hartge P, Hanchard B, Jack N, et al. Effect of human T-lymphotropic virus type I infection on non-Hodgkin's lymphoma incidence. J Natl Cancer Inst [Internet]. 1995 [cited 2017 Nov 14];87(13):1009–14. Available from: http://www.ncbi.nlm.nih.gov/pubmed/7629870.
23. Kaplan JE, Osame M, Kubota H, Igata A, Nishitani H, Maeda Y, et al. The risk of development of HTLV-I-associated myelopathy/tropical spastic paraparesis among persons infected with HTLV-I. J Acquir Immune Defic Syndr [Internet]. 1990 [cited 2017 Nov 14];3(11):1096–101. Available from: http://www.ncbi.nlm.nih.gov/pubmed/2213510.
24. Murphy EL, Hanchard B, Figueroa JP, Gibbs WN, Lofters WS, Campbell M, et al. Modelling the risk of adult T-cell leukemia/lymphoma in persons infected with human T-lymphotropic virus type I. Int J Cancer [Internet]. 1989 [cited 2017 Nov 14];43(2):250–3. Available from: http://www.ncbi.nlm.nih.gov/pubmed/2917802.
25. Yamaguchi K, Watanabe T. Human T lymphotropic virus type-I and adult T-cell leukemia in Japan. Int J Hematol [Internet]. 2002 [cited 2017 Nov 14];76 Suppl 2:240–5. Available from: http://www.ncbi.nlm.nih.gov/pubmed/12430931.
26. Bangham CRM, Ratner L. How does HTLV-1 cause adult T-cell leukaemia/lymphoma (ATL)? Curr Opin Virol [Internet]. NIH Public Access; 2015 [cited 2017 Nov 14];14:93–100. Available from: http://www.ncbi.nlm.nih.gov/pubmed/26414684.
27. Satake M, Yamada Y, Atogami S, Yamaguchi K. The incidence of adult T-cell leukemia/lymphoma among human T-lymphotropic virus type 1 carriers in Japan. Leuk Lymphoma [Internet]. 2015 [cited 2017 Nov 14];56(6):1806–12. Available from: http://www.ncbi.nlm.nih.gov/pubmed/25219595.
28. Phillips AA, Shapira I, Willim RD, Sanmugarajah J, Solomon WB, Horwitz SM, et al. A critical analysis of prognostic factors in North American patients with human T-cell lymphotropic virus type-1-associated adult T-cell leukemia/lymphoma. Cancer [Internet]. 2010 [cited 2017 Nov 14];116(14):3438–46. Available from: http://www.ncbi.nlm.nih.gov/pubmed/20564100.
29. Tajima K. The 4th nation-wide study of adult T-cell leukemia/lymphoma (ATL) in Japan: estimates of risk of ATL and its geographical and clinical features. The T- and B-cell Malignancy Study Group. Int J Cancer [Internet]. 1990 [cited 2017 Nov 14];45(2):237–43. Available from: http://www.ncbi.nlm.nih.gov/pubmed/2303290.
30. Bittencourt AL, Vieira M da G, Brites CR, Farre L, Barbosa HS. Adult T-cell leukemia/lymphoma in Bahia, Brazil. Am J Clin Pathol [Internet]. 2007 [cited 2017 Nov 14];128(5):875–82. Available from: http://www.ncbi.nlm.nih.gov/pubmed/17951212.
31. Barbeau B, Peloponese J-M, Mesnard J-M. Functional comparison of antisense proteins of HTLV-1 and HTLV-2 in viral pathogenesis. Front Microbiol [Internet]. Frontiers Media SA; 2013 [cited 2017 Nov 14];4:226. Available from: http://www.ncbi.nlm.nih.gov/pubmed/23966985.
32. Shimoyama M. Diagnostic criteria and classification of clinical subtypes of adult T-cell leukaemia-lymphoma. A report from the Lymphoma Study Group (1984–87). Br J Haematol

[Internet]. 1991 [cited 2017 Nov 14];79(3):428–37. Available from: http://www.ncbi.nlm.nih.gov/pubmed/1751370.

33. Satoh M, Toma H, Sugahara K, Etoh K, Shiroma Y, Kiyuna S, et al. Involvement of IL-2/IL-2R system activation by parasite antigen in polyclonal expansion of CD4+25+ HTLV-1-infected T-cells in human carriers of both HTLV-1 and S. stercoralis. Oncogene [Internet]. 2002 [cited 2017 Nov 14];21(16):2466–75. Available from: http://www.ncbi.nlm.nih.gov/pubmed/11971181.
34. Gonçalves DU, Proietti FA, Ribas JGR, Araújo MG, Pinheiro SR, Guedes AC, et al. Epidemiology, treatment, and prevention of human T-cell leukemia virus type 1-associated diseases. Clin Microbiol Rev [Internet]. 2010 [cited 2015 Feb 18];23(3):577–89. Available from: http://www.pubmedcentral.nih.gov/articlerender.fcgi?artid=2901658&tool=pmcentrez&rendertype=abstract.
35. Taylor GP, Matsuoka M. Natural history of adult T-cell leukemia/lymphoma and approaches to therapy. Oncogene [Internet]. 2005 [cited 2017 Nov 14];24(39):6047–57. Available from: http://www.ncbi.nlm.nih.gov/pubmed/16155611.
36. Nosaka K, Miyamoto T, Sakai T, Mitsuya H, Suda T, Matsuoka M. Mechanism of hypercalcemia in adult T-cell leukemia: overexpression of receptor activator of nuclear factor kappaB ligand on adult T-cell leukemia cells. Blood [Internet]. 2002 [cited 2017 Nov 14];99(2):634–40. Available from: http://www.ncbi.nlm.nih.gov/pubmed/11781248.
37. Ogata M, Ogata Y, Kohno K, Uno N, Ohno E, Ohtsuka E, et al. Eosinophilia associated with adult t-cell leukemia: role of interleukin 5 and granulocyte-macrophage colony-stimulating factor. Am J Hematol [Internet]. Wiley Subscription Services, Inc., A Wiley Company; 1998 [cited 2017 Nov 14];59(3):242–5. Available from: http://doi.wiley.com/10.1002/%28SICI%291096-8652%28199811%2959%3A3%3C242%3A%3AAID-AJH11%3E3.0.CO%3B2-O.
38. Stewart DM, Ramanathan R, Mahanty S, Fedorko DP, Janik JE, Morris JC. Disseminated *Strongyloides stercoralis* infection in HTLV-1-associated adult T-cell leukemia/lymphoma. Acta Haematol [Internet]. Karger Publishers; 2011 [cited 2017 Nov 14];126(2):63–7. Available from: http://www.ncbi.nlm.nih.gov/pubmed/21474923.
39. Montes M, Sanchez C, Verdonck K, Lake JE, Gonzalez E, Lopez G, et al. Regulatory T cell expansion in HTLV-1 and strongyloidiasis co-infection is associated with reduced IL-5 responses to *Strongyloides stercoralis* antigen. PLoS Negl Trop Dis [Internet]. Public Library of Science; 2009 [cited 2017 Nov 14];3(6):e456. Available from: http://www.ncbi.nlm.nih.gov/pubmed/19513105.
40. Nicot C. Current views in HTLV-I-associated adult T-cell leukemia/lymphoma. Am J Hematol [Internet]. 2005 [cited 2017 Nov 14];78(3):232–9. Available from: http://www.ncbi.nlm.nih.gov/pubmed/15726602.
41. Campuzano-Zuluaga G, Pimentel A, Chapman-Fredricks JR, Ramos J. Differential CD30 expression in adult T-cell leukemia-lymphoma subtypes. Retrovirology [Internet]. BioMed Central; 2014 [cited 2017 Nov 14];11(Suppl 1):P129. Available from: https://doi.org/10.1186/1742-4690-11-S1-P129.
42. Dittus C, Sloan JM. Adult T-cell leukemia/lymphoma. Hematol Oncol Clin N Am [Internet]. 2017 [cited 2017 Nov 14];31(2):255–72. Available from: http://www.ncbi.nlm.nih.gov/pubmed/28340877.
43. Jabbour M, Tuncer H, Castillo J, Butera J, Roy T, Pojani J, et al. Hematopoietic SCT for adult T-cell leukemia/lymphoma: a review. Bone Marrow Transplant [Internet]. Nature Publishing Group; 2011 [cited 2017 Nov 14];46(8):1039–44. Available from: https://doi.org/10.1038/bmt.2011.27.
44. Teshima T, Akashi K, Shibuya T, Taniguchi S, Okamura T, Harada M, et al. Central nervous system involvement in adult T-cell leukemia/lymphoma. Cancer [Internet]. 1990 [cited 2017 Nov 14];65(2):327–32. Available from: http://www.ncbi.nlm.nih.gov/pubmed/2295055.
45. Huang C-T, Lee Y-H, Chow K-C, Yang C-F, Chen PC-H, Hsiao L-T, et al. Adult T-cell leukaemia/lymphoma can mimic other lymphomas in a non-endemic area: dilemmas in diagnosis and

treatment. Intern Med J [Internet]. 2014 [cited 2017 Nov 14];44(4):374–83. Available from: http://www.ncbi.nlm.nih.gov/pubmed/24533861.
46. Karube K, Suzumiya J, Okamoto M, Takeshita M, Maeda K, Sakaguchi M, et al. Adult T-cell lymphoma/leukemia with angioimmunoblastic T-cell lymphomalike features: report of 11 cases. Am J Surg Pathol [Internet]. 2007 [cited 2017 Nov 14];31(2):216–23. Available from: http://www.ncbi.nlm.nih.gov/pubmed/17255766.
47. Katsuya H, Ishitsuka K, Utsunomiya A, Hanada S, Eto T, Moriuchi Y, et al. Treatment and survival among 1594 patients with ATL. Blood [Internet]. 2015 [cited 2017 Nov 14];126(24):2570–7. Available from: http://www.ncbi.nlm.nih.gov/pubmed/26361794.
48. Tsukasaki K, Hermine O, Bazarbachi A, Ratner L, Ramos JC, Harrington W, et al. Definition, prognostic factors, treatment, and response criteria of adult T-cell leukemia-lymphoma: a proposal from an international consensus meeting. J Clin Oncol [Internet]. 2009 [cited 2017 Nov 15];27(3):453–9. Available from: http://www.ncbi.nlm.nih.gov/pubmed/19064971.
49. Oken MM, Creech RH, Tormey DC, Horton J, Davis TE, McFadden ET, et al. Toxicity and response criteria of the Eastern Cooperative Oncology Group. Am J Clin Oncol [Internet]. 1982 [cited 2017 Nov 15];5(6):649–55. Available from: http://www.ncbi.nlm.nih.gov/pubmed/7165009.
50. Major prognostic factors of patients with adult T-cell leukemia-lymphoma: a cooperative study. Lymphoma Study Group (1984–1987). Leuk Res [Internet]. 1991 [cited 2017 Nov 15];15(2–3):81–90. Available from: http://www.ncbi.nlm.nih.gov/pubmed/2016910.
51. Takasaki Y, Iwanaga M, Imaizumi Y, Tawara M, Joh T, Kohno T, et al. Long-term study of indolent adult T-cell leukemia-lymphoma. Blood [Internet]. 2010 [cited 2017 Nov 15];115(22):4337–43. Available from: http://www.ncbi.nlm.nih.gov/pubmed/20348391.
52. Katsuya H, Yamanaka T, Ishitsuka K, Utsunomiya A, Sasaki H, Hanada S, et al. Prognostic index for acute- and lymphoma-type adult T-cell leukemia/lymphoma. J Clin Oncol [Internet]. 2012 [cited 2017 Nov 15];30(14):1635–40. Available from: http://www.ncbi.nlm.nih.gov/pubmed/22473153.
53. Takasaki Y, Iwanaga M, Tsukasaki K, Kusano M, Sugahara K, Yamada Y, et al. Impact of visceral involvements and blood cell count abnormalities on survival in adult T-cell leukemia/lymphoma (ATLL). Leuk Res [Internet]. 2007 [cited 2017 Nov 15];31(6):751–7. Available from: http://www.ncbi.nlm.nih.gov/pubmed/17188352.
54. Utsunomiya A, Ishida T, Inagaki A, Ishii T, Yano H, Komatsu H, et al. Clinical significance of a blood eosinophilia in adult T-cell leukemia/lymphoma: a blood eosinophilia is a significant unfavorable prognostic factor. Leuk Res [Internet]. 2007 [cited 2017 Nov 15];31(7):915–20. Available from: http://www.ncbi.nlm.nih.gov/pubmed/17123603.
55. Pimentel A, Diaz LA, Chapman-Fredricks JR, Ramos JC. CD30 expression is associated with decreased survival in patients with acute and unfavorable chronic types of adult T-cell leukemia-lymphoma. Blood [Internet]. 2013 [cited 2017 Nov 15];122(21). Available from: http://www.bloodjournal.org/content/122/21/4312?sso-checked=true.
56. Phillips A, Fields P, Hermine O, Taylor GP, Delioukina M, Horwitz S, et al. Anti-CCR4 monoclonal antibody KW-0761 (mogamulizumab) or investigator's choice in subjects with relapsed or refractory adult T-cell leukemia-lymphoma (ATL). Retrovirology [Internet]. BioMed Central; 2015 [cited 2018 Jan 25];12(Suppl 1):P31. Available from: https://doi.org/10.1186/1742-4690-12-S1-P31.
57. NCCN. Non-Hodgkin Lymphoma (NHL) treatment regimens: adult T-cell leukemia/lymphoma [Internet]. NCCN; 2016 [cited 2017 Nov 15]. Available from: http://www.nccn.org/professionals/physician_gls/pdf/nhl.pdf.
58. Kudo H, Fukushima S, Masuguchi S, Sakai K, Jinnin M, Ihn H. Cutaneous type adult T-cell leukaemia/lymphoma successfully treated with narrowband ultraviolet B phototherapy. Clin Exp Dermatol [Internet]. Blackwell Publishing Ltd; 2012 [cited 2017 Nov 15];37(2):183–4. Available from: https://doi.org/10.1111/j.1365-2230.2011.04141.x.
59. Takemori N, Hirai K, Onodera R, Saito N, Yokota K, Kinouchi M, et al. Satisfactory remission achieved by PUVA therapy in a case of crisis-type adult T-cell leukaemia/lymphoma with generalized cutaneous leukaemic cell infiltration. Br J Dermatol [Internet]. Blackwell

Publishing Ltd; 1995 [cited 2017 Nov 15];133(6):955–60. Available from: https://doi.org/10.1111/j.1365-2133.1995.tb06933.x.

60. Sawada Y, Shimauchi T, Yamaguchi T, Okura R, Hama-Yamamoto K, Fueki-Yoshioka H, et al. Combination of skin-directed therapy and oral etoposide for smoldering adult T-cell leukemia/lymphoma with skin involvement. Leuk Lymphoma [Internet]. 2013 [cited 2017 Nov 15];54(3):520–7. Available from: http://www.ncbi.nlm.nih.gov/pubmed/22830614.
61. Gill PS, Harrington W, Kaplan MH, Ribeiro RC, Bennett JM, Liebman HA, et al. Treatment of adult T-cell leukemia–lymphoma with a combination of interferon alfa and zidovudine. N Engl J Med [Internet]. 1995 [cited 2017 Nov 15];332(26):1744–8. Available from: http://www.ncbi.nlm.nih.gov/pubmed/7760890.
62. Hermine O, Allard I, Lévy V, Arnulf B, Gessain A, Bazarbachi A, et al. A prospective phase II clinical trial with the use of zidovudine and interferon-alpha in the acute and lymphoma forms of adult T-cell leukemia/lymphoma. Hematol J [Internet]. 2002 [cited 2018 Jan 25];3(6):276–82. Available from: http://www.ncbi.nlm.nih.gov/pubmed/12522449.
63. Bazarbachi A, Plumelle Y, Carlos Ramos J, Tortevoye P, Otrock Z, Taylor G, et al. Meta-analysis on the use of zidovudine and interferon-alfa in adult t-cell leukemia/lymphoma showing improved survival in the leukemic subtypes. J Clin Oncol [Internet]. 2010 [cited 2017 Nov 15];28(27):4177–4183. Available from: http://www.ncbi.nlm.nih.gov/pubmed/20585095.
64. Barbeau B, Hiscott J, Bazarbachi A, Carvalho E, Jones K, Martin F, et al. Conference highlights of the 16th international conference on human retrovirology: HTLV and related retroviruses, 26–30 June 2013, Montreal, Canada. Retrovirology [Internet]. BioMed Central. 2014 [cited 2017 Nov 15];11(1):19. Available from: http://retrovirology.biomedcentral.com/articles/10.1186/1742-4690-11-19.
65. Hodson A, Crichton S, Montoto S, Mir N, Matutes E, Cwynarski K, et al. Use of zidovudine and interferon alfa with chemotherapy improves survival in both acute and lymphoma subtypes of adult t-cell leukemia/lymphoma. J Clin Oncol [Internet]. 2011 [cited 2017 Nov 15];29(35):4696–4701. Available from: http://www.ncbi.nlm.nih.gov/pubmed/22042945.
66. Bazarbachi A, El-Sabban ME, Nasr R, Quignon F, Awaraji C, Kersual J, et al. Arsenic trioxide and interferon-alpha synergize to induce cell cycle arrest and apoptosis in human T-cell lymphotropic virus type I-transformed cells. Blood [Internet]. 1999 [cited 2017 Nov 15];93(1):278–283. Available from: http://www.ncbi.nlm.nih.gov/pubmed/9864171.
67. Hermine O, Dombret H, Poupon J, Arnulf B, Lefrère F, Rousselot P, et al. Phase II trial of arsenic trioxide and alpha interferon in patients with relapsed/refractory adult T-cell leukemia/lymphoma. Hematol J [Internet]. 2004 [cited 2017 Nov 15];5(2):130–4. Available from: http://www.ncbi.nlm.nih.gov/pubmed/15048063.
68. Oliveira PD, Farre L, Bittencourt AL, Oliveira PD, Farre L, Bittencourt AL. Adult T-cell leukemia/lymphoma. Rev Assoc Med Bras [Internet]. Associação Médica Brasileira; 2016 [cited 2017 Nov 14];62(7):691–700. Available from: http://www.scielo.br/scielo.php?script=sci_arttext&pid=S0104-42302016000700691&lng=en&tlng=en.
69. Utsunomiya A, Choi I, Chihara D, Seto M. Recent advances in the treatment of adult T-cell leukemia-lymphomas. Cancer Sci [Internet]. 2015 [cited 2017 Nov 14];106(4):344–51. Available from: http://www.ncbi.nlm.nih.gov/pubmed/25613789.
70. Di Venuti G, Nawgiri R, Foss F. Denileukin diftitox and hyper-CVAD in the treatment of human T-cell lymphotropic virus 1-associated acute T-cell leukemia/lymphoma. Clin Lymphoma [Internet]. 2003 [cited 2017 Nov 15];4(3):176–178. Available from: http://www.ncbi.nlm.nih.gov/pubmed/14715100.
71. Younes A, Bartlett NL, Leonard JP, Kennedy DA, Lynch CM, Sievers EL, et al. Brentuximab vedotin (SGN-35) for relapsed CD30-positive lymphomas. N Engl J Med [Internet]. Massachusetts Medical Society; 2010 [cited 2017 Nov 15];363(19):1812–1821. Available from: http://www.nejm.org/doi/abs/10.1056/NEJMoa1002965.
72. Pro B, Advani R, Brice P, Bartlett NL, Rosenblatt JD, Illidge T, et al. Brentuximab vedotin (SGN-35) in patients with relapsed or refractory systemic anaplastic large-cell lymphoma:

results of a phase II study. J Clin Oncol [Internet]. 2012 [cited 2017 Nov 15];30(18):2190–6. Available from: http://www.ncbi.nlm.nih.gov/pubmed/22614995.

73. Younes A, Gopal AK, Smith SE, Ansell SM, Rosenblatt JD, Savage KJ, et al. Results of a pivotal phase II study of brentuximab vedotin for patients with relapsed or refractory Hodgkin's lymphoma. J Clin Oncol [Internet]. 2012 [cited 2017 Nov 15];30(18):2183–2189. Available from: http://www.ncbi.nlm.nih.gov/pubmed/22454421.
74. Horwitz SM, Advani RH, Bartlett NL, Jacobsen ED, Sharman JP, O'Connor OA, et al. Objective responses in relapsed T-cell lymphomas with single-agent brentuximab vedotin. Blood [Internet]. 2014 [cited 2017 Nov 15];123(20):3095–3100. Available from: http://www.ncbi.nlm.nih.gov/pubmed/24652992.
75. Duvic M, Tetzlaff MT, Gangar P, Clos AL, Sui D, Talpur R. Results of a phase II trial of brentuximab vedotin for CD30 + cutaneous T-cell lymphoma and lymphomatoid papulosis. J Clin Oncol [Internet]. 2015 [cited 2017 Nov 15];33(32):3759–3765. Available from: http://www.ncbi.nlm.nih.gov/pubmed/26261247.
76. Jacobsen ED, Sharman JP, Oki Y, Advani RH, Winter JN, Bello CM, et al. Brentuximab vedotin demonstrates objective responses in a phase 2 study of relapsed/refractory DLBCL with variable CD30 expression. Blood [Internet]. 2015 [cited 2017 Nov 15];125(9):1394–1402. Available from: http://www.ncbi.nlm.nih.gov/pubmed/25573987.
77. Fanale MA, Horwitz SM, Forero-Torres A, Bartlett NL, Advani RH, Pro B, et al. Brentuximab vedotin in the front-line treatment of patients with CD30 + peripheral T-cell lymphomas: results of a phase I study. J Clin Oncol [Internet]. 2014 [cited 2017 Nov 15];32(28):3137–3143. Available from: http://www.ncbi.nlm.nih.gov/pubmed/25135998.
78. Fanale MA, Horwitz SM, Forero-Torres A, Bartlett NL, Advani RH, Pro B, et al. Five-year outcomes for frontline brentuximab vedotin with CHP for CD30-expressing peripheral T-cell lymphomas. Blood [Internet]. 2018 [cited 2018 Aug 14];131(19):2120–4. Available from: http://www.ncbi.nlm.nih.gov/pubmed/29507077.
79. Thomas Manley M. ECHELON-2: a comparison of brentuximab vedotin and CHP with standard-of-care CHOP in the treatment of patients with CD30-positive mature T-cell lymphomas - ClinicalTrials.gov [Internet]. [cited 2017 Nov 15]. Available from: https://clinicaltrials.gov/ct2/show/NCT01777152.
80. Owen A. O'Connor, Barbara Pro, Tim Illidge, Lorenz H. Trumper, Emily K. Larsen DAK. Phase 3 trial of brentuximab vedotin and CHP versus CHOP in the frontline treatment of patients (pts) with CD30+ mature T-cell lymphomas (MTCL). Abstract TPS8612. J Clin Oncol [Internet]. 2014;32:5s. Available from: http://ascopubs.org/doi/abs/10.1200/jco.2014.32.15_suppl.tps8612.
81. Alex F. Herrera M. Brentuximab vedotin and combination chemotherapy in treating patients with CD30-positive peripheral T-cell lymphoma - ClinicalTrials.gov - NCT03113500 [Internet]. [cited 2017 Nov 15]. Available from: https://clinicaltrials.gov/ct2/show/NCT03113500.
82. Ishida T, Utsunomiya A, Iida S, Inagaki H, Takatsuka Y, Kusumoto S, et al. Clinical significance of CCR4 expression in adult T-cell leukemia/lymphoma: its close association with skin involvement and unfavorable outcome. Clin Cancer Res [Internet]. 2003 [cited 2017 Nov 15];9(10 Pt 1):3625–34. Available from: http://www.ncbi.nlm.nih.gov/pubmed/14506150.
83. Subramaniam JM, Whiteside G, McKeage K, Croxtall JC. Mogamulizumab. Drugs [Internet]. 2012 [cited 2017 Nov 15];72(9):1293–1298. Available from: http://www.ncbi.nlm.nih.gov/pubmed/22686619.
84. Ishida T, Joh T, Uike N, Yamamoto K, Utsunomiya A, Yoshida S, et al. Defucosylated anti-CCR4 monoclonal antibody (KW-0761) for relapsed adult T-cell leukemia-lymphoma: a multicenter phase II study. J Clin Oncol [Internet]. 2012 [cited 2017 Nov 15];30(8):837–842. Available from: http://www.ncbi.nlm.nih.gov/pubmed/22312108.
85. Ishida T, Jo T, Takemoto S, Suzushima H, Uozumi K, Yamamoto K, et al. Dose-intensified chemotherapy alone or in combination with mogamulizumab in newly diagnosed aggressive adult T-cell leukaemia-lymphoma: a randomized phase II study. Br J Haematol [Internet]. 2015 [cited 2017 Nov 15];169(5):672–82. Available from: http://www.ncbi.nlm.nih.gov/pubmed/25733162.

86. Fuji S, Inoue Y, Utsunomiya A, Moriuchi Y, Uchimaru K, Choi I, et al. Pretransplantation anti-CCR4 antibody mogamulizumab against adult T-cell leukemia/lymphoma is associated with significantly increased risks of severe and corticosteroid-refractory graft-versus-host disease, nonrelapse mortality, and overall mortality. J Clin Oncol [Internet]. 2016 [cited 2017 Nov 15];34(28):3426–3433. Available from: http://www.ncbi.nlm.nih.gov/pubmed/27507878.
87. Rodig SJ, Abramson JS, Pinkus GS, Treon SP, Dorfman DM, Dong HY, et al. Heterogeneous CD52 expression among hematologic neoplasms: implications for the use of alemtuzumab (CAMPATH-1H). Clin Cancer Res [Internet]. 2006 [cited 2017 Nov 16];12(23):7174–7179. Available from: http://www.ncbi.nlm.nih.gov/pubmed/17145843.
88. Jiang L, Yuan CM, Hubacheck J, Janik JE, Wilson W, Morris JC, et al. Variable CD52 expression in mature T cell and NK cell malignancies: implications for alemtuzumab therapy. Br J Haematol [Internet]. 2009 [cited 2017 Nov 16];145(2):173–179. Available from: http://www.ncbi.nlm.nih.gov/pubmed/19236377.
89. Gallamini A, Zaja F, Patti C, Billio A, Specchia MR, Tucci A, et al. Alemtuzumab (Campath-1H) and CHOP chemotherapy as first-line treatment of peripheral T-cell lymphoma: results of a GITIL (Gruppo Italiano Terapie Innovative nei Linfomi) prospective multicenter trial. Blood [Internet]. 2007 [cited 2017 Nov 16];110(7):2316–2323. Available from: http://www.ncbi.nlm.nih.gov/pubmed/17581918.
90. Sharma K, Janik JE, O'Mahony D, Stewart D, Pittaluga S, Stetler-Stevenson M, et al. Phase II Study of Alemtuzumab (CAMPATH-1) in Patients with HTLV-1-Associated Adult T-cell Leukemia/lymphoma. Clin Cancer Res [Internet]. American Association for Cancer Research; 2017 [cited 2018 Aug 14];23(1):35–42. Available from: http://www.ncbi.nlm.nih.gov/pubmed/27486175.
91. Berkowitz JL, Janik JE, Stewart DM, Jaffe ES, Stetler-Stevenson M, Shih JH, et al. Safety, efficacy, and pharmacokinetics/pharmacodynamics of daclizumab (anti-CD25) in patients with adult T-cell leukemia/lymphoma. Clin Immunol [Internet]. 2014 [cited 2017 Nov 16];155(2):176–87. Available from: http://www.ncbi.nlm.nih.gov/pubmed/25267440.
92. Ceesay MM, Matutes E, Taylor GP, Fields P, Cavenagh J, Simpson S, et al. Phase II study on combination therapy with CHOP-Zenapax for HTLV-I associated adult T-cell leukaemia/lymphoma (ATLL). Leuk Res [Internet]. 2012 Jul [cited 2017 Nov 16];36(7):857–61. Available from: http://www.ncbi.nlm.nih.gov/pubmed/22209076.
93. Mehta-Shah N, Horwitz SM. Lenalidomide in adult T-cell leukemia/lymphoma. J Clin Oncol [Internet]. 2016 [cited 2017 Nov 15];34(34):4066–7. Available from: http://ascopubs.org/doi/10.1200/JCO.2016.69.4505.
94. Ogura M, Imaizumi Y, Uike N, Asou N, Utsunomiya A, Uchida T, et al. Lenalidomide in relapsed adult T-cell leukaemia-lymphoma or peripheral T-cell lymphoma (ATLL-001): a phase 1, multicentre, dose-escalation study. Lancet Haematol [Internet]. 2016 [cited 2017 Nov 15];3(3):e107–18. Available from: http://linkinghub.elsevier.com/retrieve/pii/S2352302615002847.
95. Ishida T, Fujiwara H, Nosaka K, Taira N, Abe Y, Imaizumi Y, et al. Multicenter phase II study of lenalidomide in relapsed or recurrent adult T-cell leukemia/lymphoma: ATLL-002. J Clin Oncol [Internet]. 2016 Dec [cited 2017 Nov 15];34(34):4086–93. Available from: http://ascopubs.org/doi/10.1200/JCO.2016.67.7732.
96. Andorsky DJ, Yamada RE, Said J, Pinkus GS, Betting DJ, Timmerman JM. Programmed death ligand 1 is expressed by non-hodgkin lymphomas and inhibits the activity of tumor-associated T cells. Clin Cancer Res [Internet]. American Association for Cancer Research; 2011 [cited 2017 Nov 15];17(13):4232–44. Available from: http://www.ncbi.nlm.nih.gov/pubmed/21540239.
97. Chen BJ, Chapuy B, Ouyang J, Sun HH, Roemer MGM, Xu ML, et al. PD-L1 expression is characteristic of a subset of aggressive B-cell lymphomas and virus-associated malignancies. Clin Cancer Res [Internet]. American Association for Cancer Research; 2013 [cited 2017 Nov 15];19(13):3462–73. Available from: http://www.ncbi.nlm.nih.gov/pubmed/23674495.

98. Ribas A. Tumor immunotherapy directed at PD-1. N Engl J Med [Internet]. Massachusetts Medical Society; 2012 [cited 2017 Nov 15];366(26):2517–9. Available from: http://www.nejm.org/doi/abs/10.1056/NEJMe1205943.
99. Rossille D, Gressier M, Damotte D, Maucort-Boulch D, Pangault C, Semana G, et al. High level of soluble programmed cell death ligand 1 in blood impacts overall survival in aggressive diffuse large B-Cell lymphoma: results from a French multicenter clinical trial. Leukemia [Internet]. 2014 [cited 2017 Nov 15];28(12):2367–75. Available from: http://www.ncbi.nlm.nih.gov/pubmed/24732592.
100. Kiyasu J, Miyoshi H, Hirata A, Arakawa F, Ichikawa A, Niino D, et al. Expression of programmed cell death ligand 1 is associated with poor overall survival in patients with diffuse large B-cell lymphoma. Blood [Internet]. American Society of Hematology; 2015 [cited 2017 Nov 15];126(19):2193–201. Available from: http://www.ncbi.nlm.nih.gov/pubmed/26239088.
101. Ansell SM, Lesokhin AM, Borrello I, Halwani A, Scott EC, Gutierrez M, et al. PD-1 blockade with nivolumab in relapsed or refractory Hodgkin's Lymphoma. N Engl J Med [Internet]. 2015 [cited 2017 Nov 15];372(4):311–9. Available from: http://www.ncbi.nlm.nih.gov/pubmed/25482239.
102. Shimauchi T, Kabashima K, Nakashima D, Sugita K, Yamada Y, Hino R, et al. Augmented expression of programmed death-1 in both neoplastic and non-neoplastic CD4+ T-cells in adult T-cell leukemia/lymphoma. Int J Cancer [Internet]. 2007 [cited 2017 Nov 15];121(12):2585–90. Available from: http://www.ncbi.nlm.nih.gov/pubmed/17721918.
103. Kozako T, Yoshimitsu M, Fujiwara H, Masamoto I, Horai S, White Y, et al. PD-1/PD-L1 expression in human T-cell leukemia virus type 1 carriers and adult T-cell leukemia/lymphoma patients. Leukemia [Internet]. 2009 [cited 2017 Nov 15];23(2):375–82. Available from: http://www.ncbi.nlm.nih.gov/pubmed/18830259.
104. Miyoshi H, Kiyasu J, Kato T, Yoshida N, Shimono J, Yokoyama S, et al. PD-L1 expression on neoplastic or stromal cells is respectively a poor or good prognostic factor for adult T-cell leukemia/lymphoma. Blood [Internet]. 2016 [cited 2017 Nov 15];128(10):1374–81. Available from: http://www.ncbi.nlm.nih.gov/pubmed/27418641.
105. National Cancer Institute. Nivolumab in Treating Patients With HTLV-Associated T-Cell Leukemia/Lymphoma - ClinicalTrials.gov - NCT02631746 [Internet]. [cited 2017 Nov 16]. Available from: https://clinicaltrials.gov/ct2/show/NCT02631746.
106. Ratner L, Waldmann TA, Janakiram M, Brammer JE. Rapid progression of adult T-cell leukemia–lymphoma after PD-1 inhibitor therapy. N Engl J Med [Internet]. Massachusetts Medical Society; 2018 [cited 2018 Aug 14];378(20):1947–8. Available from: http://www.nejm.org/doi/10.1056/NEJMc1803181.
107. O'Connor OA, Heaney ML, Schwartz L, Richardson S, Willim R, MacGregor-Cortelli B, et al. Clinical experience with intravenous and oral formulations of the novel histone deacetylase inhibitor suberoylanilide hydroxamic acid in patients with advanced hematologic malignancies. J Clin Oncol [Internet]. 2006 [cited 2017 Nov 16];24(1):166–73. Available from: http://www.ncbi.nlm.nih.gov/pubmed/16330674.
108. Hasegawa H, Yamada Y, Tsukasaki K, Mori N, Tsuruda K, Sasaki D, et al. LBH589, a deacetylase inhibitor, induces apoptosis in adult T-cell leukemia/lymphoma cells via activation of a novel RAIDD-caspase-2 pathway. Leukemia [Internet]. Nature Publishing Group; 2011 [cited 2017 Nov 16];25(4):575–87. Available from: http://www.ncbi.nlm.nih.gov/pubmed/21242994.
109. Dang NH, Pro B, Hagemeister FB, Samaniego F, Jones D, Samuels BI, et al. Phase II trial of denileukin diftitox for relapsed/refractory T-cell non-Hodgkin lymphoma. Br J Haematol [Internet]. 2007 [cited 2017 Nov 16];136(3):439–47. Available from: http://www.ncbi.nlm.nih.gov/pubmed/17233846.
110. Foss FM, Sjak-Shie N, Goy A, Jacobsen E, Advani R, Smith MR, et al. A multicenter phase II trial to determine the safety and efficacy of combination therapy with denileukin diftitox and cyclophosphamide, doxorubicin, vincristine and prednisone in untreated peripheral

T-cell lymphoma: the CONCEPT study. Leuk Lymphoma [Internet]. 2013 [cited 2017 Nov 16];54(7):1373–9. Available from: http://www.ncbi.nlm.nih.gov/pubmed/23278639.
111. Di Venuti G, Nawgiri R, Foss F. Denileukin diftitox and hyper-CVAD in the treatment of human T-cell lymphotropic virus 1-associated acute T-cell leukemia/lymphoma. Clin Lymphoma [Internet]. 2003 Dec [cited 2017 Nov 16];4(3):176–8. Available from: http://www.ncbi.nlm.nih.gov/pubmed/14715100.
112. Suehiro Y. HTLV-1-targeted immunotherapy. Rinsho Ketsueki [Internet]. 2016 [cited 2018 Jan 25];57(10):2250–8. Available from: http://www.ncbi.nlm.nih.gov/pubmed/27795537.
113. Youko Suehiro. Novel autologous dendritic cell vaccine therapy targeting HTLV-1 specific antigen Combined with anti-CCR4 antibody for previously treated patients with adult T-cell leukemia. A phase Ia/Ib study - UMIN Clinical Trials Registry [Internet]. Available from: https://upload.umin.ac.jp/cgi-open-bin/ctr_e/ctr_view.cgi?recptno=R000019348.
114. Tsukasaki K, Maeda T, Arimura K, Taguchi J, Fukushima T, Miyazaki Y, et al. Poor outcome of autologous stem cell transplantation for adult T cell leukemia/lymphoma: a case report and review of the literature. Bone Marrow Transplant [Internet]. 1999 [cited 2017 Nov 16];23(1):87–9. Available from: http://www.ncbi.nlm.nih.gov/pubmed/10037056.
115. Borg A, Yin JA, Johnson PR, Tosswill J, Saunders M, Morris D. Successful treatment of HTLV-1-associated acute adult T-cell leukaemia lymphoma by allogeneic bone marrow transplantation. Br J Haematol [Internet]. 1996 [cited 2017 Nov 16];94(4):713–5. Available from: http://www.ncbi.nlm.nih.gov/pubmed/8826899.
116. Japan. HCT in. Annual Report of Nationwide Survey 2013. The Japanese Data Center for Hematopoietic Cell Transp lantation/The Japan Society for Hematopoietic Cell Transplantation 2014. 2014.
117. Kanda J, Hishizawa M, Utsunomiya A, Taniguchi S, Eto T, Moriuchi Y, et al. Impact of graft-versus-host disease on outcomes after allogeneic hematopoietic cell transplantation for adult T-cell leukemia: a retrospective cohort study. Blood [Internet]. 2012 [cited 2017 Nov 16];119(9):2141–8. Available from: http://www.ncbi.nlm.nih.gov/pubmed/22234682.
118. Ishida T, Hishizawa M, Kato K, Tanosaki R, Fukuda T, Taniguchi S, et al. Allogeneic hematopoietic stem cell transplantation for adult T-cell leukemia-lymphoma with special emphasis on preconditioning regimen: a nationwide retrospective study. Blood [Internet]. 2012 [cited 2017 Nov 16];120(8):1734–41. Available from: http://www.ncbi.nlm.nih.gov/pubmed/22689862.
119. Bazarbachi A, Cwynarski K, Boumendil A, Finel H, Fields P, Raj K, et al. Outcome of patients with HTLV-1-associated adult T-cell leukemia/lymphoma after SCT: a retrospective study by the EBMT LWP. Bone Marrow Transplant [Internet]. 2014 [cited 2017 Nov 16];49(10):1266–8. Available from: http://www.ncbi.nlm.nih.gov/pubmed/25029232.
120. University Hospital Center of Martinique. High Risk Adult T-cell Leukemia/Lymphoma (ATLL-HR) and Allogeneic Transplant - ClinicalTrials.gov - NCT01941680 [Internet]. [cited 2017 Nov 16]. Available from: https://clinicaltrials.gov/ct2/show/NCT01941680.
121. Schmitz N, Trümper L, Ziepert M, Nickelsen M, Ho AD, Metzner B, et al. Treatment and prognosis of mature T-cell and NK-cell lymphoma: an analysis of patients with T-cell lymphoma treated in studies of the German High-Grade Non-Hodgkin Lymphoma Study Group. Blood [Internet]. American Society of Hematology; 2010 [cited 2018 Jan 21];116(18):3418–25. Available from: http://www.ncbi.nlm.nih.gov/pubmed/20660290.
122. Hishizawa M, Kanda J, Utsunomiya A, Taniguchi S, Eto T, Moriuchi Y, et al. Transplantation of allogeneic hematopoietic stem cells for adult T-cell leukemia: a nationwide retrospective study. Blood [Internet]. 2010 [cited 2017 Nov 16];116(8):1369–76. Available from: http://www.ncbi.nlm.nih.gov/pubmed/20479287.
123. Salles F, Bacellar A, Amorim M, Orge G, Sundberg M, Lima M, et al. Treatment of strongyloidiasis in HTLV-1 and Strongyloides stercoralis coinfected patients is associated with increased TNFα and decreased soluble IL2 receptor levels. Trans R Soc Trop Med Hyg [Internet]. 2013 [cited 2017 Nov 15];107(8):526–9. Available from: http://www.ncbi.nlm.nih.gov/pubmed/23843560.

124. Plumelle Y, Edouard A. Strongyloides stercoralis in T-cell leukemia/lymphoma in adults and acquired immunodeficiency syndrome. La Rev Med interne [Internet]. 1996 [cited 2017 Nov 15];17(2):125–9. Available from: http://www.ncbi.nlm.nih.gov/pubmed/8787083.
125. Ratner L, Grant C, Zimmerman B, Fritz J, Weil G, Denes A, et al. Effect of treatment of Strongyloides infection on HTLV-1 expression in a patient with adult T-cell leukemia. Am J Hematol [Internet]. NIH Public Access; 2007 [cited 2017 Nov 15];82(10):929–31. Available from: http://www.ncbi.nlm.nih.gov/pubmed/17617788.
126. Gabet A-S, Mortreux F, Talarmin A, Plumelle Y, Leclercq I, Leroy A, et al. High circulating proviral load with oligoclonal expansion of HTLV-1 bearing T cells in HTLV-1 carriers with strongyloidiasis. Oncogene [Internet]. 2000 [cited 2017 Nov 15];19(43):4954–60. Available from: http://www.ncbi.nlm.nih.gov/pubmed/11042682.

Chapter 10
Extranodal NK/T-Cell Lymphoma

Mary Beth Seegars and Zanetta S. Lamar

Background and Clinical Presentation

Introduction and Epidemiology

Extranodal NK/T-cell lymphoma (ENKTCL) is a rare, aggressive form of non-Hodgkin lymphoma which occurs worldwide but is more common in Asia and Central and South America. In countries such as China, Japan, and Brazil, ENKTCL accounts for 5–15% of all lymphoma cases [1]. However, in the United States and Europe, it accounts for less than 1% of all lymphoma cases [2]. ENKTCL is further divided into subtypes based on location of disease. The nasal type is the most common and frequently presents with localized disease. Sites most commonly involved include the nose, nasopharynx, oropharynx, and Waldeyer's ring; fewer than 20% of cases present with extra-nasal lesions [3]. Dissemination to sites such as the bone marrow, spleen, liver, and skin with peripheral blood involvement is considered advanced stage disease.

The immunophenotype of ENKTCL is unique, with most cases expressing NK-cell markers (CD2+, cytoplasmic CD3+, and CD56+) (Fig. 10.1). Tumor cells are almost always infected by Epstein-Barr virus (EBV), which can be detected by in situ hybridization for EBV early RNA (EBER). The malignant cells may also express perforin, granzyme B, or TIA-I. In rare cases, CD56 is negative, and in exceptionally rare cases, T-cell gene rearrangement is positive. These cases are included under the "T-cell" nomenclature of NK/T-cell lymphoma.

M. B. Seegars · Z. S. Lamar (✉)
Wake Forest Baptist Medical Center, Winston Salem, NC, USA
e-mail: mseegars@wakehealth.edu; zlamar@wakehealth.edu

C. Dittus (ed.), *Novel Therapeutics for Rare Lymphomas*,
https://doi.org/10.1007/978-3-030-25610-4_10

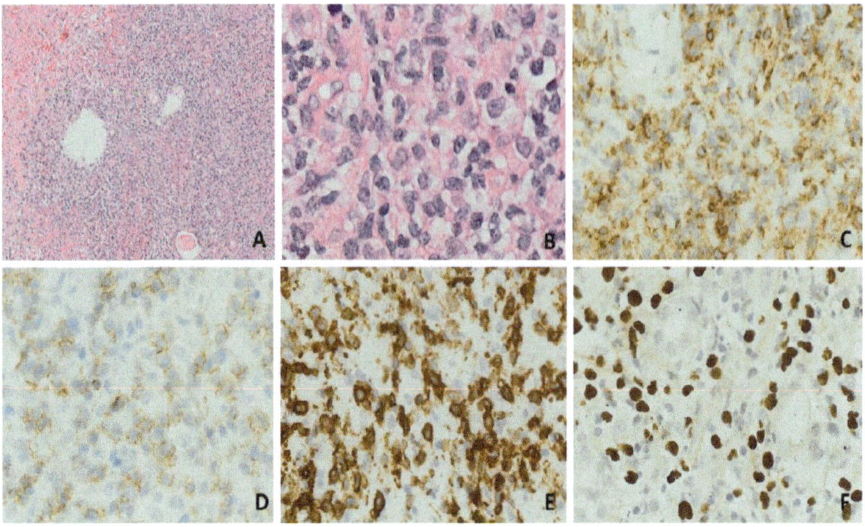

Fig. 10.1 (**a**) H&E, low-power view of the nasal septum biopsy with diffuse lymphoid infiltrate, entrapped epithelium, and areas of necrosis (top left); (**b**) H&E, high-power view of atypical lymphoid cells with intermediate-sized, irregular nuclei; (**c**) CD43 expression is present in the neoplastic lymphoid population; (**d**) CD56 is also expressed in the neoplastic lymphocytes; (**e**) CD3 highlights background mature T cells while sparing the neoplastic NK/T-cell infiltrate; (**f**) In situ hybridization for Epstein-Barr virus-encoded RNA is positive. (Imaging courtesy of Robert K. McCall, MD. Vanderbilt University Medical Center)

Clinical Presentation

ENKTCL is a primarily an extranodal disease, most often presenting as a localized lymphoma in the nasal region. Lesions may occur in the nose, nasopharynx, paranasal sinuses, tonsils, Waldeyer's ring, or oropharynx. Spread to the cerebrospinal fluid is rare [1]. Symptoms may include epistaxis, obstruction, and pain from necrotic lesions in the nose or hard palate. Patients may also present with extra-nasal masses of the skin, salivary glands, testis, and gastrointestinal tract. Positron emission tomography (PET) imaging has demonstrated that most extra-nasal lymphomas are associated with occult nasal primary tumors. This implies that the extra-nasal subtypes are likely disseminated nasal lymphomas. To meet the formal definition of extra-nasal ENKTCL, the absence of a nasal primary mass must be detected by random nasopharyngeal biopsies and PET imaging. Rarely, patients present with widespread disease. If there is involvement of the bone marrow and peripheral blood, the diagnosis can overlap with aggressive NK-cell leukemia. NK-cell leukemia carries an extremely poor prognosis, with a median survival of weeks [4].

The differential diagnosis for ENKTCL includes malignant and nonmalignant conditions such as invasive fungal and bacterial infections, Wegener's granulomatosis, NK-cell enteropathy, enteropathy-associated T-cell lymphoma, other lymphomas, and primary and secondary malignancies. Among these considerations,

NK-cell enteropathy is particularly difficult to differentiate from ENKTCL due to similar pathologic findings. Patients with NK-cell enteropathy classically have a CD56 and cytoplasmic CD3-positive infiltrate which mimics ENKTCL. EBV testing in NK-cell enteropathy, however, is negative which excludes the diagnosis of ENKTCL. Mansoor et al. published a case series in which eight patients with NK-cell enteropathy were misdiagnosed with ENKTCL. Several received unnecessary chemotherapy as a result [5]. This report highlights the challenges and diagnostic overlap between these conditions. Unlike ENKTCL, in patients with NK-cell enteropathy, the disease is limited to the gastrointestinal tract. Given the immunophenotypic overlap, it is important to work closely with pathologists to confirm ENKTCL before initiating aggressive therapy [5].

Initial Evaluation, Diagnosis, and Staging

Patients suspected of having ENKTCL should undergo a thorough initial evaluation to include nasal panendoscopy, PET/CT imaging, and plasma EBV DNA testing. Nasal panendoscopy should be performed regardless of the primary site of presentation, and random biopsies should be taken even if no suspicious lesions are seen. Biopsies should include the leading edges of the lesions because biopsy specimens are often necrotic [6]. Diagnostic delays can compromise overall survival by increasing the likelihood of disease dissemination in the interim. In one study of 25 patients with ENKTCL, the median time from symptoms to diagnosis was 5 months. Twelve patients required more than one diagnostic biopsy; delay in diagnosis was prolonged up to 36 months. Given these concerns, generous biopsy specimens should be taken when feasible to ensure more timely diagnoses [2].

Upon diagnosis, the first important distinction is whether the specimen is surface or cytoplasmic CD3 positive. If a fresh specimen is not sent, the next step is to confirm positive results on CD56, EBER (EBV by in situ hybridization), and cytotoxic molecule testing. Cytologic examination will reveal small- to medium-sized cells with azurophilic granules and pale cytoplasm. Neoplastic cells are often mixed with lymphocytes, plasma cells, and eosinophils. Thus, the term "polymorphic reticulosis" is used to describe the histology of ENKTCL. Tumor cells are classically positive for CD2, cytoplasmic CD3, and CD56.

Next-generation sequencing has identified several somatic mutations in the Janus kinase 3 (JAK3) gene leading to constitutive activation of the JAK/STAT pathway. In this scenario, increased cell growth occurs in approximately 35% of cases [7]. The most frequent cytogenetic aberration in NK malignancies is the deletion of chromosome 6q21. Notable tumor suppressor genes in this region include FOXO3, PRDM1, and HACE1. PRDM1 is integral to the maturation and homeostasis of NK cells [8]. In addition to the JAK/STAT pathway, other activated pathways resulting in tumorigenesis include AKT, Wnt, and Notch-1.

Initial imaging should include PET/CT, as lesions are invariably PET avid [9]. The SUV maximum for ENKTCL is lower than for other aggressive lymphomas such as diffuse large B-cell lymphoma. As in other types of non-Hodgkin lymphoma, the Ann Arbor System is used for staging. Plasma EBV DNA testing should be performed at diagnosis and can be serially monitored to follow response to treatment and to detect recurrence [10].

Conventional Treatment Approach for Localized Nasal-Type ENKTCL

Treatment approaches are based on subtype (nasal or extra-nasal disease) and stage (localized or advanced). For patients with stage I/II nasal-type ENKTCL who are candidates for chemotherapy, standard treatment options include chemoradiation given either in concurrent, sequential, or "sandwich" fashion defined as induction chemotherapy followed by radiation and then consolidation chemotherapy.

Concurrent Chemoradiation

Evidence for concurrent chemoradiation stems from two prospective trials. Kim et al. conducted a study using concurrent radiation therapy (40 Gy) and cisplatin followed by three cycles of etoposide, ifosfamide, cisplatin, and dexamethasone (VIPD) in patients with localized nasal NK/T-cell lymphoma. The overall response rate was 83%, and the complete response rate was 80%. Patients in this study had a 3-year overall survival of 86% and a 3-year progression-free survival of 85% [11]. In 2009, Yamaguchi et al. conducted a trial in localized nasal type using concurrent radiation therapy (50 Gy) and DeVIC chemotherapy (dexamethasone, etoposide, ifosfamide, and carboplatin). The overall response rate was 81%, and 77% of the 27 patients achieved a complete response. The 5-year overall survival rate was 70%, and the 5-year progression-free survival rate was 63%. Grade 3/4 neutropenia occurred in 93% of patients and grade 3 radiation-related mucositis in 30% of patients [12].

Sandwich Chemoradiation

Sandwich chemoradiation was efficacious in two studies of NK/T-cell lymphoma. Jiang et al. conducted a phase II trial of 26 patients with stage I/II nasal disease. Patients received six cycles of L-asparaginase, vincristine, and prednisolone (LVP) sandwiched with radiation therapy after two cycles. After completion of radiation therapy and 2–4 cycles of LVP, the ORR was 89%, and the CR rate was 81%. The 2-year OS was 88.5%, and 2-year PFS was 80.6%. Grade 3 neutropenia occurred in 2.7% of patients, and grade 3 radiation-related mucositis was seen in 23.1% of patients [13]. In another prospective trial, gemcitabine, L-asparaginase, and oxaliplatin (GELOX) were given for two cycles followed by radiation therapy (56 Gy). After radiation, GELOX was given for 2–4 more cycles. The overall response rate was 96%, and the complete remission rate was 74%, with a 2-year overall survival rate of 86%. Grade 3/4 neutropenia occurred in 33.3% and radiation-related mucositis in 15% of participants [14].

Sequential Chemoradiation

In a retrospective review, Lunning et al. described their experience with a modified SMILE chemotherapy regimen (dexamethasone, methotrexate, ifosfamide, L-asparaginase, and etoposide). In this regimen, one dose of L-asparaginase is given, rather than a dose with each cycle. Twelve patients with stage I nasal-type ENKTCL received two cycles of modified SMILE followed by 45 Gy of radiation therapy. Patients with stage II disease received three cycles followed by radiation therapy. After 1–2 cycles of the modified SMILE regimen, the overall response rate was 92%, and the complete response rate was 75% [15].

Radiation Therapy for Localized Nasal-Type ENKTCL

For patients with localized, nasal-type ENKTCL, radiation therapy is an integral component of treatment. In 2017, Yang et al. evaluated 1332 patients with localized ENKTCL treated at ten institutions between 2000 and 2014. The goal of the study was to determine if improved locoregional control translates into progression-free and overall survival gains for patients with early stage disease. Patients received radiation, chemotherapy, or combination chemoradiation. After analysis, it was found that radiation therapy had a dose-dependent effect on locoregional control, PFS, and OS. High-dose radiation therapy, defined as ≥50 Gy, led to improved locoregional control (85% vs 73%), PFS (61% vs 50%), and OS (70% vs 58%) [16]. The LRC benefit with radiation therapy in the high-dose group was independent of the sequence of chemotherapy relative to radiation therapy and was independent of response to chemotherapy. This study concluded 50 Gy is the optimal dose, and the gains in PFS and OS highlight the significant role of radiation therapy in the treatment of early stage disease. The technique of radiation therapy delivery has also changed significantly in recent years, with most institutions using intensity-modulated radiation therapy (IMRT) to improve target coverage and reduce dose to adjacent normal tissues improving toxicity outcomes [17, 18].

The benefit of chemoradiotherapy as compared to radiation therapy alone has also been investigated in past studies with conflicting results. In 2009, Ma et al. conducted a study of 64 patients with stage IE or IIE early stage ENKTCL. Of these patients, 23 received radiation therapy alone, and 41 received chemoradiation with an anthracycline-based regimen. The 5-year OS rate was 57.9% for those who received radiation therapy alone and 61.5% for those who received chemoradiation ($P = 0.47$). The study concluded that chemoradiation compared to radiation therapy alone did not lead to improved OS. Of note, anthracycline-based regimens have been proven to be inferior to asparaginase-based chemotherapy and represent an important limitation of this study [19].

A more recent study conducted by Su et al. reviewed 248 patients in the United States with localized disease from 2004 to 2014. Chemoradiation was given in 68.9%, and radiation therapy alone was given in 31.1%. After multivariable analysis, chemoradiation was associated with an improved OS compared to radiation therapy alone with a hazard ratio of 0.504. The survival benefit was also apparent in the geriatric subgroup. Based on this and other studies, the preferred approach endorsed by the NCCN is to recommend chemoradiation for patients who are fit to receive chemotherapy [20].

Summary of Treatment Recommendations for Localized Nasal Type

The decision of which regimen to use (concurrent vs. sandwich vs. sequential chemoradiotherapy) can be challenging, and various factors including adherence must be accounted for. The logistics of performing concurrent chemoradiotherapy make this a difficult treatment strategy in some patients with limited transportation. One advantage of the sequential approach is that radiation therapy is often better tolerated, as patients are more likely in a complete response. Ultimate treatment decisions must be made individually. If a patient is deemed not to be fit for chemotherapy, radiation therapy alone is a viable option for localized nasal-type ENKTCL. Treatment options are summarized in Table 10.1.

Conventional Treatment Approach for Extra-Nasal Type ENKTCL

The presence of extra-nasal disease is considered a poor prognostic factor, and patients with this subtype generally have a more difficult course. This impacts treatment recommendations, which tend to favor more aggressive regimens compared to those outlined for localized nasal-type disease. Many past studies that included patients with localized extra-nasal disease were performed before PET/CT imaging. These cases were likely to include patients with nasal primary tumors, so the results are difficult to interpret. There is a definitive association between extra-nasal disease and decreased overall survival [1]. Therefore, for all stages of extra-nasal-type ENKTCL, asparaginase-based systemic chemotherapy is recommended. Radiation therapy may be indicated, depending on the site of disease [6].

Table 10.1 Summary of treatment recommendations [12–16]

Concurrent chemoradiation		
Treatment	Number treated	Survival rates %
Cisplatin 30 mg/m^2 weekly with radiation (40 Gy) followed by [a]VIPD × 3 cycles	30	3 year PFS – 85
		3 year OS – 86
[b]DeVIC chemotherapy × 3 cycles with radiation (50 Gy)	33	2 year OS – 78
Sandwich chemotherapy		
Treatment modality	Number treated	Survival rates
[c]LVP × 2 cycles followed by radiation (56 Gy) then LVP for 2–4 cycles	26	2 year PFS – 80.6
		2 year OS – 88.5
[d]GELOX × 2 cycles followed by radiation (56 Gy) then GELOX × 2–4 cycles	27	2 year PFS and OS – 86%
Sequential chemoradiation		
[e]Modified SMILE × 2–3 cycles followed by radiation (45 Gy)	12	ORR – 92

PFS progression-free survival, *OS* overall survival, *ORR* overall response rate
[a]VIPD: etoposide 100 mg/m^2 days 1–3, ifosfamide 1200 mg/m^2 days 1–3, cisplatin 33 mg/m^2 days 1–3, and dexamethasone 40 mg days 1–4
[b]DeVIC: dexamethasone, 40 mg on days 1–3; etoposide, 67 mg/m^2 IV on days 1–3; ifosfamide, 1.0 g/m^2 on days 1–3; and carboplatin, 200 mg/m^2 IV on day 1
[c]LVP: L-asparaginase 6000 IU/m^2 IV on days 1–5, vincristine 1.4 mg/m^2 IV on day 1, and prednisone 100 mg given orally on days 1–5. Repeated every 3 weeks
[d]GELOX: gemcitabine 1000 mg/m^2 IV on days 1 and 8, oxaliplatin 130 mg/m^2 IV on day 1, and L-asparaginase 6000 IU/m^2 daily IV days 1–7 every 21 days. For those receiving pegasparaginase, the modified regimen was gemcitabine 1250 mg/m^2 IV on day 1, oxaliplatin 85 mg/m^2 IV on day 1, and pegaspargase 2500 IU/m^2 daily IM on day 1 repeated every 14 days
[e]Modified SMILE: methotrexate 2000 mg/m^2 day 1, ifosfamide 1500 mg/m^2 days 2–4, etoposide 100 mg/m^2 days 2–4, dexamethasone 40 mg days 2–4, and pegaspargase 2000–2500 units/m^2 day 8

Conventional Treatment Approach for Advanced ENKTCL

For advanced stage disease (stage III/IV nasal type and stage I–IV extra-nasal type), the primary treatment approach is chemotherapy with an asparaginase-based regimen. Anthracycline-based regimens were used in initial studies, with poor overall response rates. ENKTCL cells express high concentrations of P-glycoprotein, which translates to a multidrug- resistant phenotype [21]. P-glycoprotein is an ATP-dependent efflux pump that exports anticancer agents outside lymphoma cells. This inherent quality of ENKTCL accounts for the disappointing results seen with cyclophosphamide, doxorubicin, vincristine, and prednisone (CHOP) and other anthracycline-based regimens [21].

Several studies have demonstrated the efficacy of asparaginase-based chemotherapy regimens for advanced/relapsed/refractory ENKTCL. In a phase II trial using SMILE chemotherapy in 38 patients with advanced nasal-type disease, 20 were newly diagnosed stage IV, 14 were in their first relapse, and 4 patients had refractory disease. Two cycles were planned, and thereafter study participants could receive further cycles and/or stem cell transplant if recommended by the treating oncologist. Granulocyte colony stimulating factor was included in the protocol based on the phase I study. After two cycles of therapy, the overall response rate was 79%, and the complete remission rate was 45%. A total of 28 patients completed the treatment protocol, and 21 then received a stem cell transplant (4 autologous 17 allogeneic). The 1-year overall survival rate was 55%. Notably, 92% of patients had grade 4 neutropenia, and 61% of patients had infectious complications [22].

In addition to SMILE chemotherapy, other frontline regimens for advanced stage ENKTCL include AspaMetDex (L-asparaginase, methotrexate, and dexamethasone) and P-GEMOX (gemcitabine, pegaspargase, and oxaliplatin). The AspaMetDex regimen was investigated in a phase II prospective study of 19 patients with refractory or relapsed nasal-type ENKTCL. Study participants received three cycles of the 21-day regimen. Objective responses were observed in 73% of patients, and 61% achieved complete remission. The median response duration was 1 year. The most frequent toxicities were cytopenias, abnormal liver function tests, and allergic reactions [23].

The P-GEMOX regimen was investigated in a retrospective study by Wang et al. [20]. Among a cohort of 117 patients, 96 had newly diagnosed disease, and 21 had refractory/relapsed disease. Patients received 2–8 cycles of therapy. The overall response rate was 88.8%, and the 3-year overall survival rate was 72.7%. The most common toxicities were cytopenias, elevated liver function test, and hypertriglyceridemia. Overall, the regimen was tolerated well [16].

Role of Stem Cell Transplantation for Treatment of Advanced ENKTCL

For advanced stage disease, frontline chemotherapy regimen options include SMILE, AspaMetDex, and P-GEMOX. These three regimens have similar overall response rates and toxicity profiles. If patients achieve a complete remission with frontline treatment, stem cell transplantation should be considered. There are no definitive data to guide whether autologous or allogeneic stem cell transplantation should be pursued; decisions must be made individually. If patients only achieve a partial response to chemotherapy, biopsy should be repeated. If negative, stem cell transplantation may be pursued. When patients have a poor response to first-line treatment or if a repeat biopsy is positive, several second-line options may be investigated, including clinical trials. These options for refractory and relapsed disease will be discussed in detail in Sect. II.

Prognosis

The prognosis for all stages of ENKTCL has significantly improved with the use of asparaginase-based chemotherapy. Former scoring systems reflected the prognosis

Table 10.2 Prognostic index of PINK [21]

PINK score risk factors	*3-year overall survival rate*
Age > 60 years	Low – no risk factors – 81%
Stage III/IV	Intermediate – 1 risk factor – 62%
Distant lymph node involvement	High – 2 or more risk factors – 25%
Non-nasal disease	
PINK-E risk factors	*3-year overall survival rate*
All of the above and	Low – zero or 1 risk factor – 81%
EBV DNA	Intermediate – 2 risk factors – 55%
	High – 3 or more risk factors – 28%

for patients treated with inferior anthracycline-based regimens. In recent years, a new prognostic index has been developed to more accurately predict patient outcomes.

Kim et al. retrospectively reviewed 527 newly diagnosed patients who received non-anthracycline-based treatments, with the goal of developing a prognostic scoring system. Four factors (age over 60, stage III/IV disease, distant lymph node involvement, and non-nasal disease) correlated with overall and progression-free survival. These factors were used to develop the prognostic index of natural killer lymphoma (PINK) and are shown in Table 10.2. Patients are grouped into one of the three following groups: low-risk disease with no risk factors, intermediate-risk with one risk factor, or high-risk with two or more risk factors. The 3-year overall survival rates for these groups were 81%, 62%, and 25%, respectively [24].

In this study, having a detectable EBV titer was also found to be a prognostic factor for overall survival. The PINK-E model incorporates detectable EBV titer along with the other four risk factors. Patients are divided into three groups: low-risk with one risk factor, intermediate-risk with two risk factors, and high-risk with three or more risk factors. Both models have been validated and are endorsed by the National Comprehensive Cancer Network guidelines. In the future, as therapy options increase and novel agents are introduced, these prognostic models may influence treatment algorithms [24].

Novel Treatment Options for Advanced Disease

For the management of advanced ENKTCL, asparaginase-based chemotherapy is the recommended frontline therapy. Novel agents are currently being investigated in the relapsed and refractory setting with promising results. These therapies include immunotherapy, Janus-associated kinase (JAK) inhibitors, monoclonal antibodies, pan-class I phosphoinositide 3-kinase (PI3K) inhibitors, and histone deacetylase inhibitors. Given the rarity of ENKTCL and lack of a standard efficacious treatment regimen for those with relapsed or refractory disease, all patients should be evaluated for clinical trials. In this section, novel agents and ongoing clinical trials will be reviewed. A proposed algorithm for management of ENKTCL in both the frontline and relapsed/refractory section will conclude the chapter.

Immunotherapy

Immunotherapy enhances the immune system to fight cancer. Targeted therapies such as checkpoint inhibitors of the programmed death ligand 1 (PDL1) and chimeric antigen receptor T (CART)-cell therapy are two forms of immunotherapy under active investigation for ENKTCL. PDL1 binds to the PD1 receptor on T cells which provides a mechanism for ENKTCL to evade T-cell targeting. ENKTCL expresses PDL1 in 50–80% of tumor cells and infiltrating immune cells, while expression of PD1 is less robust [25, 26]. ENKTCL is characterized by EBV infection, and chronic EBV infection suppresses T-cell cytotoxicity by upregulating PDL1 [27]. Pembrolizumab, a PDL1 inhibitor, which is approved for many solid and hematologic malignancies, is considered an attractive treatment strategy for ENKTCL.

A retrospective study of seven patients who received pembrolizumab after disease progression on asparaginase-based regimen was recently published [28]. Pembrolizumab was given at 2 mg/kg every 3 weeks. All patients were male with a median age of 49 years. The majority of patients (six out of seven) had stage IV disease prior to receiving pembrolizumab. Two of the seven patients had received allogeneic stem cell transplant. Clinical, radiographic, morphologic, and molecular parameters were followed to assess response. All patients had an objective response, and five patients remained in a complete remission after a median follow-up of 6 months. Pembrolizumab was well tolerated. PDL1 expression was found to correlate with treatment responses [28].

Researchers at the Mayo Clinic are currently recruiting patients for a phase II study investigating the efficacy of nivolumab for patients with relapsed or refractory disease. Nivolumab will be given every 14 days for up to eight cycles. Patients who respond will continue therapy every 28 days for up to 24 cycles. The primary outcome measure is the proportion of complete or partial responses assessed according to the revised Lugano Classification Response Criteria (ClinicalTrials.gov Identifier: NCT03075553). Another area of active investigation includes cellular immunotherapy. A phase II trial is underway to evaluate the efficacy of autologous EBV-specific T cells in relapsed/refractory ENKTCL (ClinicalTrials.gov Identifier: NCT01948180).

JAK Inhibitors

As previously detailed in Sect. I, the JAK/STAT pathway is an active oncogenic pathway in ENKTCL. Approximately 35% of all ENKTCL patients have somatic mutations in the JAK3 gene which lead to constitutive activity of the JAK/STAT pathway. Currently, several centers are recruiting patients for a phase II study of ruxolitinib, a JAK inhibitor, in those with relapsed or refractory T- or NK-cell lymphoma. Patients will receive ruxolitinib at a dose of 20 mg twice daily for 28-day cycles. The primary outcome measure is objective response rate (ClinicalTrials.gov Identifier: NCT02974647).

Monoclonal Antibodies

CD38 is a transmembrane protein with expression in several hematologic malignancies. The clinical data of 94 patients with ENKTCL was reviewed by Wang et al., and showed that 95% of patients expressed CD38, but half ($n = 47$) had strong expression of CD38. Further strong expression of CD38 was an independent adverse prognostic feature [29]. In 2016, Hari et al. published a case report using daratumumab, a monoclonal antibody which induces apoptosis of CD38 expressing cells, in a patient with refractory ENKTCL [29]. The case report described a 56-year-old female with relapsed advanced stage ENKTCL who was treated with SMILE chemotherapy. After completing chemotherapy, she went on to receive an allogeneic stem cell transplantation but relapsed within 1 month. Five months following transplant, she was noted to have persistent disease with positive plasma PCR for EBV DNA and received single agent daratumumab at a dose of 16 mg/kg given on a weekly basis. EBV DNA titers increased by a factor of ten during the first 4 weeks of daratumumab treatment, but PCR became undetectable by week 6. She achieved a complete clinical, molecular, and radiographic remission which was sustained at 21-week follow-up. This case report has prompted clinical trials investigating the role of monoclonal antibodies in ENKTCL [27].

PI3K Inhibitors

Latent membrane protein (LMP) 1 is an oncoprotein essential for EBV-driven lymphomas and leads to the activation of signaling pathways which include nuclear factor kB and phosphoinositide 3-kinase (PI3K) [30]. PI3K inhibitors such as copanlisib are currently being studied in relapsed/refractory ENKTCL [31]. Copanlisib is FDA approved for patients with relapsed follicular lymphoma who have failed two prior lines of systemic therapy. It has great promise for a wide range of malignancies from ENKTCL to stage IV cholangiocarcinoma. A phase I/II multicenter study incorporating PI3K inhibitors into the treatment for relapsed/refractory ENKTCL is expected to start recruiting in the near future. Patients will receive copanlisib in combination with gemcitabine. The primary outcome measures are to determine the maximum tolerated dose, dose-limiting toxicities, and the objective response rate.

Histone Deacetylase Inhibitors

In 2017, Zhou et al. investigated chidamide, an oral histone deacetylase inhibitor, in ENKTCL cell lines. Two cell lines were exposed to varying concentrations of chidamide, and proteins involved in multiple signaling pathways were measured using Western blot. Chidamide was found to suppress cell proliferation in a dose- and time-dependent manner. PCR was also employed to measure expression of EBV genes. Chidamide induced expression of lytic phase EBV genes. This novel agent had various antitumor effects via multiple signaling pathways [32].

Histone deacetylase inhibitors are being investigated in multiple phase I and II clinical trials. For instance, a phase II trial investigating panobinostat is underway for patients with relapsed or refractory non-Hodgkin lymphoma. Another promising study is the multicenter phase II trial of panobinostat and bortezomib in patients with relapsed/refractory peripheral T-cell lymphoma or ENKTCL (ClinicalTrials.gov Identifier: NCT00901147).

Summary of Treatment Approach

The management of ENKTCL is evolving with many promising novel agents currently under investigation in clinical trials. Frontline management is dependent on stage and subtype. Figure 10.2a, b provides a summary of the standard treatment

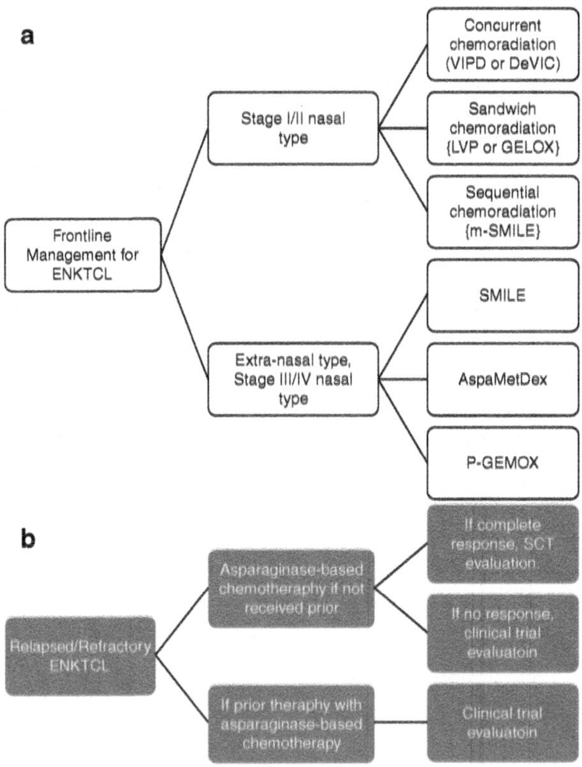

Fig. 10.2 (**a**) Treatment algorithm for localized, advanced, and extra-nasal ENKTCL. *VIPD* etoposide, ifosfamide, cisplatin, and dexamethasone; *DeVIC* dexamethasone, etoposide, ifosfamide, and carboplatin; *LVP* asparaginase, vincristine, and prednisone; *GELOX* gemcitabine, oxaliplatin, and L-asparaginase; *SMILE* methotrexate, ifosfamide, etoposide, dexamethasone, and pegasparaginase; *AspaMetDex* L-asparaginase, methotrexate, and dexamethasone; *P-GEMOX* pegasparaginase, gemcitabine, and oxaliplatin. (**b**) Treatment algorithm for relapsed/refractory ENKTCL. *CR* complete response, *SCT* stem cell transplant

approach. The role of autologous and allogeneic stem cell transplantation remains controversial. In general, if patients with advanced disease achieve a complete remission with frontline chemotherapy, stem cell transplantation should be considered. In the relapsed and refractory setting, patients should be evaluated for clinical trials. Current therapies being investigated include immunotherapy, JAK inhibitors, immunomodulators, PI3K inhibitors, and histone deacetylase inhibitors.

References

1. Tse E, Kwong YL. How I treat NK/T-cell lymphomas. Blood. 2013;121(25):4997–5005.
2. Haverkos BM, et al. Extranodal NK/T cell lymphoma, nasal type (ENKTL-NT): an update on epidemiology, clinical presentation, and natural history in North American and European cases. Curr Hematol Malig Rep. 2016;11(6):514–27.
3. Tse E, Kwong YL. The diagnosis and management of NK/T-cell lymphomas. J Hematol Oncol. 2017;10(1):85.
4. Au WY, et al. Clinical differences between nasal and extranasal natural killer/T-cell lymphoma: a study of 136 cases from the International Peripheral T-Cell Lymphoma Project. Blood. 2009;113(17):3931–7.
5. Mansoor A, et al. NK-cell enteropathy: a benign NK-cell lymphoproliferative disease mimicking intestinal lymphoma: clinicopathologic features and follow-up in a unique case series. Blood. 2011;117(5):1447–52.
6. Horwitz SM, et al. NCCN guidelines insights: T-cell lymphomas, version 2.2018. J Natl Compr Cancer Netw. 2018;16(2):123–35.
7. Koo GC, et al. Janus kinase 3-activating mutations identified in natural killer/T-cell lymphoma. Cancer Discov. 2012;2(7):591–7.
8. Liang L, et al. The genetic deletion of 6q21 and PRDM1 and clinical implications in extranodal NK/T cell lymphoma, nasal type. Biomed Res Int. 2015;2015:435423.
9. Moon SH, et al. The role of 18F-FDG PET/CT for initial staging of nasal type natural killer/T-cell lymphoma: a comparison with conventional staging methods. J Nucl Med. 2013;54(7):1039–44.
10. Suzuki R, et al. Prospective measurement of Epstein-Barr virus-DNA in plasma and peripheral blood mononuclear cells of extranodal NK/T-cell lymphoma, nasal type. Blood. 2011;118(23):6018–22.
11. Kim SJ, et al. Phase II trial of concurrent radiation and weekly cisplatin followed by VIPD chemotherapy in newly diagnosed, stage IE to IIE, nasal, extranodal NK/T-Cell Lymphoma: Consortium for Improving Survival of Lymphoma study. J Clin Oncol. 2009;27(35):6027–32.
12. Yamaguchi M, et al. Phase I/II study of concurrent chemoradiotherapy for localized nasal natural killer/T-cell lymphoma: Japan Clinical Oncology Group Study JCOG0211. J Clin Oncol. 2009;27(33):5594–600.
13. Jiang M, et al. Phase 2 trial of "sandwich" L-asparaginase, vincristine, and prednisone chemotherapy with radiotherapy in newly diagnosed, stage IE to IIE, nasal type, extranodal natural killer/T-cell lymphoma. Cancer. 2012;118(13):3294–301.
14. Wang L, et al. First-line combination of gemcitabine, oxaliplatin, and L-asparaginase (GELOX) followed by involved-field radiation therapy for patients with stage IE/IIE extranodal natural killer/T-cell lymphoma. Cancer. 2013;119(2):348–55.
15. Lunning M, et al. Modified SMILE (mSMILE) is active in the treatment of extranodal natural killer/T-cell lymphoma: a single center US experience. Clin Lymphoma Myeloma Leuk. 2014;14:S143–4.
16. Wang JH, et al. Analysis of the efficacy and safety of a combined gemcitabine, oxaliplatin and pegaspargase regimen for NK/T-cell lymphoma. Oncotarget. 2016;7(23):35412–22.

17. Wang H, et al. Mild toxicity and favorable prognosis of high-dose and extended involved-field intensity-modulated radiotherapy for patients with early-stage nasal NK/T-cell lymphoma. Int J Radiat Oncol Biol Phys. 2012;82(3):1115–21.
18. Tomita N, et al. A comparison of radiation treatment plans using IMRT with helical tomotherapy and 3D conformal radiotherapy for nasal natural killer/T-cell lymphoma. Br J Radiol. 2009;82(981):756–63.
19. Ma H-H, et al. Treatment outcome of radiotherapy alone versus radiochemotherapy in early stage nasal natural killer/T-cell lymphoma. Med Oncol. 2010;27(3):798–806.
20. Su C, et al. Comparison of chemoradiotherapy with radiotherapy alone for early-stage extranodal natural killer/T-cell lymphoma, nasal type in elderly patients. Leuk Lymphoma. 2018;59(6):1406–12.
21. Suzuki R. Pathogenesis and treatment of extranodal natural killer/T-cell lymphoma. Semin Hematol. 2014;51(1):42–51.
22. Yamaguchi M, et al. Phase II study of SMILE chemotherapy for newly diagnosed stage IV, relapsed, or refractory extranodal natural killer (NK)/T-cell lymphoma, nasal type: the NK-Cell Tumor Study Group study. J Clin Oncol. 2011;29(33):4410–6.
23. Jaccard A, et al. Efficacy of L-asparaginase with methotrexate and dexamethasone (AspaMetDex regimen) in patients with refractory or relapsing extranodal NK/T-cell lymphoma, a phase 2 study. Blood. 2011;117(6):1834–9.
24. Kim SJ, et al. A prognostic index for natural killer cell lymphoma after non-anthracycline-based treatment: a multicentre, retrospective analysis. Lancet Oncol. 2016;17(3):389–400.
25. Chen BJ, et al. PD-L1 expression is characteristic of a subset of aggressive B-cell lymphomas and virus-associated malignancies. Clin Cancer Res. 2013;19(13):3462–73.
26. Jo JC, et al. Expression of programmed cell death 1 and programmed cell death ligand 1 in extranodal NK/T-cell lymphoma, nasal type. Ann Hematol. 2017;96(1):25–31.
27. Kim WY, et al. Expression of programmed cell death ligand 1 (PD-L1) in advanced stage EBV-associated extranodal NK/T cell lymphoma is associated with better prognosis. Virchows Arch. 2016;469(5):581–90.
28. Kwong YL, et al. PD1 blockade with pembrolizumab is highly effective in relapsed or refractory NK/T-cell lymphoma failing l-asparaginase. Blood. 2017;129(17):2437–42.
29. Wang L, et al. CD38 expression predicts poor prognosis and might be a potential therapy target in extranodal NK/T cell lymphoma, nasal type. Ann Hematol. 2015;94(8):1381–8.
30. Sun L, et al. LMP-1 induces survivin expression to inhibit cell apoptosis through the NF-kappaB and PI3K/Akt signaling pathways in nasal NK/T-cell lymphoma. Oncol Rep. 2015;33(5):2253–60.
31. Markham A. Copanlisib: first global approval. Drugs. 2017;77(18):2057–62.
32. Zhou J, et al. Histone deacetylase inhibitor chidamide induces growth inhibition and apoptosis in NK/T lymphoma cells through ATM-Chk2-p53-p21 signalling pathway. Invest New Drugs. 2018;36(4):571–80.

Chapter 11
Anaplastic Large Cell Lymphoma

Austin Kim and Eric Jacobsen

Introduction/Epidemiology

Peripheral T-cell lymphomas (PTCLs) make up around 10–15% of all adult non-Hodgkin lymphomas (NHL) and, in most circumstances, have a worse prognosis than B-cell NHL. Primary systemic anaplastic large cell lymphoma (ALCL) is the second most common PTCL subset in North America and comprises about 2% of all adult non-Hodgkin lymphomas (NHL) [1]. ALCL has a bimodal peak in age at presentation with an initial peak in the childhood/adolescent years and a second peak around the age of 60. It has a male predominance with a male to female ratio as high as 3:1 in young patients [2].

The four distinct subsets of ALCL include anaplastic lymphoma kinase-positive (ALK-positive) ALCL, anaplastic lymphoma kinase-negative (ALK-negative) ALCL, breast implant-associated ALCL, and primary cutaneous ALCL. This chapter will only focus on primary systemic ALK-positive and ALK-negative ALCL. The *ALK* gene is located on chromosome 2p23, and ALK-positive ALCL is most commonly associated with a t(2;5)(p23;q35) chromosome translocation causing the *ALK* gene on chromosome 2 to fuse with the *NPM* (nucleophosmin) gene on chromosome 5 although other partner translocations do occur. The NPM-ALK fusion gene encodes the NPM-ALK hybrid protein thought to play a key role in lymphomagenesis [3].

A. Kim (✉) · E. Jacobsen
Harvard Medical School, Dana-Farber Cancer Institute, Boston, MA, USA
e-mail: austini_kim@dfci.harvard.edu; edjacobsen@partners.org

C. Dittus (ed.), *Novel Therapeutics for Rare Lymphomas*,
https://doi.org/10.1007/978-3-030-25610-4_11

Clinical Presentation

Systemic ALCL presents similarly to other aggressive lymphomas with rapidly progressive lymphadenopathy and "B" symptoms: fevers, drenching night sweats, and unintentional weight loss in almost 60% of patients. Nearly two-thirds of patients present with advanced stage disease and/or extranodal involvement of the bone, skin, liver, bone marrow, and lung. The overall risk of central nervous system involvement is 2–6% [4]; however ALK-positive ALCL patients with >1 extranodal site of involvement have been reported to have a higher cumulative risk of 17% at 1 year [5]. ALK-positive ALCL constitutes approximately 50% of cases and is more common in young patients than ALK-negative ALCL (median age at diagnosis 34 versus 58) [6].

Diagnosis, Staging, and Workup

Excisional or incisional biopsy of a lymph node or affected tissue is preferred to establish the diagnosis of ALCL. Core needle biopsy should only be used if an incisional/excisional biopsy is contraindicated. Fine-needle aspirate is inadequate to make the diagnosis. Classically, ALCL histology shows "hallmark cells," large cells with eccentric, horseshoe-shaped nuclei with prominent nucleoli and a prominent pale cytoplasm with paranuclear hof (Fig. 11.1). Mature T-cell markers such as CD3, CD4, CD5, and CD7 are variably expressed on ALCL, and it can have a "null" phenotype with no surface T-cell markers. CD30 is universally expressed in ALCL though its function is unclear. ALCL can be confused with Hodgkin lymphoma or primary mediastinal B-cell lymphoma as these entities also have high-level CD30 expression. However, CD15 and Pax5 are commonly expressed in Hodgkin lymphoma but not in ALCL, and CD20 and other B-cell markers are expressed in PMBL but not ALCL. ALK is variably expressed in ALCL but never in Hodgkin lymphoma or PMBL. The lack of clinical or radiologic evidence of systemic involvement and epithelial membrane antigen (EMA) positivity can be helpful in distinguishing systemic ALCL from primary cutaneous ALCL [7]. Pathology should always be reviewed by an experienced hematopathologist.

ALK-positive ALCL has a rearrangement of the *ALK* gene that can be reliably detected by FISH or cytogenetics, but positive staining for ALK is sufficient to make the diagnosis. ALK-negative ALCL lacks ALK protein expression and does not have a rearrangement of the *ALK* gene [8]. However, in the updated 2016 WHO classification of lymphoid neoplasms, up to 30% of ALK-negative ALCL have t(6;7)(p25.3;q32.3), *DUSP22-IRF4* rearrangement, and 8% have rearrangements in *TP63* that are mutually exclusive with *DUSP22* rearrangements [9]. Staging and workup of ALCL is similar to other lymphomas and includes either PET/CT scan

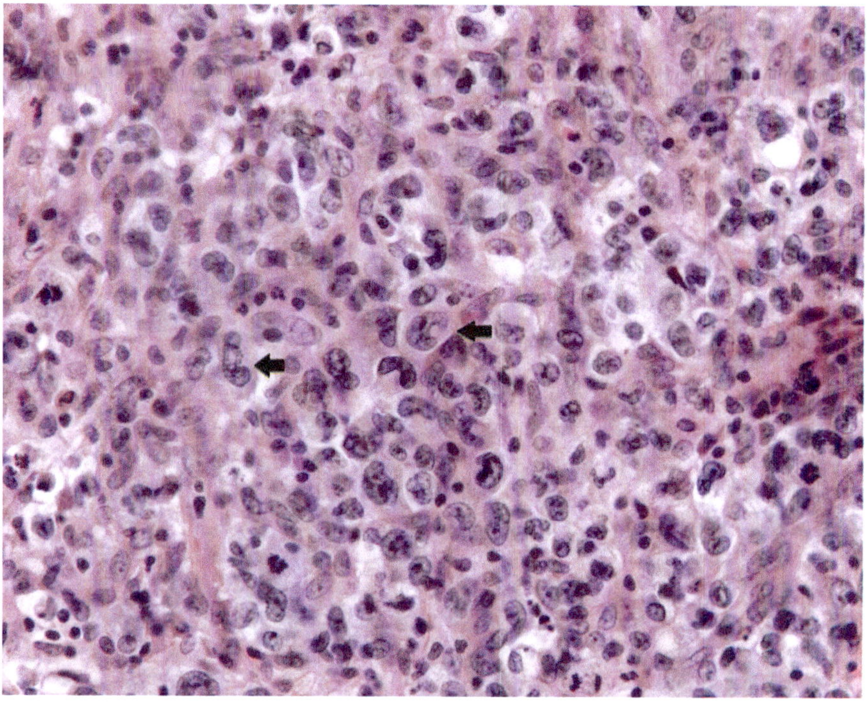

Fig. 11.1 Anaplastic large cell lymphoma, classical variant. Large, anaplastic lymphoma cells with prominent nucleoli are seen in cohesive clusters. Characteristic "hallmark cells" with horseshoe-shaped nuclei and perinuclear hof are present (arrows). Hematoxylin and eosin, 50× magnification. (Photo credit: Elizabeth A. Morgan, MD., Brigham and Women's Hospital. Assistant Professor, Harvard Medical School)

(preferred) without bone marrow biopsy or neck/chest/abdomen/pelvis CT with contrast and bone marrow aspiration and biopsy.

Prognosis and Conventional Treatment Approach

The International Prognostic Index (IPI) score is one of the main prognostic indicators despite the recent development of T-cell lymphoma-specific prognostic indices. In ALCL, an IPI ≥ 3 is associated with shorter overall survival [10]. ALK status of the tumor is the other important prognostic factor in ALCL with ALK-positive ALCL having an improved overall survival compared to ALK-negative ALCL. The International Peripheral T-cell Lymphoma (IPTL) project, the largest retrospective analysis of peripheral T-cell lymphomas, showed a 70% 5-year overall survival in

ALK-positive ALCL compared to 49% 5-year overall survival in ALK-negative ALCL, although patients with ALK+ ALCL and an IPI ≥ 3 had an inferior prognosis [1]. There are also data to suggest that the improved outcome in ALK-positive ALCL is limited to patients under the age of 40 with beta-2-microglobulin <3 [11]. *DUSP22-IRF4* rearrangement, t(6;7)(p25.3;q32.3), involving the DUSP22 gene and the FRA7H fragile site, is associated with a favorable prognosis in ALK-negative ALCL, similar to outcomes seen in ALK-positive ALCL. However, *TP63* rearrangement on 3q28 in ALK-negative ALCL is associated with an inferior prognosis, with a 5-year overall survival rate of 17% [12].

For decades, standard first-line therapy for ALCL included an anthracycline-based combination chemotherapy regimen, CHOP (cyclophosphamide, doxorubicin, vincristine, prednisone) with or without etoposide (CHOEP). In general, patients ≤60 years old benefited from CHOEP, whereas patients >60 years old received CHOP induction therapy based on retrospective data from the German and Swedish study groups showing improved event-free survival (EFS) and PFS in patients under the age of 60 receiving CHOEP compared to CHOP [13, 14]. However, recently published data from the ECHELON-2 trial, a randomized phase III study in untreated CD30-positive peripheral T-cell lymphomas comparing brentuximab vedotin (BV), an antibody-drug conjugate of an anti-CD30 monoclonal antibody linked to the anti-microtubule agent monomethyl auristatin E (MMAE), and cyclophosphamide, doxorubicin, and prednisone (CHP) to CHOP, suggests that BV + CHP should be the new standard frontline therapy in both ALK-positive and ALK-negative ALCL [15]. The primary endpoint of the study, median PFS, was met with 48.2 months in the BV + CHP arm versus 20.8 months in the CHOP arm. Overall survival was improved in the BV + CHP arm compared to CHOP with a hazard ratio (HR) 0.66, $p = 0.024$. Based on these data, BV + CHP was FDA approved in November 2018 for previously untreated systemic ALCL and other CD30-expressing peripheral T-cell lymphomas.

Radiation therapy (RT) can be considered for patients with early stage (stage I/II) ALCL, preferably in combination with chemotherapy. Three or four cycles of BV + CHP followed by RT are acceptable in patients who cannot tolerate six cycles of chemotherapy. However, abbreviated chemotherapy followed by RT cannot be recommended for all early stage ALCL. Six cycles of BV + CHP are recommended for most early stage ALCL patients. Patients with early stage ALCL who achieve a partial response (PR) after chemotherapy and patients with advanced stage ALCL with localized residual disease who are not transplant candidates can also be considered for consolidation with RT. Consolidative RT following six cycles of chemotherapy is not recommended due to lack of evidence showing PFS or OS benefit.

Consolidation with high-dose chemotherapy and autologous stem cell transplant (HDT/ASCT) in first complete remission (CR1) is considered for patients with a high risk of relapse, generally ALK-positive patients >40 years old with an IPI score ≥ 3 and most ALK-negative patients, particularly those with IPI score ≥ 2 [10]. Patients with relapsed or refractory ALCL generally receive second-line salvage therapy. Patients who attain a complete remission and are candidates for stem cell transplantation should be considered for autologous SCT (if not performed in CR1) or allogeneic SCT (if the patient had a prior autoSCT).

Novel Agents in the Relapsed Setting

The only novel agent that is approved by the US FDA specifically for the treatment of relapsed/refractory ALCL is brentuximab vedotin (BV), based on the pivotal phase II multicenter trial of BV in relapsed/refractory ALCL. Single-agent BV had an overall response rate (ORR) of 86% with a 57% complete response (CR) rate [16]. After 5 years of follow-up, 14% of patients treated with BV alone for up to 1 year remained in a sustained remission without ASCT or subsequent anticancer therapy [17]. The main toxicities of BV include neutropenia, peripheral sensory neuropathy, thrombocytopenia, and anemia. The combination of a high response rate, favorable toxicity profile, and ease of outpatient administration has led BV to be the preferred second-line therapy in ALCL. Despite this excellent efficacy, the role for BV in the second-line setting will now change as it is used more frequently in the frontline setting.

The ALK inhibitors, crizotinib and ceritinib, are approved by the US FDA for the treatment of ALK-positive metastatic non-small cell lung cancers (NSCLC). Therefore, there has been interest in using these agents in the treatment of other ALK-positive tumors, such as ALCL. Crizotinib was the first ALK inhibitor available for clinical use and is an oral small-molecule tyrosine kinase inhibitor of ALK, MET, and ROS1. Nine out of nine patients with ALK-positive ALCL who had failed at least one previous line of combination chemotherapy obtained a CR with single-agent crizotinib. Two-year progression-free survival (PFS) was 63.7%, and 2-year overall survival (OS) was 72.7%. Two of the ALK-positive ALCL patients who relapsed while on crizotinib had their tumors evaluated in vitro and were found to have mutations in the *NPM/ALK* kinase domain that were thought to confer resistance to crizotinib [18]. Caution must be used when interrupting crizotinib therapy for ALK-positive ALCL; there are reports of abrupt relapse within 3 weeks of discontinuing crizotinib in ALK-positive ALCL patients in CR for over 3 years on crizotinib [19].

Ceritinib is a second-generation ALK inhibitor that is approximately 20 times more potent than crizotinib in vitro and is active in ALK-positive NSCLC patients who progressed on crizotinib. The ASCEND-1 trial included three patients with relapsed ALK-positive ALCL. Two out of the three patients achieved CR, while the third patient achieved a partial response (PR) with 95% reduction in maximal tumor volume. All three patients had durable responses ranging between ≥20 and ≥26 months [20].

Pralatrexate, romidepsin, and belinostat are all approved by the US FDA for relapsed/refractory peripheral T-cell lymphoma (PTCL), including ALCL. Pralatrexate is an antifolate analog that is actively transported into malignant cells by RFC-1 and decreases intracellular concentrations of thymidylate and purines, leading to errors in DNA replication and apoptosis. The international phase II PDX-008 study in 109 patients with relapsed/refractory PTCL, of which 17 patients had ALCL, showed a 27% ORR and 9% CR or CR, unconfirmed rate [21]. The primary side effects of pralatrexate were mucositis and thrombocytopenia. Romidepsin is a histone deacetylase inhibitor (HDAC) that induces acetylation of histones and other proteins, resulting in antitumor activity by growth arrest, cellular differentiation, and apoptosis. The international phase II trial of romidepsin leading to US FDA approval in 2011 in relapsed/refractory PTCL included 130 patients, 22 patients with ALCL, and ORR was 25% with CR rate 15% [22]. A single institution, phase I trial of pralatrexate in combination with romidepsin showed an ORR 71% and CR rate 29% in 14 patients with relapsed/refractory PTCL, of which 3 patients had ALK-negative ALCL [23]. However, this combination is not recommended outside of a clinical trial.

Belinostat is another HDAC inhibitor thought to inhibit all zinc-dependent HDAC enzymes. The international phase II (BELIEF) trial of belinostat in 120 patients with relapsed/refractory PTCL included 15 patients with ALCL, and showed a 26% ORR and 11% CR rate [24]. Results from this study led to the US FDA approval in 2014 for belinostat in relapsed/refractory PTCL. Bendamustine is a nitrogen mustard alkylating agent commonly used in frontline therapy for indolent B-cell non-Hodgkin lymphomas. Bendamustine was studied in a phase II trial (BENTLY trial) in relapsed/refractory PTCL and found to have an ORR 50% though responses were short-lived [25].

Ongoing Clinical Trials

The combination of ceritinib and BV is in a phase I/II trial for frontline treatment of ALK-positive ALCL [26]. Lenalidomide is an immunomodulatory agent and thalidomide analog that is FDA approved for use in multiple myeloma, myelodysplastic syndrome with deletion 5q, and relapsed/refractory mantle cell lymphoma. Lenalidomide in addition to the HDAC inhibitor romidepsin is in a phase II trial for previously untreated PTCL, including ALCL [27].

There are more ongoing clinical trials in the relapsed/refractory setting for ALCL with novel agents that have different mechanisms of action from those mentioned previously. Duvelisib is a dual phosphoinositide-3-kinase (PI3K)-δ and PI3K-γ inhibitor. PI3K-δ and PI3K-γ are necessary for adaptive and innate immunity and thus play an important role in hematologic malignancies. PI3K-γ is particularly important in T-cell proliferation and development. Single-agent duvelisib had a response rate of 50% in a phase I/II trial [28]. A larger phase II study of duvelisib in relapsed/refractory PTCL is planned. A second PI3K-δγ inhibitor, tenalisib, has also shown encouraging activity in a small number of patients in a phase I/II trial

[29]. Additionally, duvelisib in combination with romidepsin or bortezomib is currently in a phase I/II trial for relapsed/refractory PTCL [30]. Bortezomib is a small-molecule proteasome inhibitor that has limited single-agent activity in PTCL but may provide synergy with other agents.

Onalespib (AT13387) is a small-molecule inhibitor of HSP90 (heat shock protein 90), a molecular chaperone participating within multifactor complexes to stabilize client proteins and prevent ubiquitination and proteasomal degradation. Inhibition of HSP90 results in dissociation of the client proteins from the chaperone complex resulting in proteasomal degradation [31]. Onalespib is currently in a phase II trial for transplant-ineligible patients with relapsed ALK-positive ALCL following progression on BV [32].

Ruxolitinib is an oral Janus-associated kinase (JAK) inhibitor that is currently approved by the FDA for myelofibrosis and polycythemia vera. JAK1 and JAK2 mediate signaling of cytokines responsible for hematopoiesis and immune function. JAK1 and JAK3 mediate signaling of signal transducers and activators of transcription (STAT) to cytokine receptors that leads to modulation of gene expression and survival of T- or NK-cell lymphomas, among other tumors. Increased signaling through the JAK/STAT pathway is common in PTCL, particularly ALCL, and can occur with or without defined mutations in the pathway. In fact, intact signaling through this pathway is necessary for lymphomagenesis even in the presence of JAK/STAT mutations. Ruxolitinib monotherapy is in a multicenter phase II trial for relapsed/refractory T-cell or NK-cell lymphomas, and the pan-JAK inhibitor tofacitinib may also be active [33]. SYK, though not typically expressed in normal T cells, is expressed in >90% of PTCL and is important in TCR signaling. A phase II trial of the SYK inhibitor fostamatinib in PTCL was stopped early when 0 of the first 17 patients responded. The SYK/JAK/TYK2 inhibitor cerdulatinib has shown promising early phase activity in PTCL though the full activity of this agent and its relative efficacy compared to JAK inhibitors alone remains to be defined [34].

Immunotherapy with checkpoint inhibitors, monoclonal antibodies binding to the programmed cell death-1 (PD-1) receptor or programmed death ligand 1 (PD-L1) to restore antitumor T-cell function, has been FDA approved for treatment of several solid tumor subtypes as well as relapsed classical Hodgkin lymphoma. The anti-PD-L1 antibody, avelumab, and anti-PD-1 antibodies, nivolumab, pembrolizumab, and durvalumab, are all being studied as monotherapy in phase II trials to evaluate response rates in relapsed or refractory PTCL [35–37]. These checkpoint inhibitors are also being combined with other agents with the hope of improving efficacy and response rates. For example, the anti-PD-1 antibody, pembrolizumab, will be combined with the antifolate analog, pralatrexate, and a hypomethylating agent, decitabine, in relapsed/refractory PTCL [38]. However, preclinical data suggests that PD-1 may be a haploinsufficient tumor suppressor in PTCL, and therefore PD-1 inhibitors may worsen PTCL as evidence by case reports of explosive disease in adult T-cell leukemia/lymphoma (ATLL) patients treated with the PD-1 inhibitor nivolumab [39, 40].

Promising Early Phase/Preclinical Agents

ALRN-6924 is a stapled peptide that reactivates p53-mediated tumor suppression by inhibiting the two primary p53 suppressor proteins murine double minute 2 (MDM2) and murine double minute X (MDMX). Preclinical data of ALRN-6924 showed tumor growth suppression, p53-dependent cell cycle arrest, and apoptosis in an MDMX-/MDM2-overexpressing wild-type p53 xenograft model and is currently in a multicenter phase II trial for relapsed/refractory PTCL [41].

ADCT-301 (camidanlumab tesirine) is an antibody-drug conjugate (ADC) comprised of an anti-CD25 monoclonal antibody conjugated to a pyrrolobenzodiazepine (PBD) dimer toxin. CD25 is a protein expressed primarily on activated T cells, forming part of the IL-2 receptor complex that conveys growth and immunological signals from outside into the cell. Once ADCT-301 binds to a CD25-expressing cell, it is internalized, and enzymes release the PBD toxin where it binds in the minor groove of DNA and forms DNA interstrand cross-links that cause cell death. In a phase I study of ADCT-301 that included relapsed/refractory PTCL, ORR was 33% [42].

Recommended Treatment Approach for Frontline and Relapsed Disease

Based on the new ECHELON-2 data, BV + CHP is recommended as frontline therapy for ALK-positive and ALK-negative ALCL. High-risk patients in CR1 following induction chemotherapy should still be considered for consolidation with high-dose chemotherapy and autoSCT. Generally, this includes ALK-positive patients >40 years old with an IPI score ≥ 3 and most ALK-negative patients but particularly those with IPI score > 1.

Patients with relapsed or refractory ALCL generally receive second-line salvage chemotherapy to attain a complete remission in preparation for an autologous SCT if they are transplant-eligible. The preferred second-line salvage regimen has been brentuximab vedotin (BV) due to its high efficacy, outpatient administration, and reasonable side effect profile, but with BV now approved for frontline therapy, other salvage regimens such as GDP (gemcitabine, dexamethasone, cisplatin), DHAP (dexamethasone, high-dose cytarabine, cisplatin), and ICE (ifosfamide, carboplatin, etoposide) will be used more frequently. GDP is our cytotoxic salvage regimen of choice given its outpatient administration, favorable toxicity profile, and similar overall response rate compared to DHAP.

For relapsed/refractory ALCL, patients who are transplant-ineligible due to age and/or comorbidities, BV is still the preferred second-line agent due to the reasons listed above.

Crizotinib is a reasonable second- or third-line option for patients with ALK + ALCL. Ceritinib can be reserved for progression on crizotinib as responses to ceritinib have been seen in ALK-positive non-small cell lung cancer following progression on crizotinib. For ALK-negative ALCL patients who do not respond to BV or GDP, other agents approved for relapsed/refractory PTCL can be used such as pralatrexate, romidepsin, and belinostat. Finally, we reserve allogeneic stem cell transplant for patients who are medically fit and relapse following previous autoSCT, have a partial remission (PR) after second-line therapy, or require several lines of therapy at relapse to achieve CR.

References

1. Vose JM, Armitage J, Weisenburger D. International peripheral T-cell and natural killer/T-cell lymphoma study: pathology findings and clinical outcomes. J Clin Oncol. 2008;26:4124–30.
2. Falini B, Pileri S, Zinzani PL, et al. ALK+ lymphoma: clinico-pathological findings and outcome. Blood. 1999;93(8):2697–706.
3. Amin HM, Lai R. Pathobiology of ALK+ anaplastic large-cell lymphoma. Blood. 2007;110(7):2259–67.
4. Ellin F, Landström J, Jerkeman M, et al. Central nervous system relapse in peripheral T-cell lymphomas: a Swedish Lymphoma Registry study. Blood. 2015;126(1):36–41.
5. Chihara D, Fanale MA, Miranda RN, et al. The risk of central nervous system relapses in patients with peripheral T-cell lymphoma. PLoS One. 2018;13(3):e0191461.
6. Jacobsen E. Anaplastic large-cell lymphoma, T-/null-cell type. Oncologist. 2006;11:831–40.
7. Filippa DA, Ladanyi M, Wollner N, et al. CD30 (Ki-1)-positive malignant lymphomas: clinical, immunophenotypic, histologic, and genetic characteristics and differences with Hodgkin's disease. Blood. 1996;87(7):2906–17.
8. Swerdlow SH, Campo E, Harris NL, et al. World Health Organization classification of tumours of haematopoietic and lymphoid tissues, vol. 2. 4th ed. Geneva: International Agency for Research on Cancer; 2008.
9. Swedlow SH, Campo E, Pileri SA, et al. The 2016 revision of the World Health Organization classification of lymphoid neoplasms. Blood. 2016;127(20):2375–90.
10. Savage KJ, Harris NL, Vose JM, et al. ALK- anaplastic large-cell lymphoma is clinically and immunophenotypically different from both ALK+ ALCL and peripheral T-cell lymphoma, not otherwise specified: report from the International Peripheral T-Cell Lymphoma Project. Blood. 2008;111(12):5496–504.
11. Sibon D, Fournier M, Briere J, et al. Long-term outcome of adults with systemic anaplastic large-cell lymphoma treated within the Groupe d'Etude des Lymphomes de l'Adulte trials. J Clin Oncol. 2012;30(32):3939–46.
12. Parrilla Castellar ER, Jaffe ES, Said JW, et al. ALK-negative anaplastic large cell lymphoma is a genetically heterogeneous disease with widely disparate clinical outcomes. Blood. 2014;124(9):1473–80.
13. Schmitz N, Trümper L, Ziepert M, et al. Treatment and prognosis of mature T-cell and NK-cell lymphoma: an analysis of patients with T-cell lymphoma treated in studies of the German High-Grade Non-Hodgkin Study Group. Blood. 2010;116(18):3418–25.
14. Ellin F, Landström J, Jerkeman M, et al. Real-world data on prognostic factors and treatment in peripheral T-cell lymphomas: a study from the Swedish Lymphoma Registry. Blood. 2014;124(10):1570–7.
15. Horwitz S, O'Connor OA, Pro B, et al. Brentuximab vedotin with chemotherapy for CD30-positive peripheral T-cell lymphoma (ECHELON-2): a global, double-blind, randomized, phase 3 trial. Lancet. 2019;393(10168):229–40. https://doi.org/10.1016/S0140-6736(18)32984-2.

16. Pro B, Advani R, Brice P, et al. Brentuximab vedotin (SGN-35) in patients with relapsed or refractory systemic anaplastic large-cell lymphoma: results of a phase II study. J Clin Oncol. 2012;30(18):2190–6.
17. Pro B, Advani R, Brice P, et al. Five-year results of brentuximab vedotin in patients with relapsed or refractory systemic anaplastic large cell lymphoma. Blood. 2017;130(25):2709–17.
18. Gambacorti Passerini C, Farina F, Stasia A, et al. Crizotinib in advanced, chemoresistant anaplastic lymphoma kinase-positive lymphoma patient. J Natl Cancer Inst. 2014;106(2):djt378.
19. Gambacorti Passerini C, Mussolin L, Brugieres L, et al. Abrupt relapse of ALK-positive lymphoma after discontinuation of crizotinib. N Engl J Med. 2016;374(1):95–6.
20. Richly H, Kim TM, Schuler M, et al. Ceritinib in patients with advanced anaplastic lymphoma kinase-rearranged anaplastic large-cell lymphoma. Blood. 2015;126(10):1257–8.
21. Malik SM, Liu K, Qiang X, et al. Folotyn (pralatrexate injection) for the treatment of patients with elapsed or refractory peripheral T-cell lymphoma: U.S. Food and Drug Administration drug approval summary. Clin Cancer Res. 2010;16(20):4921–7.
22. Coiffier B, Pro B, Prince HM, et al. Results from a pivotal, open-label, phase II study of romidepsin in relapsed or refractory peripheral T-cell lymphoma after prior systemic therapy. J Clin Oncol. 2012;30:631–6.
23. Amengual JE, Lichtenstein R, Lue J, et al. A phase I study of romidepsin and pralatrexate reveals marked activity in relapsed and refractory T-cell lymphoma. Blood. 2018;131(4):397–407.
24. O'Connor OA, Horwitz S, Masszi T, et al. Belinostat in patients with relapsed or refractory peripheral T-cell lymphoma: results of the pivotal phase II BELIEF (CLN-19) study. J Clin Oncol. 2015;33:2492–9.
25. Damaj G, Gressin R, Bouabdallah K, et al. Results from a prospective, open-label, phase II trial of bendamustine in refractory or relapsed T-cell lymphomas: the BENTLY trial. J Clin Oncol. 2012;31:104–10.
26. Ceritinib with brentuximab vedotin in treating patients with ALK-positive anaplastic large cell lymphoma [Internet] 2016 Apr 6 [updated 2018 Jan 12; cited 2018 Apr 5]. Available from: https://clinicaltrials.gov/ct2/show/study/NCT02729961.
27. Romidepsin and lenalidomide in treating patients with previously untreated peripheral T-cell lymphoma [Internet] 2014 Sept 5 [updated 2018 Jan 9; cited 2018 Apr 5]. Available from: https://clinicaltrials.gov/ct2/show/record/NCT02232516.
28. Horwitz SM, Koch R, Porcu P, et al. Activity of the PI3K- δ, γ inhibitor duvelisib in a phase I trial and preclinical models of T-cell lymphoma. Blood. 2018;131(8):888–98.
29. Oki Y, Haverkos B, Zain JM, et al. Tenalisib, a dual PI3K δ/γ inhibitor: safety and efficacy results from an on-going phase I/Ib study in relapsed/refractory T-cell lymphoma. J Clin Oncol. 2018;36(suppl):abstr 7510.
30. Trial of duvelisib in combination with either romidepsin or bortezomib in relapsed/refractory T-cell lymphomas [Internet] 2016 May 26 [updated 2018 Feb 23; cited 2018 Apr 5]. Available from: https://clinicaltrials.gov/ct2/show/NCT02783625.
31. Jacobson C, Kopp N, Layer JV, et al. HSP90 inhibition overcomes ibrutinib resistance in mantle cell lymphoma. Blood. 2016;128(21):2517–26.
32. Onalespib in treating patients with relapsed or refractory anaplastic large cell lymphoma, mantle cell lymphoma, or diffuse large B-cell lymphoma [Internet] 2015 Oct 9 [updated 2018 Mar 5; cited 2018 Apr 5]. Available from: https://clinicaltrials.gov/ct2/show/NCT02572453.
33. Study of ruxolitinib in relapsed or refractory T or NK cell lymphoma [Internet] 2016 Nov 28 [updated 2018 Mar 29; cited 2018 Apr 5]. Available from: https://clinicaltrials.gov/ct2/show/NCT02974647.
34. Hamlin PA, Cheson BD, Farber CM, et al. The dual SYK/JAK inhibitor cerdulatinib demonstrates rapid tumor responses in a phase 2 study in patients with relapsed/refractory B- and T-cell non-Hodgkin lymphoma (NHL). J Clin Oncol. 2018;36(suppl):abstr 7511.
35. Avelumab in relapsed and refractory peripheral T-cell lymphoma (AVAIL-T) [Internet] 2017 Feb 8 [updated 2017 Nov 28; cited 2018 Apr 5]. Available from: https://clinicaltrials.gov/ct2/show/NCT03046953.

36. Nivolumab in treating patients with relapsed or refractory peripheral T-cell lymphoma [Internet] 2017 Mar 9 [updated 2017 Dec 2; cited 2018 Apr 5]. Available from: https://clinicaltrials.gov/ct2/show/NCT03075553.
37. Durvalumab with or without lenalidomide in treating patients with relapsed or refractory cutaneous or peripheral T cell lymphoma [Internet] 2017 Jan 5 [updated 2017 Nov 30; cited 2018 Apr 5]. Available from: https://clinicaltrials.gov/ct2/show/NCT03011814.
38. Study of pembrolizumab combined with decitabine and pralatrexate in PTCL and CTCL [Internet] 2017 Aug 7 [updated 2018 Mar 8; cited 2018 Apr 5]. Available from: https://clinicaltrials.gov/ct2/show/NCT03240211.
39. Wartewig T, Kurgyis Z, Keppler S, et al. PD-1 is a haploinsufficient suppressor of T cell lymphomagenesis. Nature. 2017;552(7683):121–5.
40. Ratner L, Waldmann TA, Janakiram M, et al. Rapid progression of adult T-cell leukemia–lymphoma after PD-1 inhibitor therapy. N Engl J Med. 2018;378(20):1947–8.
41. ALRN-6924 in patients with advances solid tumors or lymphomas [Internet] 2014 Oct 15 [updated 2017 Jun 27; cited 2018 Apr 9]. Available from: https://clinicaltrials.gov/ct2/show/study/NCT02264613.
42. Horwitz SM, Hamadani M, Fanale MA, et al. Interim results from a phase 1 study of ADCT-301 (camidanlumab tesirine) show promising activity of a novel pyrrolobenzodiazepine-based antibody drug conjugate in relapsed/refractory Hodgkin/non-Hodgkin lymphoma. Blood. 2017;130:1510.

Chapter 12
Enteropathy-Associated T-Cell Lymphomas

Stephanie Teja and Neha Mehta-Shah

Introduction: Classic Enteropathy-Associated T-Cell Lymphoma and Monomorphic Epitheliotropic Intestinal T-Cell Lymphoma

Enteropathy-associated T-cell lymphoma (EATL) and monomorphic epitheliotropic intestinal T-cell lymphoma (MEITL) are two forms of T-cell lymphoma that primarily present in the intestine. In 2016, the diagnoses of EATL and MEITL were formally distinguished by the World Health Organization Classification of Tumors of Hematopoietic and Lymphoid Tissues based on histopathology and immunophenotype [1] (see Table 12.1). Antecedent to this, clinical series of EATL and MEITL were often referred to as EATL which can make the interpretation of historical data challenging.

EATL, formerly known as EATL type 1 or classic EATL, is strongly associated with a history of celiac disease and is the more common form of enteropathy-associated T-cell lymphoma in North America and Northern Europe where the prevalence of celiac disease is high (relative to Asia). Histologically, EATL is observed to have a large cell, pleomorphic cytology. The malignant cells are positive for CD3, CD7, and CD13 and negative for CD4 and CD5 and have variable expression of CD8. They often carry a clonal rearrangement of TCRβ [2]. For a more detailed discussion of the pathologic features of EATL, please see section on "Pathology."

Based on clinical presentation, EATL can be further classified into two subgroups: primary and secondary EATL. Primary EATL develops without a preceding history of celiac disease; patients often present emergently with perforation or

S. Teja
Washington University School of Medicine in St. Louis, St. Louis, MO, USA

N. Mehta-Shah (✉)
Division of Oncology, Washington University Medical School, St. Louis, MO, USA
e-mail: mehta-n@wustl.edu

C. Dittus (ed.), *Novel Therapeutics for Rare Lymphomas*,
https://doi.org/10.1007/978-3-030-25610-4_12

Table 12.1 Comparison of EATL and MEITL

	EATL	MEITL
Immunohistochemistry	Positive for CD3, CD103 Negative for CD4, CD5, CD8 May be positive for CD30	Positive for CD3, CD8, CD56, cytoplasmic expression of SYK Negative for CD4, CD5, CD8, CD30
Relation to celiac disease	Associated with history of celiac disease	Not associated with history of celiac disease
Racial distribution	More common in Caucasians	More common in Asian and non-Caucasian population
Mutational predominance	JAK1, STAT3, SOCS1	STATB5, SETD2, JAK3

obstruction, leading to the diagnoses of both EATL and celiac disease. In secondary EATL, patients have known celiac diseases that are well-established or refractory (see section "Celiac Disease and Refractory Celiac Disease").

Monomorphic epitheliotropic intestinal T-cell lymphoma (MEITL), formerly known as EATL type 2, is now formally distinguished from EATL given its unique histopathology and clinical course. It forms about 10–20% of all cases of enteropathy-associated T-cell lymphoma. It is less strongly associated with celiac disease and is more common in Asia, where the prevalence of celiac disease is low, with studies strongly suggesting that intestinal T-cell lymphomas affecting Asian patients might be predominantly MEITL [3]. MEITL is characterized by expression of CD3+, CD8+, and CD56+ and lack of expression of CD4. It often carries a clonal TCRβ [2, 4, 5]. For a more detailed discussion of the pathologic features of MEITL, please see section on "Pathology."

Epidemiology

Enteropathy-associated T-cell lymphomas make up less than 1% of non-Hodgkin lymphomas and 5.4% of all T-cell lymphomas [5, 6]. Incidence of EATL is 0.10–0.14/100000 per year [7]. Approximately two-thirds of cases of intestinal/enteropathy-associated T-cell lymphomas are EATL and one-third represent MEITL. In Northern Europe, EATL makes up approximately 80% of cases of enteropathy-associated T-cell lymphomas [5]. The average patient with EATL presents in the sixth decade with some studies reporting a male predominance (61–74%) and others suggesting a nearly equal gender distribution [5–8]. The Asia Lymphoma Study Group, reporting on the analysis of 38 patients with MEITL, found that men were affected twice as frequently as women, with a median age of 59 [3].

The prevalence of EATL varies geographically; a study of a cohort of 62 patients with EATL among 1153 patients with peripheral T-cell lymphoma (PTCL) from 22 centers found the highest frequency in Europe (9.1%), followed by North America (5.8%) and then Asia (1.9%) [5]. Another institution-based study of 74 enteropathy-type T-cell lymphoma cases in Taiwan showed an 8.1% frequency [9]. Indeed, it now appears that most cases of enteropathy-type lymphoma in Asian countries, where there is a low prevalence of celiac disease, such as Japan, China, and Taiwan, are in fact MEITL [3, 10–12].

The disease incidence differs by race as well. A study using the Surveillance, Epidemiology, and End Results (SEER) database and the National Cancer Database (NCDB), the two largest public cancer databases in the United States, compared the incidence of EATL by self-reported race. In the years 2000–2010, the overall age-adjusted incidence rate of EATL in the United States was 0.111 per 1,000,000. Asians/Pacific Islanders had a higher incidence rate (0.236) compared with other races (Caucasian (0.101), African American (0.107), American Indian/Alaska native (0.128)) [13].

Celiac Disease and Refractory Celiac Disease

EATL is a neoplastic complication of celiac disease, which is a chronic gluten-sensitive enteropathy more prevalent in patients with European ancestry. Those with refractory celiac disease, defined as failure to respond to at least 12 months of a gluten-free diet, are at higher risk of EATL. Refractory celiac disease can be further subclassified as refractory celiac disease 1 or 2, on the basis of histological findings. Refractory celiac disease 1 features villous atrophy despite adherence to a gluten-free diet, and though it has increased populations of intraepithelial lymphocytes, they are still phenotypically normal. Refractory celiac disease 2 is characterized by a clonal expansion of abnormal intraepithelial lymphocytes lacking the normal surface markers.

Refractory celiac disease 2 is strongly associated with the development of EATL. It has been reported that 60–80% of patients with refractory celiac disease 2 will develop EATL within 5 years [3]. The time from the diagnosis of celiac disease to the development of lymphoma can range widely between months and years [14]. Those with refractory celiac disease 1 had a 5-year survival between 80% and 96%, but those with refractory celiac disease 2 had a 5-year survival of only 40–58%. Those with refractory celiac disease 2 who developed EATL had the worst prognosis, with a 5-year survival of 8–20% [15].

There is evidence that adherence to a gluten-free duet can reduce the risk of intestinal lymphomas. In a large Italian registry that studied complications in 1757 patients with celiac disease over 3 years, the morbidity ratio associated with the development of intestinal lymphoma dropped from 6.42 to 0.22 with adherence to a strict gluten-free diet [16]. However, at least one study found continued persistent risk of non-Hodgkin's lymphoma, both T-cell and B-cell types, in patients with celiac disease, despite a gluten-free diet. These patients also have been demonstrated to have an increased risk of small intestinal adenocarcinoma, esophageal cancer, and melanoma [17].

Diagnosis

Clinical Presentation

Many patients with both EATL and MEITL present with abdominal perforation or obstruction requiring emergent treatment, as well as symptoms associated with such complications, including pain, nausea/vomiting, weight loss, anorexia, and fatigue [7, 18]. In one study, more than a third of patients diagnosed with these intestinal lymphomas required enteral or parenteral feeding [6]. Other common presenting symptoms are diarrhea and B-symptoms (fever and night sweats) [19, 20]. Most patients present with reduced performance status (ECOG > 1) due to acute abdominal symptoms and/or chronically poor nutritional status (caused by both malabsorption and hypermetabolism) [18, 21].

Regarding lab values, a majority of patients present with anemia and hypoalbuminemia, likely due to malnutrition. Elevated LDH values and elevated CRP are also common owing to the aggressive nature of enteropathy-associated lymphoma [6, 7, 19]. Hemophagocytic lymphohistiocytosis (HLH) has been reported in several studies occurring at presentation or later on in the disease course of both EATL and MEITL, which carries a very poor prognosis [22–25].

A significant proportion of patients present with disseminated disease, with the most common sites of involvement being the bone marrow, lung, mediastinal lymph nodes, and liver [23]. CNS involvement is rare at presentation but may be the only site of relapse and carries poor prognosis [18, 26, 27]. There are unusual cases of patients with EATL presenting with eosinophilia, Sweet's syndrome, cavitating mesenteric lymph node syndrome, and subacute polyradiculopathy [28–32].

In contrast to EATL, where the small bowel is almost always the primary site (due to its origin from pre-existing celiac disease), MEITL might involve any part of the gut as well as multiple extraintestinal sites [33]. Additionally, several studies report patients with MEITL presenting with isolated large bowel or stomach lesions, a phenomenon that is exceedingly rare in EATL [3, 33]. At the time of relapse, patients with MEITL may have multiple extraintestinal metastases, commonly in the thorax and central nervous system [34]. There are cases of MEITL presenting as pleural effusions, pyoid ascites, cutaneous deposits, chronic diarrhea, and bilateral ovarian masses [35–41].

Differential Diagnosis

Differential diagnoses that must be considered include refractory celiac disease, B-cell lymphomas, indolent T-cell lymphoproliferative disease, extra-nodal NK/T--cell lymphoma, gamma-delta T-cell lymphoma, anaplastic large cell lymphoma, malignant melanoma, and tumors of histiocytic origin [42]. Notably, patients with celiac disease are more likely to be diagnosed with B-cell non-Hodgkin lymphoma or lymphomas of non-intestinal origin than with EATL or MEITL [43].

In particular, there are two indolent lymphoproliferative processes of the GI tract that can be mistaken for EATL: (1) indolent T-cell lymphoproliferative disease of the gastrointestinal tract and (2) NK-enteropathy. Neither of these disorders typically requires or responds to systemic therapy, and both typically follow an indolent course [44].

Pathology

Histologically, EATL is observed to have a large cell, pleomorphic cytology, and the cells are positive for CD3, CD7, and CD13 and negative for CD4 and CD5 and have variable expression of CD8 and TCRβ [2]. A significant majority of EATL are CD30+, with 2 studies finding positivity in 25/25 cases and 12/14 cases respectively [4, 23]. Most patients with EATL have the genotype HLA-DQA1∗0501 and DBQ∗0201 and they more commonly have 1q32.2-q41 and 5q34-q35.2 gains [45, 46]. A limited study of eight EATL cases found recurrent mutations in JAK1(50%) and STAT3 (25%), but no SETD2, STAT5B or JAK3 mutations. H3K36 trimethylation is generally preserved [47].

In contrast, MEITL is characterized by atypical T-cells that express CD3, CD8, and CD56 and are negative for CD4. They can be clonal for TCRβ+ [2, 4, 5]. This cytotoxic T-cell phenotype differentiates MEITL from EATL histologically. Furthermore, MEITL is rarely positive for CD30 and has a predominance of CD8 and CD56 [1, 4].

Patients with MEITL more commonly have chromosome 8q24 gains and less commonly 1q and 5q gains. The tumor suppressor gene SETD2 has been found to be recurrently silenced in EATL. A study of 15 MEITL samples found SETD2 inactivation in 93% of cases [47]. Additionally, the JAK-STAT pathway was the most frequently mutated pathway, with mutations in STAT5B (60%) as well as JAK1, JAK3(46%), STAT3, SOCS1, and SH2B3 (20%) [47, 48]. Mutations in KRAS, TP53, BRAF, and TERT have also been observed [47, 49].

A recent study found that the cytoplasmic expression of spleen tyrosine kinase (SYK) seemed to be a distinctive marker for MEITL [46]. In contrast, both MEITL and EATL predominantly express ZAP-70 (92.5% and 96%, respectively). In addition, the composition of the T-cell receptor (TCR) was found to be different between MEITL and EATL. MEITL was predominantly found to have a positive TCR phenotype (85% cases). In contrast, EATL demonstrated a clonal TCR in 35% cases.

Work-Up

Though most EATL patients obtain a diagnosis from surgical pathology specimens taken during emergency laparotomies, there are times when radiologic and endoscopic procedures are helpful [6, 15].

18F-fluorodeoxyglucose positron emission tomography (^{18}F-FDG PET) is preferred to CT scans for work-up; in general, the majority of lesions of EATL and MEITL are hypermetabolic [33, 50]. In a study of 38 patients, ^{18}F-FDG PET, when compared to CT alone, had better sensitivity, particularly for extra-nodal disease [50]. Nevertheless, up to 8% of cases may not demonstrate FDG avid lesions [19].

As an adjunct to PET, magnetic resonance enterography (MRE) is able to detect EATL confined to the epithelial layer of the bowel wall as well as assess response to treatment. The diagnostic accuracy of MRE in detecting refractory celiac disease 2 or EATL is approximately 90% [15].

Prognosis and Prognostic Factors

The 5-year overall survival of 62 patients with "enteropathy-type PTCL" identified in the International PTCL Project (ITCP) was only 20% [5]. Similarly, in the published data from the Swedish Lymphoma Registry, among 68 patients with EATL, the 5-year overall survival (OS) and progression-free survival (PFS) was 20% and 18%, respectively [51].

A large tumor size of >5 cm at diagnosis, a non-ambulatory condition, elevated serum LDH, and elevated CRP were adversely correlated with OS and PFS. Disease stage (3 or 4), age >60 years, and IHC markers (CD8, CD56, CD30, or TIA1) did not correlate with OS and PFS [5].

Another study from the Netherlands, by Nijeboer et al., analyzing a total of 61 patients with EATL (30 in the setting of refractory celiac disease, 31 with EATL and occult celiac disease diagnosed at presentation) found that the overall 5-year survival was only 10% [19]. In general, patients with EATL diagnosed in the setting of refractory celiac disease had worse median overall survivals (4 vs. 14 months). In this study, the median overall survival was found to be 7.4 months with 1- and 5-year overall survival rates of 40% and 11%, respectively. It is important to note that 10 of the 61 patients could not be treated due to poor clinical status or advanced disease. These patients who were not candidates for systemic therapy had a particularly poor prognosis with a median survival of 10 days. Other series have replicated similar findings [6, 52]. Patients with EATL in the setting of refractory celiac disease had higher rates of relapse in 5 years after achieving a complete remission (CR) (60% vs. 40%). IPI score significantly correlated with the rate of CR to initial therapy but did not affect relapse risk afterward.

In series where patients were treated with combination chemotherapy with the intent to pursue an autologous transplant in first remission, the median survival and progression-free survival of patients with EATL mimics those of other T-cell lymphomas. In the Nordic study, the largest prospective multicenter trial of CHOP with etoposide (CHOEP) followed by ASCT in peripheral T-cell lymphoma, 21 patients had EATL. On an intent to treat basis, those with EATL fared similarly to those with PTCL-NOS and AITL with a 5-year PFS and OS of 38% and 48%, respectively. This demonstrates that for patients who are fit to receive chemotherapy with EATL, prognosis is likely superior to those who were not candidates for systemic, anthracycline-based therapy. Unfortunately, a large fraction of patients with EATL are diagnosed in the setting of refractory abdominal pain, nutritional deficiencies, and recent abdominal surgery, which makes the overall prognosis for this disease worse than other types of T-cell lymphoma.

Prognostic indices used for aggressive lymphomas such as the International Prognostic Index (IPI) and the Prognostic Index for PTCL (PIT) have not shown as much prognostic stratification in EATL. A retrospective multicenter study based on 92 patients with EATL in the Netherlands, England, and Scotland found a new and validated prognostic model that better stratifies patients according to survival outcomes [20]. Interestingly, the presence of B symptoms (defined as a fever with temperature of ≥38 °C (100.4 °F) and/or night sweats) was found to be a strong adverse predictor for overall survival. The new EATL prognostic index (EPI), composed of IPI variables and the presence of B-symptoms, stratifies patients into three risk groups, (A) a high-risk group, characterized by the presence of B-symptoms, irrespective of IPI score (median overall survival of 2 months); (B) an intermediate-risk group, comprising patients without B-symptoms and an IPI score ≥2 (7 months); and (C) a low-risk group, representing patients without B-symptoms and an IPI score of 0–1 (34 months). In contrast with the IPI and PIT, the EPI better classified patients in risk groups according to their clinical outcomes.

Regarding the prognosis and prognostic factors for MEITL, the largest analysis to date is of 38 patients with MEITL from the Asia Lymphoma Study Group [3]. The overall median survival was only 7 months (range 0.5–108 months) and median PFS was 1 month (range 0–42 months). Ten of the thirty-eight patients were not able to initiate therapy with chemotherapy, and these patients had a median survival of 1 month from diagnosis. In contrast, patients who achieved remission and went on to transplants had superior outcomes (OS 26 vs. 67 months; disease-free-survival 7 vs. 38 months). The only other factors found to impact outcomes were good performance status, defined as ECOG of 0 or 1 (OS improved, PFS unchanged), and the ability to receive and respond to initial chemotherapy (OS and PFS improved).

Conventional Treatment Approach

There is no established standard treatment for EATL/MEITL owing to the rarity of the disease and a lack of high-quality randomized controlled trials. Most of the data comes from case reports, single-institution studies, and sub-analyses of larger studies in which only a handful of patients with EATL/MEITL are included.

It must be noted that a significant proportion of the patients present in poor nutritional status due to their chronic celiac disease or because they present with an obstruction or perforation. After undergoing the first therapeutic procedure, which is generally de-bulking surgery, many patients are unable to proceed with further therapy. In 1 study, 5 out of 62 patients could not undergo any treatment due to their poor performance status at diagnosis [5]. As discussed earlier, this subset of patients with very low performance status must be kept in mind when looking at outcomes from prospective studies or series of more aggressive treatment strategies for which these patients would likely not have been eligible [52].

As mentioned earlier, often patients' first treatment is surgical de-bulking. Unfortunately, surgery might delay the start of chemotherapy, especially in cases with surgical complications, poor wound healing, or worsening post-op poor performance status [15]. Early surgical complications include leakage at the anastomotic site with resulting sepsis. Later complications include stenosis at the anastomotic site. Mortality is higher when the procedure is done emergently.

With regard to systemic therapy, the CHOP regimen is the most widely used with an overall 5-year survival rate of 9–22% [6, 7, 53–55]. Other chemotherapy regimens that have been used are BACOP (bleomycin, doxorubicin, cyclophosphamide, vincristine, and prednisone), ProMACE-MOPP (prednisone, doxorubicin, cyclophosphamide, etoposide, mechlorethamine, vincristine, and procarbazine), VAMP (vincristine, doxorubicin, high-dose methotrexate, and prednisolone), PEACE-BOM (prednisolone, etoposide, doxorubicin, cyclophosphamide-bleomycin, vincristine, and methotrexate), CHOEP (CHOP with etoposide), EPOCH-ICE (etoposide, prednisone, vincristine, cyclophosphamide, and doxorubicin-ifosfamide, carboplatin, and etoposide), MACOP-B (methotrexate, doxorubicin, cyclophosphamide, vincristine, prednisone, and bleomycin), and CHOP-ESHAP (Table 12.2). Intestinal perforation is not uncommon following chemotherapy and can occur even after multiple prior cycles. The few remissions that were observed, two with complete remission and three with partial remissions, were short-lived with only two

Table 12.2 Upfront chemotherapeutic options in enteropathy-associated T-cell lymphomas

Reference	Study type	No. of patients	Type of chemotherapy	Overall response rate %/complete response rate %	Median survival in months (range)
[7]	Retrospective	54	CHOP, CHOP-derived	32/32	7 (0–140)
[6]	Retrospective	31	CHOP, VAMP, PEACE-BOM	58/32	7.5 (0–83)
[61]	Retrospective	24	CHOP, BACOP, ProMACE-MOPP	Unk/Unk	10 (0–196)
[63]	Retrospective	10	CHOP	Unk/50	5 (1–12)
[62]	Retrospective	1	Hyper-CVAD	100/100	34 (Unk)
[64]	Prospective	23	CHOP	Unk/35	7 (Unk)
[63]	Prospective	10	CHOEP	60/30	7 (2–16)

BACOP bleomycin, doxorubicin, cyclophosphamide, vincristine, prednisone; *CHOP* cyclophosphamide, doxorubicin, vincristine, prednisone; *CHOEP* CHOP plus etoposide; *Hyper-CVAD* cyclophosphamide, vincristine, dexamethasone, methotrexate, cytarabine; *PEACE-BOM* prednisolone, etoposide, doxorubicin, cyclophosphamide-bleomycin, vincristine, methotrexate; ProMACE-MOPP prednisone, doxorubicin, cyclophosphamide, etoposide, mechlorethamine, vincristine, procarbazine; *Unk* unknown; *VAMP* vincristine, doxorubicin, high-dose methotrexate, prednisolone

patients alive at a median follow-up of 7 months [56]. Even when patients responded to a regimen, the remissions were not durable. In another study by Gale et al. of 31 patients in the United Kingdom, out of 19 patients who responded to initial therapy, 15 relapsed at a median of 6 months with 12 relapsing at small bowel sites [6].

Using the ability to receive anthracycline-containing combination chemotherapy as a practical surrogate for treatment with curative intent, data from the International T-cell Project show that ~20% of those who received anthracycline-containing chemotherapy were alive and failure-free at 2 years, whereas none among those who could not receive such therapy were alive without progression at 1 year [52]. It is important to note that chemotherapy cannot be given to about 50% of newly diagnosed patients due to their poor performance status; a further 50% of patients who initiate chemotherapy are unable to complete it. Only 35–40% of patients who complete the full course of chemotherapy achieve a CR [6, 53, 56, 57]. Interestingly, some patients survived more than 1 year despite failing to attain CR [19].

The role of consolidation with an autologous transplant in first remission is controversial, as are other dose-intensified strategies. A large multicenter clinical trial was done by the Nordic Lymphoma Group (NLG-T-01) evaluating the efficacy of induction treatment (six cycles of CHOEP) followed by ASCT in newly diagnosed PTCL that contained 21 patients with EATL [58]. The 5-year OS and PFS values for patients with EATL were 48% and 38%, respectively. In another study, the Scotland and Newcastle Lymphoma Group (SNLG) performed a prospective study of 54 patients with EATL and found an overall median PFS of 3.4 months and overall survival of 7.1 months [7]. In the study, 26 patients were tried on a pilot regimen of intensive chemotherapy, IVE (ifosfamide, etoposide, epirubicin) with high-dose methotrexate (MTX), followed by ASCT, and this group had significantly improved outcomes (5 year PFS of 52% and OS of 60%) compared to the historical group of patients treated with conventional anthracycline-based chemotherapy. In another promising report, six patients with EATL were treated with intensive chemotherapy (IVE plus high-dose MTX) followed by ASCT resulting in five CRs and one PR; two patients relapsed at 2.5 and 20.5 months, but four patients remained in complete remission for 22–52 months [59]. Similarly, results of studies by the European Society for Blood and Marrow Transplantation (EBMT) and by Sieniawski et al. suggest that ASCT could be a curative approach in the majority of EATL patients who receive high-dose therapy in first CR or PR [7, 60]. While these results are pooled from small series, the results are favorable when viewed in comparison to historical data. These data provide hope that intensive chemotherapy followed by ASCT in eligible patients may lead to a durable remission.

On the other hand, studies like the retrospective analysis of patients with EATL by Nijeboer et al. found that even though transplanted patients had the best outcomes (1- and 5-year overall survival rates of 100% and 33%, respectively), some of these patients relapsed within 1–2 months posttransplant [19, 61].

For MEITL, the largest existing series consists of 38 patients retrospectively analyzed by the Asia Lymphoma Study Group [3]. Thirty one patients (86%) had surgical resection either due to an emergent presentation or the need for a histologic diagnosis. Afterward, due to poor general condition, eight could not receive further chemotherapy, and two could only receive steroids. Out of the 26 patients (72%) who could receive chemotherapy, the overall response rate was 46%, and 10 achieved a complete remission. The two most common regimens were anthracycline-based and L-asparaginase-based, but choice of regimen did not affect the overall response rate. Five patients were able to proceed to a transplant after chemotherapy, and all were still alive at the time of publication (overall survival 26–67 months, disease-free survival 7–38 months). There are case reports of patients with MEITL with long remissions following ASCT [62].

There is no standard second-line chemotherapy for relapsed/refractory patients, and clinical trials should be strongly encouraged. In a retrospective single-center analysis of 19 patients with EATL undergoing second-line chemotherapy, 3 patients achieved a complete remission lasting 4, 7+, and 64+ months with 2 patients having no evidence of disease. The regimens used were ifosfamide, carboplatin, and etoposide (ICE); fludarabine and cyclophosphamide (FC); dexamethasone, cisplatin, and cytarabine (DHAP); and cladribine as a single agent [63]. Non-chemotherapy options have primarily been extrapolated from relapsed/refractory PTCL (see section on "Novel Treatments"). These include standard salvage chemotherapies, histone deacetylase inhibitors, lenalidomide-based therapies, and brentuximab vedotin. A multi-institutional retrospective series of patients who underwent allogeneic transplant in T-cell lymphoma contained five patients with EATL or MEITL [64]. Of these patients, who were deemed to be candidates for transplant, 40% were disease free at 2 years from transplant.

Novel Treatments

It is clear that better treatments for patients with EATL are needed. In particular, given the poor performance status of many patients with EATL, identification of well-tolerated nontraditional chemotherapeutic agents that can be incorporated into frontline therapies will be an important component of improving therapy for these patients. As it is hard to recruit patients owing to the rarity of EATL, most trials enroll patients with a range of diagnoses and very few studies focus exclusively on patients with EATL.

Targeting CD30+

Brentuximab vedotin (BV) is an antibody drug conjugate which targets CD30, a transmembrane glycoprotein. BV is FDA-approved for use in anaplastic large cell lymphoma, Hodgkin lymphoma, and CD30+ mycosis fungoides, which are all characterized by CD30 positivity. Most cases of EATL express CD30 on a proportion of tumor cells making BV a promising agent. Adverse events are also tolerable with peripheral neuropathy being most frequently reported [65]. It must be noted that MEITL is rarely CD30+ and thus would likely require an alternative treatment.

In a case report, a 64-year-old man with EATL had a complete remission with eight cycles of BV (1.8 mg/m^2 every 3 weeks for four cycles, then 1.0 mg/m^2 thereafter due to the resulting neuropathy) after failing CHOP, ICE, gemcitabine and vinorelbine, and romidepsin [66]. In another case, a patient was started on BV after relapsing 8 months after completion of CHOP therapy [67]. His disease was controlled for 18 cycles.

Brentuximab-based therapy is being evaluated as a single agent or combination with other therapies. For example, there is a current study of BV in combination with nivolumab (NCT02581631), open to patients with recurrent EATL. Additionally, there are other studies that are currently open that allow patients with EATL (e.g., NCT02588651, NCT03217643, NCT03113500). Furthermore, patients with EATL were eligible for ECHELON-2 which is a randomized, double-blinded study of CHOP compared to BV-CHP (cyclophosphamide, doxorubicin, prednisone) (NCT01777152). We look forward to these results to inform us about the use of BV in this patient population.

Histone Deacetylase Inhibitors

Histone deacetylase (HDAC) plays multiple roles in cancer pathogenesis, targeting signaling pathways regulating cellular processes involved in cancer-cell differentiation, proliferation, migration, and survival. The principal mode of action is thought to be the mediation of posttranslational modifications of various histone and nonhistone proteins. Inhibitors of HDAC (HDACi) induce acetylation of histones, upregulate expression of tumor suppressor genes, and cause cell cycle arrest. HDAC1, in particular, has higher expression in PTCL, suggesting a sensitivity to HDAC inhibitors [68]. Examples of HDAC inhibitors are romidepsin, vorinostat, belinostat, and panobinostat. These are promising agents for EATL because of the many mutations in chromatin modifying genes in the disease.

Romidepsin is an HDACi approved by the FDA in 2011 for treatment of PTCL. In a phase 2 study of single-agent romidepsin in patients with relapsed/refractory PTCL and CTCL, the one enrolled patient with EATL had a PR lasting 8 months [69]. Other early trials seem to suggest that romidepsin in combination with other agents would have higher efficacy than single-agent romidepsin. Romidepsin has been, or is currently being, investigated in patients with PTCL in various combinations, including with ICE, liposomal doxorubicin, lenalidomide, gemcitabine, pralatrexate, bortezomib, and azacitidine [70, 71].

Two patients with EATL were included in the registration study of belinostat, a pan-HDACi, and one achieved a clinical response [72].

PI3K Inhibition

Phosphoinositide-3-kinases (PI3K) are crucial in cell signaling, and they regulate multiple cellular functions. The PI3K-δ and PI3K-γ isoforms are important to the growth and survival of certain T-cell malignancies, and inhibition of PI3K is a therapeutic strategy for PTCL and CTCL. Duvelisib is an oral inhibitor of PI3K-δ and PI3K-γ that has proven efficacious in various trials for PTCL [73, 74]. In the phase 1 study of duvelisib, a CR was seen in the one patient with EATL [75]. Another promising trial is ongoing testing duvelisib in combination with either romidepsin or bortezomib in relapsed/refractory PTCL including EATL (NCT02783625).

Proteasome Inhibitors

Preliminary data in EATL shows an increased expression of NF-KB target genes, likely resulting in upregulation of NF-KB activity in EATL cells. Bortezomib is a proteasome inhibitor that inhibits NF-KB activity and can induce apoptosis by upregulating the pro-apoptotic BH3-only protein Noxa. In a study by De Baaij et al., it was found that expression of Noxa was significantly downregulated in EATL cells compared to healthy donor samples [76]. Bortezomib resulted in induction of apoptosis in all the EATL samples tested, which was shown to be due to upregulation of Noxa. Therefore, bortezomib has been studied as a single agent and in combination with agents such as duvelisib (see section "PI3K Inhibition").

Immunomodulatory Agents

Lenalidomide is a thalidomide analog that acts by inhibition of vascular endothelial growth factor (VEGF), activation of NK cells and T lymphocytes, and modulation of various cytokines [77]. Through these mechanisms, it is able to target both neoplastic cells and the tumor microenvironment. A Canadian phase 2 study of 39 patients with systemic T-cell lymphoma, including 2 patients with EATL, reported a response rate of 26% [77]. Unfortunately, the two patients with EATL did not have an evaluable response. Trials of lenalidomide, as monotherapy or in combination with other regimens, are ongoing in PTCL (e.g., NCT02561273).

Targeting CD52

CD52 is an antigen present with minimal expression in the most common PTCL subtypes [78]. Alemtuzumab, a humanized monoclonal antibody against CD52, has been tried in patients with PTCL with some success. In a trial of alemtuzumab plus CHOP, the sole patient with EATL initially achieved a complete response but then died of progressive disease shortly thereafter [79]. There is a case report of a patient with EATL responding to alemtuzumab, but no data from large prospective trials is available to date [80].

Checkpoint Inhibitors

Nivolumab, a human IgG4 anti-PD-1 monoclonal antibody that works as a checkpoint inhibitor, has already been approved in multiple solid tumors and relapsed/refractory Hodgkin lymphoma. Trials are ongoing in PTCL, which include EATL (e.g., NCT03075553). The efficacy of checkpoint inhibitors in EATL and MEITL remains unknown.

Other Agents

PEG-asparaginase is a modified enzyme that has been evaluated successfully in case reports and is part of a regimen being trialed for PTCL, including EATL (e.g., NCT03071822) [81].

Syk inhibitors are currently being tested clinically and has shown efficacy in a phase 2 study in patients with relapsed/refractory B-cell malignancies [82]. Overexpression of Syk has been shown in PTCL with inhibition of Syk inducing apoptosis and blocking proliferation in T-cell lymphomas [83, 84]. Given the overexpression of Syk in MEITL (see section on "Pathology"), this is a promising pathway to target in future studies of MEITL.

Recommended Treatment Approach for Frontline and Relapsed Disease

There is no standard of care for patients with MEITL and EATL given the rare nature of the disease. Given the relatively poor performance status of these patients at the time of diagnosis, which is often complicated by nutritional deficiencies, history of celiac disease, and recent surgeries, therapeutic decisions regarding initial management can be complicated. It is our approach to initiate cytotoxic, anthracycline-based chemotherapy as soon as allowable. As many patients are diagnosed in the setting of bowel obstructions requiring surgery, close communication with the surgeons, nutritional support, and pathologists is critical. If the patient is a candidate for an appropriate clinical trial, a clinical trial is our preferred upfront approach. Given the favorable outcomes demonstrated by the Nordic Lymphoma Group, we favor using CHOEP for initial therapy with consideration of consolidation with an autologous stem cell transplant [58]. In selected, fit, younger patients, one may consider the Newcastle regimen as an upfront approach [7]. Based on the status of the GI tract at the time of diagnosis, one may consider omitting vincristine in cycle 1. The results of patients with EATL in ECHELON-2 may help inform future upfront therapy regarding the role of brentuximab vedotin in this disease as well.

In the relapsed/refractory setting, there is no standard approach. However, one should consider allogeneic transplant for consolidation in patients who achieve adequate disease control and are otherwise candidates for this approach.

References

1. Swerdlow SH, Campo E, Pileri SA, Harris NL, Stein H, Siebert R, et al. The 2016 revision of the World Health Organization classification of lymphoid neoplasms. Blood. 2016;127(20):2375–90.
2. Ferreri AJM, Zinzani PL, Govi S, Pileri SA. Enteropathy-associated T-cell lymphoma. Crit Rev Oncol Hematol. 2011;79(1):84–90.
3. Tse E, Gill H, Loong F, Kim SJ, Ng SB, Tang T, et al. Type II enteropathy-associated T-cell lymphoma: a multicenter analysis from the Asia Lymphoma Study Group. Am J Hematol. 2012;87(7):663–8.
4. Deleeuw RJ, Zettl A, Klinker E, Haralambieva E, Trottier M, Chari R, et al. Whole-genome analysis and HLA genotyping of enteropathy-type T-cell lymphoma reveals 2 distinct lymphoma subtypes. Gastroenterology. 2007;132(5):1902–11.
5. Delabie J, Holte H, Vose JM, Ullrich F, Jaffe ES, Savage KJ, et al. Enteropathy-associated T-cell lymphoma: clinical and histological findings from the international peripheral T-cell lymphoma project. Blood. 2011;118(1):148–55.
6. Gale J, Simmonds PD, Mead GM, Sweetenham JW, Wright DH. Enteropathy-type intestinal T-cell lymphoma: clinical features and treatment of 31 patients in a single center. J Clin Oncol. 2000;18(4):795–803.
7. Sieniawski M, Angamuthu N, Boyd K, Chasty R, Davies J, Forsyth P, et al. Evaluation of enteropathy-associated T-cell lymphoma comparing standard therapies with a novel regimen including autologous stem cell transplantation. Blood. 2010;115(18):3664–70.
8. Verbeek WHM, Van De Water JMW, Al-Toma A, Oudejans JJ, Mulder CJJ, Coupe VMH. Incidence of enteropathy - associated T-cell lymphoma: a nation-wide study of a population-based registry in the Netherlands. Scand J Gastroenterol. 2008;43(11):1322–8.
9. Lee MY, Tsou MH, Tan TD, Lu MC. Clinicopathological analysis of T-cell lymphoma in Taiwan according to WHO classification: high incidence of enteropathy-type intestinal T-cell lymphoma. Eur J Haematol. 2005;75(3):221–6.
10. Chan JKC, Chan ACL, Cheuk W, Wan SK, Lee WK, Lui YH, et al. Type II enteropathy-associated T-cell lymphoma: a distinct aggressive lymphoma with frequent gamma delta T-cell receptor expression. Am J Surg Pathol. 2011;35(10):1557–69.
11. Sun J, Lu ZH, Yang D, Chen J. Primary intestinal T-cell and NK-cell lymphomas: a clinicopathological and molecular study from China focused on type II enteropathy-associated T-cell lymphoma and primary intestinal NK-cell lymphoma. Mod Pathol. 2011;24(7):983–92.
12. Takeshita M, Nakamura S, Kikuma K, Nakayama Y, Nimura S, Yao T, et al. Pathological and immunohistological findings and genetic aberrations of intestinal enteropathy-associated T cell lymphoma in Japan. Histopathology. 2011;58(3):395–407.
13. Karanam PK, Al-Hamadani M, Go RS. Enteropathy-associated T-cell lymphoma in the US: higher incidence and poorer survival among Asians. Br J Haematol. 2016;172(6):990–2.
14. Ilyas M, Niedobitek G, Agathanggelou A, Barry RE, Read AE, Tierney R, et al. Non-Hodgkins-lymphoma, celiac-disease, and Epstein-Barr-virus – a study of 13 cases of enteropathy-associated t-cell and b-cell lymphoma. J Pathol. 1995;177(2):115–22.
15. Di Sabatino A, Biagi F, Gobbi PG, Corazza GR. How I treat enteropathy-associated T-cell lymphoma. Blood. 2012;119(11):2458–68.
16. Silano M, Volta U, De Vincenzi A, Dessi M, De Vincenzi M, Collaborating Centers of the Italian Registry of the Complications of Coeliac Disease. Effect of a gluten-free diet on the risk of enteropathy-associated T-cell lymphoma in celiac disease. Dig Dis Sci. 2008;53(4):972–6.

17. Green PHR, Fleischauer AT, Bhagat G, Goyal R, Jabri B, Neugut AI. Risk of malignancy in patients with celiac disease. Am J Med. 2003;115(3):191–5.
18. Sieniawski MK, Lennard AL. Enteropathy-associated T-cell lymphoma: epidemiology, clinical features, and current treatment strategies. Curr Hematol Malig Rep. 2011;6(4):231–40.
19. Nijeboer P, de Baaij LR, Visser O, Witte BI, Cillessen SA, Mulder CJ, et al. Treatment response in enteropathy associated T-cell lymphoma; survival in a large multicenter cohort. Am J Hematol. 2015;90(6):493–8.
20. de Baaij LR, Berkhof J, van de Water JM, Sieniawski MK, Radersma M, Verbeek WH, et al. A new and validated clinical prognostic model (EPI) for enteropathy-associated T-cell lymphoma. Clin Cancer Res. 2015;21(13):3013–9.
21. Wierdsma NJ, Nijeboer P, de van der Schueren MAE, Berkenpas M, van Bodegraven AA, Mulder CJJ. Refractory celiac disease and EATL patients show severe malnutrition and malabsorption at diagnosis. Clin Nutr. 2016;35(3):685–91.
22. Amiot A, Allez M, Treton X, Fieschi C, Galicier L, Joly F, et al. High frequency of fatal haemophagocytic lymphohistiocytosis syndrome in enteropathy-associated T cell lymphoma. Dig Liver Dis. 2012;44(4):343–9.
23. Malamut G, Chandesris O, Verkarre V, Meresse B, Callens C, Macintyre E, et al. Enteropathy associated T cell lymphoma in celiac disease: a large retrospective study. Dig Liver Dis. 2013;45(5):377–84.
24. Lu L, Ning SY, Kassam Z, Puglia M. Gluten gambit: a case of Hemophagocytic Lymphohistiocytic syndrome and enteropathy-associated T-cell lymphoma in a patient with refractory celiac disease. Am J Gastroenterol. 2012;107:S373–S4.
25. Varghese D, Koya HH, Cherian SV, Mead K, Sharma A, Sharma N, et al. Hemophagocytic lymphohistiocytosis: an uncommon presentation of enteropathy-associated T-cell lymphoma. J Clin Oncol. 2013;31(13):E226–E30.
26. Berman EL, Zauber NP, Rickert RR, Diss TC, Isaacson PG. Enteropathy-associated T cell lymphoma with brain involvement. J Clin Gastroenterol. 1998;26(4):337–41.
27. Gobbi C, Buess M, Probst A, Ruegg S, Schraml P, Herrmann R, et al. Enteropathy-associated T-cell lymphoma with initial manifestation in the CNS. Neurology. 2003;60(10):1718–9.
28. Bewig B, Wacker HH, Parwaresch MR, Nitsche R, Folsch UR. Eosinophilia-leading symptom of an enteropathy-associated T-cell lymphoma of high malignancy. Z Gastroenterol. 1993;31(11):666–70.
29. Hovenga S, de Graaf H, Joosten P, van den Berg GA, Storm H, Langerak AW, et al. Enteropathy-associated T-cell lymphoma presenting with eosinophilia. Neth J Med. 2003;61(1):25–7.
30. Soon CW, Kirsch IR, Connolly AJ, Kwong BY, Kim J. Eosinophil-rich acute febrile neutrophilic dermatosis in a patient with enteropathy-associated T-cell lymphoma, type 1. Am J Dermatopathol. 2016;38(9):704–8.
31. Schwock J, Hyjek EM, Torlakovic EE, Geddie WR. Enteropathy-associated intestinal T-cell lymphoma in cavitating mesenteric lymph node syndrome: fine-needle aspiration contributes to the diagnosis. Diagn Cytopathol. 2015;43(2):125–30.
32. Jousserand G, Poujois A, Antoine JC, Camdessanché JP. [Polyradiculopathy revealing an enteropathy associated T-cell lymphoma in a patient with celiac disease]. Rev Neurol (Paris). 2009;165(1):89–91.
33. Chan T, Lee E, Khong PL, Kwong YL, Tse E. Positron emission tomography computed tomography features of type ii enteropathy associated t cell lymphoma. Haematologica. 2016;101:689.
34. Mudhar HS, Fernando M, Rennie IG, Evans LS. Enteropathy-associated T-cell lymphoma, lacking MHC class II, with immune-privileged site recurrence, presenting as bilateral ocular vitreous humour involvement – a case report. Histopathology. 2012;61(6):1227–30.
35. Antoniadou F, Dimitrakopoulou A, Voutsinas PM, Vrettou K, Vlahadami I, Voulgarelis M, et al. Monomorphic epitheliotropic intestinal T-cell lymphoma in pleural effusion: a case report. Diagn Cytopathol. 2017;45(11):1050–4.
36. Tanaka H, Ambiru S, Nakamura S, Itabashi T, Furuya S, Shimura T, et al. Successful diagnosis of type II enteropathy-associated T-cell lymphoma using flow cytometry and the cell block

technique of celomic fluid manifesting as massive pyoid ascites that could not be diagnosed via emergency laparotomy. Intern Med. 2014;53(2):129–33.
37. Webster A, Crea P, Bamford MW, Hew R, Griffin Y, Miall F. Enteropathy-associated T-cell lymphoma presenting as cutaneous deposits. Br J Haematol. 2017;176(1):7.
38. Chen JH, Bai D, Dabhi V, Wood BL, Kussick SJ. Clinicopathologic features of primary colonic enteropathy-associated T cell lymphoma type II in an elderly Asian male with diarrhea. J Hematop. 2015;8(1):37–41.
39. Tomizawa Y, Van Slambrouck C, Kavitt RT. A rare cause of diarrhea and weight loss type II (monomorphic) enteropathy-associated T-cell lymphoma. Gastroenterology. 2015;148(7):1288–9.
40. Kaif M, Fitzmorris P, Weber F. A rare case of chronic diarrhea enteropathy-associated T-cell lymphoma, type II. Gastroenterology. 2015;148(3):510–2.
41. Jacob PM, Nair RA, Mehta J, Borges AM, Suchetha S. Enteropathy associated T cell lymphoma-monomorphic variant, presenting as bilateral ovarian masses. Indian J Pathol Microbiol. 2014;57(2):326–8.
42. Chott A, Vesely M, Simonitsch I, Mosberger I, Hanak H. Classification of intestinal T-cell neoplasms and their differential diagnosis. Am J Clin Pathol. 1999;111(1):S68–74.
43. Smedby KE, Akerman M, Hildebrand H, Glimelius B, Ekbom A, Askling J. Malignant lymphomas in coeliac disease: evidence of increased risks for lymphoma types other than enteropathy-type T cell lymphoma. Gut. 2005;54(1):54–9.
44. Perry AM, Warnke RA, Hu QL, Gaulard P, Copie-Bergman C, Alkan S, et al. Indolent T-cell lymphoproliferative disease of the gastrointestinal tract. Blood. 2013;122(22):3599–606.
45. Arps DP, Smith LB. Classic versus type II enteropathy-associated T-cell lymphoma: diagnostic considerations. Arch Pathol Lab Med. 2013;137(9):1227–31.
46. Mutzbauer G, Maurus K, Buszello C, Pischimarov J, Roth S, Rosenwald A, et al. SYK expression in monomorphic epitheliotropic intestinal T-cell lymphoma. Mod Pathol. 2018;31(3):505–16.
47. Roberti A, Dobay MP, Bisig B, Vallois D, Boéchat C, Lanitis E, et al. Type II enteropathy-associated T-cell lymphoma features a unique genomic profile with highly recurrent SETD2 alterations. Nat Commun. 2016;7:12602.
48. Nairismagi ML, Tan J, Lim JQ, Nagarajan S, Ng CCY, Rajasegaran V, et al. JAK-STAT and G-protein-coupled receptor signaling pathways are frequently altered in epitheliotropic intestinal T-cell lymphoma. Leukemia. 2016;30(6):1311–9.
49. Moffitt AB, Ondrejka SL, McKinney M, Rempel RE, Goodlad JR, Teh CH, et al. Enteropathy-associated T cell lymphoma subtypes are characterized by loss of function of SETD2. J Exp Med. 2017;214(5):1371–86.
50. Hadithi M, Mallant M, Oudejans J, van Waesberghe J, Mulder CJ, Comans EFI. F-18-FDG PET versus CT for the detection of enteropathy-associated T-cell lymphoma in refractory celiac disease. J Nucl Med. 2006;47(10):1622–7.
51. Ellin F, Landstrom J, Jerkeman M, Relander T. Real-world data on prognostic factors and treatment in peripheral T-cell lymphomas: a study from the Swedish Lymphoma Registry. Blood. 2014;124(10):1570–7.
52. Mehta-Shah N, Horwitz S. Zebras and hen's teeth: recognition and management of rare T and NK lymphomas. Hematology Am Soc Hematol Educ Program. 2015;2015:545–9.
53. Novakovic BJ, Novakovic S, Frkovic-Grazio S. A single-center report on clinical features and treatment response in patients with intestinal T cell non-Hodgkin's lymphomas. Oncol Rep. 2006;16(1):191–5.
54. Egan LJ, Walsh SV, Stevens FM, Connolly CE, Egan EL, McCarthy CF. Celiac-associated lymphoma – a single institution experience of 30 cases in the combination chemotherapy era. J Clin Gastroenterol. 1995;21(2):123–9.
55. Honemann D, Prince HM, Hicks RJ, Seymour JF. Enteropathy-associated T-cell lymphoma without a prior diagnosis of coeliac disease: diagnostic dilemmas and management options. Ann Hematol. 2005;84(2):118–21.

56. Wohrer S, Chott A, Drach J, Puspok A, Hejna M, Hoffmann M, et al. Chemotherapy with cyclophosphamide, doxorubicin, etoposide, vincristine and prednisone (CHOEP) is not effective in patients with enteropathy-type intestinal T cell lymphoma. Ann Oncol. 2004;15(11):1680–3.
57. Daum S, Ullrich R, Heise W, Dederke B, Foss HD, Stein H, et al. Intestinal non-Hodgkin's lymphoma: a multicenter prospective clinical study from the German Study Group on Intestinal non-Hodgkin's Lymphoma. J Clin Oncol. 2003;21(14):2740–6.
58. d'Amore F, Relander T, Lauritzsen GF, Jantunen E, Hagberg H, Anderson H, et al. Up-front autologous stem-cell transplantation in peripheral T-cell lymphoma: NLG-T-01. J Clin Oncol. 2012;30(25):3093–9.
59. Bishton MJ, Haynes AP. Combination chemotherapy followed by autologous stem cell transplant for enteropathy-associated T cell lymphoma. Br J Haematol. 2007;136(1):111–3.
60. Jantunen E, Boumendil A, Finel H, Luan JJ, Johnson P, Rambaldi A, et al. Autologous stem cell transplantation for enteropathy-associated T-cell lymphoma: a retrospective study by the EBMT. Blood. 2013;121(13):2529–32.
61. Nijeboer P, Malamut G, Mulder CJ, Cerf-Bensussan N, Sibon D, Bouma G, et al. Enteropathy-associated T-cell lymphoma: improving treatment strategies. Dig Dis. 2015;33(2):231–5.
62. Ikebe T, Miyazaki Y, Abe Y, Urakami K, Ohtsuka E, Saburi Y, et al. Successful treatment of refractory enteropathy-associated T-cell lymphoma using high-dose chemotherapy and autologous stem cell transplantation. Intern Med. 2010;49(19):2157–61.
63. Raderer M, Troch M, Kiesewetter B, Puspok A, Jaeger U, Hoffmann M, et al. Second line chemotherapy in patients with enteropathy-associated T cell lymphoma: a retrospective single center analysis. Ann Hematol. 2012;91(1):57–61.
64. Mehta-Shah N, Teja ST, Tao Y, Cashen A, Beaven A, Alpdoogan O, et al. Successful treatment of mature T-cell lymphoma with allogeneic stem cell transplantation: the largest multicenter retrospective analysis. American Society of Hematology 59th Annual Meeting & Exposition; 12/11/2017; Atlanta, Georgia. 2017.
65. Foyil KV, Bartlett NL. Brentuximab vedotin for the treatment of CD30(+) lymphomas. Immunotherapy. 2011;3(4):475–85.
66. Khalaf WF, Caldwell ME, Reddy N. Brentuximab in the treatment of CD30-positive enteropathy-associated T-cell lymphoma. J Natl Compr Cancer Netw. 2013;11(2):137–40.
67. Haslbauer F. Brentuximab vedotin in a patient with enteropathy-associated T-cell lymphoma of the small bowel. Memo-Mag Eur Med Oncol. 2017;10(2):111–4.
68. Marquard L, Poulsen CB, Gjerdrum LM, Brown PD, Christensen IJ, Jensen PB, et al. Histone deacetylase 1, 2, 6 and acetylated histone H4 in B- and T-cell lymphomas. Histopathology. 2009;54(6):688–98.
69. Piekarz RL, Frye R, Prince HM, Kirschbaum MH, Zain J, Allen SL, et al. Phase 2 trial of romidepsin in patients with peripheral T-cell lymphoma. Blood. 2011;117(22):5827–34.
70. Zhang YP, Xu W, Liu H, Li JY. Therapeutic options in peripheral T cell lymphoma. J Hematol Oncol. 2016;9:37.
71. Iyer SP, Foss FF. Romidepsin for the treatment of peripheral T-cell lymphoma. Oncologist. 2015;20(9):1084–91.
72. O'Connor OA, Horwitz S, Masszi T, Van Hoof A, Brown P, Doorduijn J, et al. Belinostat in patients with relapsed or refractory peripheral T-cell lymphoma: results of the pivotal phase II BELIEF (CLN-19) study. J Clin Oncol. 2015;33(23):2492–U21.
73. Horwitz SM, Porcu P, Flinn I, Kahl BS, Sweeney J, Stern HM, et al. Duvelisib (IPI-145), a phosphoinositide-3-kinase-delta,gamma inhibitor, shows activity in patients with relapsed/refractory T-cell lymphoma. Blood. 2014;124(21):803.
74. Porcu P, Flinn I, Kahl BS, Horwitz SM, Oki Y, Byrd JC, et al. Clinical activity of duvelisib (IPI-145), a phosphoinositide-3-kinase-delta, gamma inhibitor, in patients previously treated with ibrutinib. Blood. 2014;124(21):Abstract 3335.
75. Horwitz SM, Koch R, Porcu P, Oki Y, Moskowitz A, Perez M, et al. Activity of the PI3K-delta,gamma inhibitor duvelisib in a phase 1 trial and preclinical models of T-cell lymphoma. Blood. 2018;131(8):888–98.

76. de Baaij LR, Radersma M, van de Water JM, Hijmering NJ, Moesbergen L, Visser O, et al. Bortezomib restores defective apoptosis by upregulation of Noxa in enteropathy-associated T-cell lymphoma. Gastroenterology. 2013;144(5):S250–S.
77. Toumishey E, Prasad A, Dueck G, Chua N, Finch D, Johnston J, et al. Final report of a phase 2 clinical trial of lenalidomide monotherapy for patients with T-cell lymphoma. Cancer. 2015;121(5):716–23.
78. Rodig SJ, Abramson JS, Pinkus GS, Treon SP, Dorfman DM, Dong HY, et al. Heterogeneous CD52 expression among hematologic neoplasms: implications for the use of alemtuzumab (CAMPATH-1H). Clin Cancer Res. 2006;12(23):7174–9.
79. Gallamini A, Zaja F, Patti C, Billio A, Specchia MR, Tucci A, et al. Alemtuzumab (Campath-1H) and CHOP chemotherapy as first-line treatment of peripheral T-cell lymphoma: results of a GITIL (Grappo Italiano Terapie Innovative nei Linfomi) prospective multicenter trial. Blood. 2007;110(7):2316–23.
80. Soldini D, Mora O, Cavalli F, Zucca E, Mazzucchelli L. Efficacy of alemtuzumab and gemcitabine in a patient with enteropathy-type T-cell lymphoma. Br J Haematol. 2008;142(3):484–6.
81. Gentille C, Qin Q, Barbieri A, Ravi PS, Iyer S. Use of PEG-asparaginase in monomorphic epitheliotropic intestinal T-cell lymphoma, a disease with diagnostic and therapeutic challenges. Ecancermedicalscience. 2017;11:771.
82. Hamlin P, Farber C, Fenske T, Khatcheressian J, Miller C, Munoz J, et al. The dual SYK/JAK inhibitor cerdulatinib demonstrates complete inhibition of SYK and JAK and rapid tumor responses in a phase 2 study in patients with relapsed/refractory b cell malignancies. Haematologica. 2017;102:312–3.
83. Feldman AL, Sun DX, Law ME, Novak AJ, Attygalle AD, Thorland EC, et al. Overexpression of Syk tyrosine kinase in peripheral T-cell lymphomas. Leukemia. 2008;22(6):1139–43.
84. Wilcox RA, Sun DX, Novak A, Dogan A, Ansell SM, Feldman AL. Inhibition of Syk protein tyrosine kinase induces apoptosis and blocks proliferation in T-cell non-Hodgkin's lymphoma cell lines. Leukemia. 2010;24(1):229–32.

Chapter 13
Hepatosplenic T-Cell Lymphoma

Shekeab Jauhari and Matt McKinney

Introduction

Hepatosplenic T-cell lymphomas (HSTL) are exceedingly rare, accounting for ~1.4% of cases of peripheral T-cell or NK/T-cell lymphomas in the United States and Europe [1]. To date, several hundred cases of hepatosplenic T-cell lymphoma have been reported in the literature in single case reports and patient series. Using cases reported in the SEER database, the calculated incidence of hepatosplenic T-cell lymphoma in the United States was 1.8 cases per 100 million person-years in 2000 and had gradually risen to 15.2 cases per 100 million person-years by 2012 [2]. The median overall survival of patients in this report was 8.8 months and a 5-year overall survival rate of 14.6%, reflecting the high burden of disease-related mortality [2].

Based on large epidemiologic reviews, particular clinical risk factors for the development of hepatosplenic T-cell lymphoma have been identified. Approximately 18% of patients have immunocompromised status, characterized by a history of autoimmune disease, solid organ transplantation, or hematologic malignancy, while another 8% of patients have a history of inflammatory bowel disease and use of immunosuppressants [2, 3]. The report of eight patients with inflammatory bowel disease and concomitant use of infliximab who developed HSTL led the FDA to issue a black box warning in August 2006 [4, 5]. Since then, it has been better appre-

S. Jauhari
Medical Oncology and Cellular Therapy, Duke University Medical Center, Durham, NC, USA
e-mail: shekeab.jauhari@duke.edu

M. McKinney (✉)
Division of Hematologic Malignancies, Department of Medicine, Duke University School of Medicine, Durham, NC, USA
e-mail: mckin028@mc.duke.edu

C. Dittus (ed.), *Novel Therapeutics for Rare Lymphomas*,
https://doi.org/10.1007/978-3-030-25610-4_13

ciated that the risk of hepatosplenic T-cell lymphoma is higher in IBD patients using thioguanines alone or in combination with anti-TNF agents, including infliximab [2]. The risk of HSTL is higher in young males but is still a rare event; even in those receiving the higher risk combination therapy, the risk of HSTL is estimated to occur in 1:3000–1:7000 cases [6]. This risk of hepatosplenic T-cell lymphoma must be balanced with the significant clinical benefit that may be derived from the use of immunosuppressants in IBD.

Clinical Features

Hepatosplenic T-cell lymphomas are characterized by prototypical clinical features and aggressive courses. Patients are usually young at the time of presentation, with a median age of 23–42 years reported in the largest single-patient case series [7–12]. Most are male, reported as 60–83% across these case series. African Americans have been shown to have a higher incidence than other ethnic groups [2]. While predisposing conditions for HSTL (autoimmune disease, prior organ transplantation, use of immunosuppression, or malignancy) are important, most patients do not have these underlying risk factors [2, 3]. Disease-related morbidity in these otherwise young, healthy individuals can lead to significant functional compromise, with 38% of patients reported to have an ECOG performance status of 2–4 in one series [12].

Characteristic patterns of organ involvement, signs, and symptoms have been described among patients with HSTL [7–12]. Splenomegaly is a near-universal feature, identified in 95–100% of cases across patient series. Massive splenomegaly (weight ≥1000 g, spleen tip ≥6 cm below costal margin) was identified in 76% of patients in a series from MD Anderson Cancer Center (MDACC) [11]. Hepatomegaly occurs in most patients, reported in 58–88% of cases [7–12]. Bone marrow involvement has also been reported in approximately 70–100% of cases [7–12]. Median bone marrow involvement in one series was reported at 30% among patients, typically featuring an interstitial and sinusoidal pattern involvement [11]. Notably, lymphadenopathy is an uncommon feature, reported in only 0–25% of cases [7–12]. B symptoms are frequently observed, however, in up to 70–100% of patients. In our experience with HSTL, we have noted intermittent fevers in the setting of lack of documented infection, as well as elevated sedimentation rates and bouts of hypotension as a common presentation. It is possible that this constellation of symptoms and inflammatory markers is related to tumor-related cytokine release; these findings generally resolve with effective treatment.

The presence of specific laboratory abnormalities may further distinguish HSTL from other lymphoma subtypes. Cytopenias are frequently observed: among patients across series, thrombocytopenia has been reported in 61–95%, anemia in 71–88%, and leukopenia in 43–58% [7–12]. The etiology of cytopenias in these patients remains unclear. Splenomegaly is hypothesized to contribute, although cytopenias appear to correspond with disease progression, even among patients with prior splenectomy [7]. While bone marrow involvement is common, infiltration is typically low and does not appear to correspond with the degree of cytopenias observed. Soluble factors elaborated by malignant lymphocytes, including IFN-γ, may otherwise mediate bone marrow suppression. Elevations of AST, ALT, or alkaline phosphatase are typically mild, observed in 38–71% of cases. Patients commonly present with jaundice, with elevated bilirubin reported in 50% of patients in a single series [7–12]. Other markers of inflammation are often elevated as well, including beta-2 microglobulin in 90% of patients in one series and LDH in 50–91% of patients [7–12].

Other clinical features, including circulating disease, central nervous system involvement, or other sites of extranodal spread, are infrequently reported in HSTL [13]. Lymphocytosis is rare, observed in less than 10% of cases. Presentations mimicking acute lymphoblastic leukemia have been reported, with large populations of blast-like cells found on bone marrow biopsy among patients with pancytopenia [14, 15]. Hemophagocytic lymphohistiocytosis (HLH) also mimics the presentation of HSTL, but the pathologic finding of hemophagocytosis is rare in the latter [13]. CNS involvement was reported in only one patient in a large, single-center retrospective series, while cutaneous involvement [16, 17] and other atypical presentations of pathologic phenotype or clinical presentation have been reported as case reports or case series. Figure 13.1 summarizes radiologic, laboratory findings and the clinical course of a patient who was treated for chemorefractory HSTL, and our experience is that this case is representative of most HSTL patient experiences.

Approximately 20% of cases of hepatosplenic T-cell lymphoma feature clonality of the αβ T-cell receptor [12, 18]. The clinical, pathologic, and genetic features of hepatosplenic αβ T-cell lymphoma resemble the γδ subtype [19]. In some series, there is the suggested association of the αβ subtype with female gender and reduced survival compared with the γδ subtype, although it is unclear whether these are true associations or reflect selective reporting.

The median time from onset of symptoms to diagnosis is 60–75 days across series [7–12]. The diagnosis of HSTL is often delayed, as the most common findings, including hepatosplenomegaly, B symptoms, and thrombocytopenia, may form a broad differential. This may include viral syndromes, primary liver disease, or other hematologic malignancies, including myeloproliferative neoplasms or acute leukemia. Splenectomy may lead to improvement in thrombocytopenia, leading to the mistaken diagnosis of immune thrombocytopenic purpura [7]. The absence of lymphadenopathy in most cases and rarity of HSTL may also delay consideration of lymphoma.

Diagnosis, Staging, and Workup

Due to the lack of extensive nodal involvement at presentation in HSTL cases, diagnostic samples are most often obtained via bone marrow aspirate/trephine samples or liver biopsies. The neoplastic cells in HSTL are typically positive for CD3 and

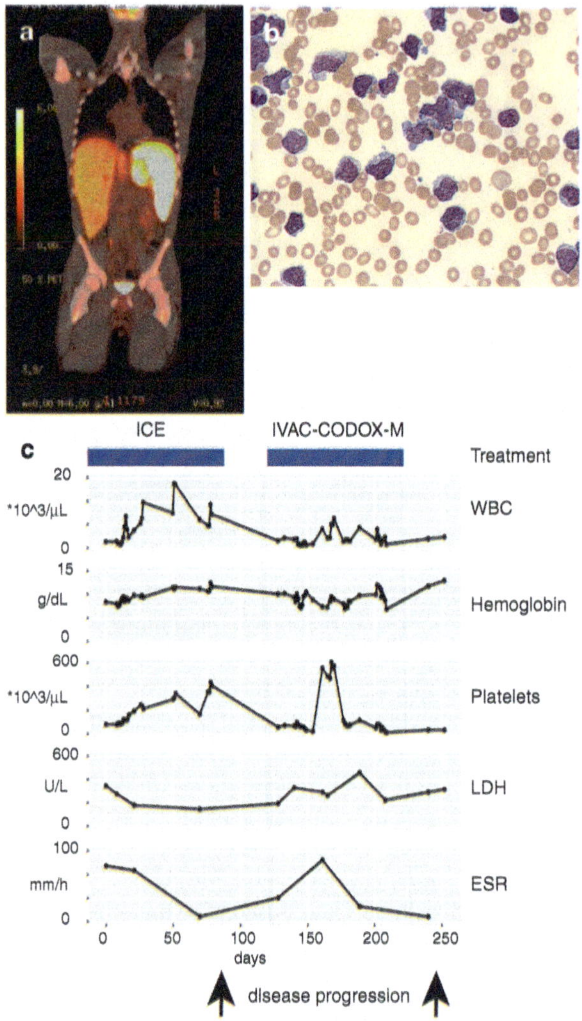

Fig. 13.1 Clinical presentation and course of a hepatosplenic T cell lymphoma patient (HSTL). Initial PET CT showing massive hepatosplenomegaly as HSTL diagnosis (**a**). Peripheral blood film of HSTL leukemia involvement (**b**). Clinical course and variation in blood counts and inflammatory biomarkers in HSTL treated with multiple therapies (**c**). *ICE* ifosfamide, carboplatin, etoposide, *CODOX-M/IVAC* cyclophosphamide, vincristine, doxorubicin, high-dose methotrexate/ ifosfamide, etoposide, and high-dose cytarabine

TCRd1, while TCRab is generally negative (although cases have been reported with a CD3+ TCRab+ phenotype). Cells are variably positive for CD56 and CD8 and are typically negative for CD4 and CD5 [20]. Cytotoxic granules can be found in HSTL, and often TIA1 or granzyme M is positive but negative for granzyme B and perforin [21]. HSTL cell may exhibit staining for other markers found on mature nonactivated cytotoxic T cells such as KIRs and CD94 [22]. Additionally, HSTL cells generally have rearranged TRG@ genes, consistent with a T-cell origin [22]. The most frequent cytogenetic rearrangements found in HSTL include isochromosome 7q or ring chromosome 7q with additional structural abnormalities, occurring in 30–50% of cases, followed by trisomy 8 [23–26]. HSTL is not generally associated with Epstein-Barr virus positivity or other oncogenic viruses [27].

Conventional Treatment Approach

A variety of combination chemotherapy approaches have been utilized in the treatment of hepatosplenic T-cell lymphoma. In the earliest patient series, CHOP or CHOP-like regimens were reported as the most frequently used for induction treatment. In one series, 12/19 or 63% of patients receiving one of these regimens had clinical responses, including half with complete remissions [28]. In another series, 6/12 or 50% of patients receiving CHOP or CHOP-like regimens had responses, with one complete remission reported [10]. More intensive chemotherapy regimens have been used as well. In a series reported from MDACC, 15/27 patients received HyperCVAD or HyperCVAD-like regimens for induction treatment [18]. On univariate analysis, this was associated with a HR of 0.6 compared to other regimens and trended toward significance with respect to overall survival. Platinum- and cytarabine-containing regimens have also been utilized for induction treatment with good effect. In a series from Memorial Sloan Kettering Cancer Center (MSKCC), 8/14 patients received ICE or IVAC for induction treatment, with 75% achieving clinical responses and a 50% rate of complete remission [29]. In the same series, 4/14 patients received CHOP, with 3/4 (75%) achieving clinical responses but 1/4 (25%) achieving complete remission. Two thirds of patients who received ICE after partial responses or disease progression with CHOP went on to achieve complete remissions. Overall, this suggests that high proportions of patients may achieve responses with induction chemotherapy. Further, more intensive combinations of chemotherapy, including platinum- and cytarabine-containing regimens, may yield higher responses than CHOP or CHOP-like regimens, but with limited data, no single regimen or approach is clearly superior.

Other treatment approaches for HSTL have yielded variable success. Splenectomy may allow for transient recovery of platelets, but does not provide for more meaningful responses [7]. Pentostatin has been reported to yield complete remissions as a single agent in case reports [30, 31]. Alemtuzumab, either with or without cladribine, has also been reported to yield complete remissions in case reports [32, 33]. Whether these agents should be utilized in novel combinations, their optimal sequence of administration, and their efficacy relative to combination chemotherapy for hepatosplenic T-cell lymphoma, remains unclear and warrants further investigation.

Despite high rates of response with induction therapy, relapses occur often and early and are a common cause of mortality. In one series, the median time to relapse among patients achieving a complete response to induction therapy with CHOP or CHOP-like regimens was 3–16 months [28]. In the same series, although all patients received induction therapy, 17/21 or 81% of ultimately died of disease. Among patients with partial responses, disease progression, or relapses after induction therapy, intensified treatment may allow for further disease control, although this has not been systematically evaluated [29].

Consolidative stem cell transplantation has allowed for the possibility of durable remissions for a subset of patients with HSTL. In a series from MSKCC, patients achieving at least a partial response after chemotherapy went on to receive consolidative stem cell transplantation. High-dose chemotherapy and autologous stem cell transplantation were performed in four patients, with two achieving durable remissions. Allogeneic stem cell transplantation was administered to eight patients, with two patients relapsing and another two having transplant-related mortality [29]. In a retrospective review performed by the European Society for Bone and Marrow Transplantation Lymphoma Working Party, 25 patients receiving consolidative stem cell transplantation were evaluated. With a median follow-up of 3 years, 5 of 7 patients relapsed after autologous stem cell transplantation, while 2 of 18 patients relapsed after allogeneic stem cell transplantation, suggesting the utility of the latter approach. In a separate review of 44 patients receiving allogeneic stem cell transplantation, 35% of patients relapsed, but none were observed 1.5 years after transplant. The estimated 3-year overall survival was 56%, while the cause of death was non-relapse mortality in 68% and relapse in 32% [34]. Interestingly, disease status at the time of transplant (whether complete or partial response) was not associated with outcome. Overall, these reports suggest the utility of consolidative allogeneic stem cell transplantation for this disease.

Novel Agents

Frontline Novel Agents With or Without Chemotherapy

As in other peripheral T-cell lymphoma entities, frontline treatment of HSTL generally employs agents found to be most active in B-cell lymphoma induction or salvage treatment with or without novel molecularly targeted or immunotherapy agents. Potential targeted agents with proven safety and efficacy when added to chemotherapy backbone programs include histone deacetylase (HDAC) inhibitors such as romidepsin [35–37] or belinostat [38] and immunomodulatory drugs such as lenalidomide [39–42]. Ongoing studies utilizing such approaches may yield evidence for this type of approach in HSTL and other PTCLs soon. It is unclear what role novel agents may play when administered with frontline high-intensity chemotherapeutic strategies. Other agents such as mogamulizumab [43] or other novel targeted agents or immunotherapy approaches may also prove useful in some HSTL patients, but these approaches are untested in HSTL.

Novel Agents in the Relapsed Setting

Unfortunately, due to the rarity of HSTL, it is unclear how best to approach relapsed or refractory HSTL. Based upon reports studying the biology of the disease, potential therapeutics of interest include ones targeting the SYK signaling access, IL-2 signaling modulators including JAK-STAT or PI-3 kinase inhibitors, or dysregulated epigenetic signaling in the disease.

In the initial report of microarray-based gene expression from Travert et al., Syk overexpression was noted among HSTL samples as compared to normal control γδ-T cells, and treatment with a model Syk inhibitor effected cellular apoptosis in cell line assays. Additionally, in this study, HSTL cells were found to be sensitive to demethylase inhibitors in vitro, and it was postulated this may have been associated with changes in expression of the epigenetic regulator AIM1 [44]. However, this report showcased a small number of HSTL tumors ($n = 9$) and used the only known patient-derived cell line representing HSTL [44].

Additional reports describing the results of targeted or whole-genome-/exome-based approaches to discover driver genes in HSTL have additionally uncovered potential targets for novel therapies in HSTL. *STAT5B* and *STAT3* are frequently mutated in HSTL [12, 45], and these genetic alterations occur in a constitutively activating fashion, thus serving to produce autonomous or amplified JAK-STAT signaling in HSTL cells. In the report by McKinney et al. documenting the genetic landscape of mutations in HSTL, JAK-STAT and PI-3 kinase signaling mediators were shown to be mutated frequently in HSTL with approximately 40% of cases having an activating mutation in one of these genes. Gene mutations in these signaling mediators appear to be activating based on experiments done in this and other studies, and the pattern of mutations documented in HSTL suggests these alterations may play an important role in producing constitutively active or amplified receptor-based IL-2 signaling in HSTL cells [12].

In preclinical models, HSTL cells are dependent upon IL-2 for growth in vitro, and STAT5B mutations appear to synergize with PI-3 kinase (PIK3CD gene) mutations, thus creating the possibility of a synergistic approach using combination JAK-STAT and PI-3 kinase inhibition. Indeed, using specific STAT5B inhibitors in combination with inhibitors specific for the δ-isoform of PI-3 kinase appears to synergistically suppress HSTL cell growth and may be an opportunity for clinical translation using available agents such as ruxolitinib [46, 47] and idelalisib [12, 48].

Analysis of somatic mutations in HSTL has elucidated other potential synthetic lethal targets. The histone-lysine methyltransferase SETD2 is mutated in more than 30% of cases of HSTL [12] (as well as enteropathy associated T-cell lymphoma [49, 50]) and, similar to mutation of JAK-STAT signal modifiers, is one of the most common genetic alterations in the disease. SETD2 mutations occur in a pattern suggestive of causing gene loss of function (frequent biallelic mutations of stop gain producing frameshift mutations are common). SETD2 loss in HSTL is thus frequent and confirms a tumor suppressor role in these tumors; cancer cells may benefit from SETD2 loss via deregulation of cell cycle control and loss of response to DNA damage/homologous repair among other mechanisms [51–56]. Interestingly, SETD2-mutated cells may be vulnerable to WEE1 inhibition or other synthetic lethal strategies based upon loss of SETD2 and the alteration of myriad cellular functions mediated by SETD2 including histone and actin methylation and downstream effects [57]. WEE1 inhibitors such as AZD1775 are currently under clinical investigation in several different tumor types, and this may represent an opportunity for a novel therapy in tumors with SETD2 as frequently occurs in HSTL.

Despite the progress in the molecular understanding of HSTL, few translational studies have been initiated. The overall low incidence of HSTL as compared to other lymphomas has limited the ability to create HSTL-specific clinical trial protocols. Perhaps the development of HSTL-specific research consortia within academic medical centers can help to study the clinical relevance of aberrant signaling pathways in HSTL. Similarly, the adoption of molecularly targeted approaches is limited given the sparse incidence of HSTL, unless cases are incorporated as part of broader investigative efforts in PTCLs or other broader clinical trials.

Recommended Treatment Approach

Our standard approach is to use platinum- and cytarabine-containing chemotherapy such as the dexamethasone, high-dose solumedrol, platinum regimen (DHAP), or other similar regimens such as ESHAP [58] for frontline induction treatment of HSTL with autologous or allogeneic transplant consolidation for patients who achieve a good response and who are eligible. IVAC chemotherapy, or a metronomic anthracycline-containing program with modifications such as the CALGB 10002 regimen [59] (dosed without rituximab), contains agents active against HSTL and may have the advantage of alternating non-cross-resistant chemotherapy. With initial treatment, responding patients often have rapid improvement or correction of cytopenias and symptoms such as fever and hepatosplenomegaly. In responding patients fit for intensive chemotherapy and consolidative transplant, we immediately refer for consideration of high-dose therapy with stem cell support, and our preference is to recommend allogeneic transplant if feasible including dual umbilical cord transplantation in patients that lack well-matched conventional donor grafts. In patients that fail initial chemotherapy induction, we generally will try an alternative non-cross-resistant cytotoxic chemotherapy regimen; however, HSTL patients are often highly chemotherapy-refractory after failing cytotoxic agents and initial responses to induction treatment can be transient. In the case of chemotherapy-refractory disease, our approach is to try novel agents as off-label therapy to attempt to achieve a response. In our experience, responses, including complete remissions, have been reached with pralatrexate and other agents, and pralatrexate in combination with romidepsin [60] showed excellent activity and an acceptable toxicity profile in a phase I/II study of PTCL cases including a few patients with HSTL. In patients with CD52-expressing HSTL, we additionally consider alemtuzumab in combination with cladribine or other chemotherapy agents as per small case reports [32, 33, 61, 62]. Patients treated in such fashion that respond should then be reconsidered for hematopoietic stem cell transplantation-based consolidation treatments.

Other potential novel agents for off-label use in relapsed/refractory HSTL, based upon studies of the molecular biology of the disease, could also be considered. These include other epigenetic modifiers or targeted molecular agents that inhibit molecular pathways of interest in HSTL. JAK-STAT inhibitors such as ruxolitinib or PI-3 kinase inhibitors such as copanlisib are in use for other hematologic malignancies and may be useful as single agents or combination with other targeted small molecule inhibitors or conventional chemotherapy for off-label compassionate use outside of a clinical trial protocol.

Summary

HSTL is a rare lymphoma that often affects young adults. HSTL cases exhibit a dire prognosis, even when compared to other T-cell lymphomas. Distinct from other PTCL entities, HSTL exhibits a unique molecular/genomic phenotype that may be utilized for improved diagnostic and treatment algorithms in the future. Currently, while treatment algorithms applied to other lymphoma subtypes are used to treat HSTL cases, the unacceptably poor outcomes with this approach confirms we need new treatments in order to potentially stop this scourge.

References

1. Vose J, Armitage J, Weisenburger D. International peripheral T-cell and natural killer/T-cell lymphoma study: pathology findings and clinical outcomes. J Clin Oncol. 2008;26:4124–30.
2. Durani U, Go RS. Incidence, clinical findings, and survival of hepatosplenic T-cell lymphoma in the United States. Am J Hematol. 2017;92:E99–e101.
3. Thai A, Prindiville T. Hepatosplenic T-cell lymphoma and inflammatory bowel disease. J Crohn's Colitis. 2010;4:511–22.
4. Mackey AC, Green L, Leptak C, Avigan M. Hepatosplenic T cell lymphoma associated with infliximab use in young patients treated for inflammatory bowel disease: update. J Pediatr Gastroenterol Nutr. 2009;48:386–8.
5. Mackey AC, Green L, Liang LC, Dinndorf P, Avigan M. Hepatosplenic T cell lymphoma associated with infliximab use in young patients treated for inflammatory bowel disease. J Pediatr Gastroenterol Nutr. 2007;44:265–7.
6. Kotlyar DS, Osterman MT, Diamond RH, et al. A systematic review of factors that contribute to hepatosplenic T-cell lymphoma in patients with inflammatory bowel disease. Clin Gastroenterol Hepatol. 2011;9:36–41.e1.
7. Weidmann E. Hepatosplenic T cell lymphoma. A review on 45 cases since the first report describing the disease as a distinct lymphoma entity in 1990. Leukemia. 2000;14:991–7.
8. Belhadj K, Reyes F, Farcet JP, et al. Hepatosplenic gammadelta T-cell lymphoma is a rare clinicopathologic entity with poor outcome: report on a series of 21 patients. Blood. 2003;102:4261–9.
9. Falchook GS, Vega F, Dang NH, et al. Hepatosplenic gamma-delta T-cell lymphoma: clinicopathological features and treatment. Ann Oncol. 2009;20:1080–5.
10. Lu CL, Tang Y, Yang QP, et al. Hepatosplenic T-cell lymphoma: clinicopathologic, immunophenotypic, and molecular characterization of 17 Chinese cases. Human Pathol. 2011;42:1965–78.
11. Yabe M, Medeiros LJ, Tang G, et al. Prognostic factors of hepatosplenic T-cell lymphoma: clinicopathologic study of 28 cases. Am J Surg Pathol. 2016;40:676–88.

12. McKinney M, Moffitt AB, Gaulard P, et al. The genetic basis of hepatosplenic T-cell lymphoma. Cancer Discov. 2017;7:369–79.
13. Yabe M, Miranda RN, Medeiros LJ. Hepatosplenic T-cell Lymphoma: a review of clinicopathologic features, pathogenesis, and prognostic factors. Hum Pathol. 2018;74:5–16.
14. Arnoux I, Loosveld M. Hepatosplenic T-cell lymphoma: an acute leukemia presentation. Blood. 2016;127:269.
15. Pizzi M, Covey S, Mathew S, et al. Hepatosplenic T-Cell lymphoma mimicking acute myeloid leukemia. Clin Lymphoma Myeloma Leuk. 2016;16:e47–50.
16. Hocker TL, Wada DA, McPhail ED, Porrata LF, el-Azhary RA, Gibson LE. Relapsed hepatosplenic T-cell lymphoma heralded by a solitary skin nodule. J Cutan Pathol. 2011;38:899–904.
17. Karpate A, Barcena C, Hohl D, Bisig B, de Leval L. Cutaneous presentation of hepatosplenic T-cell lymphoma-a potential mimicker of primary cutaneous gamma-delta T-cell lymphoma. Virchows Arch. 2016;469:591–6.
18. Yabe M, Medeiros LJ, Wang SA, et al. Clinicopathologic, immunophenotypic, cytogenetic, and molecular features of gammadelta T-Cell large granular lymphocytic leukemia: an analysis of 14 patients suggests biologic differences with alphabeta T-Cell large granular lymphocytic leukemia. [corrected]. Am J Clin Pathol. 2015;144:607–19.
19. Macon WR, Levy NB, Kurtin PJ, et al. Hepatosplenic alphabeta T-cell lymphomas: a report of 14 cases and comparison with hepatosplenic gammadelta T-cell lymphomas. Am J Surg Pathol. 2001;25:285–96.
20. Gaulard P, Bourquelot P, Kanavaros P, et al. Expression of the alpha/beta and gamma/delta T-cell receptors in 57 cases of peripheral T-cell lymphomas. Identification of a subset of gamma/delta T-cell lymphomas. Am J Pathol. 1990;137:617–28.
21. Felgar RE, Macon WR, Kinney MC, Roberts S, Pasha T, Salhany KE. TIA-1 expression in lymphoid neoplasms. Identification of subsets with cytotoxic T lymphocyte or natural killer cell differentiation. Am J Pathol. 1997;150:1893–900.
22. Cooke CB, Krenacs L, Stetler-Stevenson M, et al. Hepatosplenic T-cell lymphoma: a distinct clinicopathologic entity of cytotoxic gamma delta T-cell origin. Blood. 1996;88:4265–74.
23. Wang CC, Tien HF, Lin MT, et al. Consistent presence of isochromosome 7q in hepatosplenic T gamma/delta lymphoma: a new cytogenetic-clinicopathologic entity. Genes Chromosomes Cancer. 1995;12:161–4.
24. Jonveaux P, Daniel MT, Martel V, Maarek O, Berger R. Isochromosome 7q and trisomy 8 are consistent primary, non-random chromosomal abnormalities associated with hepatosplenic T gamma/delta lymphoma. Leukemia. 1996;10:1453–5.
25. Alonsozana E, Stamberg J, Kumar D, et al. Isochromosome 7q: the primary cytogenetic abnormality in hepatosplenic T cell lymphoma. Leukemia. 1997;11:1367–72.
26. Shetty S, Mansoor A, Roland B. Ring chromosome 7 with amplification of 7q sequences in a pediatric case of hepatosplenic T-cell lymphoma. Cancer Genet Cytogenet. 2006;167:161–3.
27. Lavergne A, Brocheriou I, Delfau MH, Copie-Bergman C, Houdart R, Gaulard PH. Primary intestinal gamma-delta T-cell lymphoma with evidence of Epstein-Barr virus. Histopathology. 1998;32:271–6.
28. Belhadj K, Reyes F, Farcet J-P, et al. Hepatosplenic γδ T-cell lymphoma is a rare clinicopathologic entity with poor outcome: report on a series of 21 patients. Blood. 2003;102:4261–9.
29. Voss MH, Lunning MA, Maragulia JC, et al. Intensive induction chemotherapy followed by early high-dose therapy and hematopoietic stem cell transplantation results in improved outcome for patients with hepatosplenic T-cell lymphoma: a single institution experience. Clin Lymphoma Myeloma Leuk. 2013;13:8–14.
30. Iannitto E, Barbera V, Quintini G, Cirrincione S, Leone M. Hepatosplenic gammadelta T-cell lymphoma: complete response induced by treatment with pentostatin. Br J Haematol. 2002;117:995–6.
31. Corazzelli G, Capobianco G, Russo F, Frigeri F, Aldinucci D, Pinto A. Pentostatin (2'-deoxycoformycin) for the treatment of hepatosplenic gammadelta T-cell lymphomas. Haematologica. 2005;90:Ecr14.

32. Mittal S, Milner BJ, Johnston PW, Culligan DJ. A case of hepatosplenic gamma-delta T-cell lymphoma with a transient response to fludarabine and alemtuzumab. Eur J Haematol. 2006;76:531–4.
33. Jaeger G, Bauer F, Brezinschek R, Beham-Schmid C, Mannhalter C, Neumeister P. Hepatosplenic gammadelta T-cell lymphoma successfully treated with a combination of alemtuzumab and cladribine. Ann Oncol. 2008;19:1025–6.
34. Rashidi A, Cashen AF. Outcomes of allogeneic stem cell transplantation in hepatosplenic T-cell lymphoma. Blood Cancer J. 2015;5:e318.
35. Piekarz RL, Frye R, Prince HM, et al. Phase 2 trial of romidepsin in patients with peripheral T-cell lymphoma. Blood. 2011;117:5827–34.
36. Coiffier B, Pro B, Prince HM, et al. Results from a pivotal, open-label, phase II study of romidepsin in relapsed or refractory peripheral T-cell lymphoma after prior systemic therapy. J Clin Oncol. 2012;30:631–6.
37. Dupuis J, Morschhauser F, Ghesquieres H, et al. Combination of romidepsin with cyclophosphamide, doxorubicin, vincristine, and prednisone in previously untreated patients with peripheral T-cell lymphoma: a non-randomised, phase 1b/2 study. Lancet Haematol. 2015;2:e160–5.
38. O'Connor OA, Horwitz S, Masszi T, et al. Belinostat in patients with relapsed or refractory peripheral T-Cell lymphoma: results of the pivotal phase II BELIEF (CLN-19) study. J Clin Oncol. 2015;33:2492–9.
39. Zinzani PL, Pellegrini C, Broccoli A, et al. Lenalidomide monotherapy for relapsed/refractory peripheral T-cell lymphoma not otherwise specified. Leukemia Lymphoma. 2011;52:1585–8.
40. Morschhauser F, Fitoussi O, Haioun C, et al. A phase 2, multicentre, single-arm, open-label study to evaluate the safety and efficacy of single-agent lenalidomide (Revlimid) in subjects with relapsed or refractory peripheral T-cell non-Hodgkin lymphoma: the EXPECT trial. Eur J Cancer. 2013;49:2869–76.
41. Hopfinger G, Nosslinger T, Lang A, et al. Lenalidomide in combination with vorinostat and dexamethasone for the treatment of relapsed/refractory peripheral T cell lymphoma (PTCL): report of a phase I/II trial. Ann Hematol. 2014;93:459–62.
42. Ogura M, Imaizumi Y, Uike N, et al. Lenalidomide in relapsed adult T-cell leukaemia-lymphoma or peripheral T-cell lymphoma (ATLL-001): a phase 1, multicentre, dose-escalation study. Lancet Haematol. 2016;3:e107–18.
43. Duvic M, Pinter-Brown LC, Foss FM, et al. Phase 1/2 study of mogamulizumab, a defucosylated anti-CCR4 antibody, in previously treated patients with cutaneous T-cell lymphoma. Blood. 2015;125:1883–9.
44. Travert M, Huang Y, de Leval L, et al. Molecular features of hepatosplenic T-cell lymphoma unravels potential novel therapeutic targets. Blood. 2012;119:5795–806.
45. Nicolae A, Xi L, Pittaluga S, et al. Frequent STAT5B mutations in gammadelta hepatosplenic T-cell lymphomas. Leukemia. 2014;28:2244–8.
46. Quintas-Cardama A, Vaddi K, Liu P, et al. Preclinical characterization of the selective JAK1/2 inhibitor INCB018424: therapeutic implications for the treatment of myeloproliferative neoplasms. Blood. 2010;115:3109–17.
47. Verstovsek S. Therapeutic potential of JAK2 inhibitors. Hematology/the Education Program of the American Society of Hematology American Society of Hematology Education Program 2009:636–42.
48. Fruman DA, Rommel C. PI3Kdelta inhibitors in cancer: rationale and serendipity merge in the clinic. Cancer Discov. 2011;1:562–72.
49. Moffitt AB, Ondrejka SL, McKinney M, et al. Enteropathy-associated T cell lymphoma subtypes are characterized by loss of function of SETD2. J Exp Med. 2017;214:1371–86.
50. Roberti A, Dobay MP, Bisig B, et al. Type II enteropathy-associated T-cell lymphoma features a unique genomic profile with highly recurrent SETD2 alterations. Nat Commun. 2016;7:12602.
51. Fahey CC, Davis IJ. SETting the stage for cancer development: SETD2 and the consequences of lost methylation. Cold Spring Harbor Perspect Med. 2017;7
52. Li J, Duns G, Westers H, Sijmons R, van den Berg A, Kok K. SETD2: an epigenetic modifier with tumor suppressor functionality. Oncotarget. 2016;7:50719–34.

53. Kanu N, Gronroos E, Martinez P, et al. SETD2 loss-of-function promotes renal cancer branched evolution through replication stress and impaired DNA repair. Oncogene. 2015;34:5699–708.
54. Zhang Y, Xie S, Zhou Y, et al. H3K36 histone methyltransferase Setd2 is required for murine embryonic stem cell differentiation toward endoderm. Cell Rep. 2014;8:1989–2002.
55. Pfister SX, Ahrabi S, Zalmas LP, et al. SETD2-dependent histone H3K36 trimethylation is required for homologous recombination repair and genome stability. Cell Rep. 2014;7:2006–18.
56. Park IY, Powell RT, Tripathi DN, et al. Dual chromatin and cytoskeletal remodeling by SETD2. Cell. 2016;166:950–62.
57. Pfister SX, Markkanen E, Jiang Y, et al. Inhibiting WEE1 selectively Kills Histone H3K36me3-Deficient cancers by dNTP starvation. Cancer Cell. 2015;28:557–68.
58. Chalmers AW, Katz DA, Miller IJ, Gregory SA. Successful treatment of hepatosplenic T-cell lymphoma with ESHAP followed by autologous stem cell transplant. Clin Adv Hematol Oncol. 2013;11:109–13.
59. Rizzieri DA, Johnson JL, Byrd JC, et al. Improved efficacy using rituximab and brief duration, high intensity chemotherapy with filgrastim support for Burkitt or aggressive lymphomas: cancer and Leukemia Group B study 10 002. British J Haematol. 2014;165:102–11.
60. Amengual JE, Lichtenstein R, Lue J, et al. A phase 1 study of romidepsin and pralatrexate reveals marked activity in relapsed and refractory T-cell lymphoma. Blood. 2018;131:397–407.
61. Jiang L, Yuan CM, Hubacheck J, et al. Variable CD52 expression in mature T cell and NK cell malignancies: implications for alemtuzumab therapy. British J Haematol. 2009;145:173–9.
62. Al-Toma A, Goerres MS, Meijer JW, et al. Cladribine therapy in refractory celiac disease with aberrant T cells. Clin Gastroenterol Hepatol. 2006;4:1322–7; quiz 00.

Chapter 14
Cutaneous T-Cell Lymphoma: Mycosis Fungoides and Sézary Syndrome

Timothy J. Voorhees, Edith V. Bowers, Christopher R. Kelsey, Yara Park, and Anne W. Beaven

Disease Overview

Cutaneous T-cell lymphomas (CTCLs) include a heterogeneous group of rare, extranodal, non-Hodgkin lymphomas (NHLs), primarily defined by malignant T-lymphocyte invasion of the skin. The clinical presentation ranges from a single patch or plaque to erythroderma involving over 80% of the body or widespread cutaneous tumors. They are almost always pruritic in nature, which can be associated with interrupted sleep, weight loss, and depression [1]. CTCL is a chronic disease for which, in most instances, there is no cure; therefore, patients typically require long-term therapy often with a combination of topical and systemic medications.

The 2017 World Health Organization (WHO) classification of lymphoid neoplasms expanded the CTCL classification to include 13 distinct clinical entities [2, 3]. Here we will focus on the most common: mycosis fungoides (MF) and its

T. J. Voorhees · A. W. Beaven (✉)
Division of Hematology and Oncology, Lineberger Comprehensive Cancer Center, The University of North Carolina at Chapel Hill, Chapel Hill, NC, USA
e-mail: Timothy.Voorhees@unchealth.unc.edu; anne_beaven@med.unc.edu

E. V. Bowers
Department of Dermatology, The University of North Carolina at Chapel Hill, Chapel Hill, NC, USA
e-mail: edith_bowers@med.unc.edu

C. R. Kelsey
Department of Radiation Oncology, Duke University Medical Center, Durham, NC, USA
e-mail: kelse003@mc.duke.edu

Y. Park
Department of Pathology and Laboratory Medicine, The University of North Carolina at Chapel Hill, Chapel Hill, NC, USA
e-mail: Yara.Park@unchealth.unc.edu

C. Dittus (ed.), *Novel Therapeutics for Rare Lymphomas*,
https://doi.org/10.1007/978-3-030-25610-4_14

leukemic variant, Sézary syndrome (SS). The cutaneous CD30+ lymphoproliferative disorders (primary cutaneous anaplastic large-cell lymphoma and lymphomatoid papulosis) are important to distinguish from MF but are not fully addressed here.

Mycosis fungoides (MF) was first described in 1825 in a patient with diffuse patches, plaques, and mushroomlike tumors of the skin [4]. Almost a century later, Sézary and Bouvrain described a patient with generalized exfoliative erythroderma and abnormal lymphoid cells in the blood, a condition that eventually became known as Sézary syndrome [5]. It was not until 1975 that CTCLs were defined as a distinct clinical entity rather than a cutaneous manifestation of systemic peripheral T-cell lymphomas [6].

CTCLs are rare lymphomas with a reported annual incidence in the United States of 5.6–6.4 cases per million persons [7]. It has been hypothesized that persistent antigenic stimulation by allergens may be associated with the development of CTCL, particularly MF [8], but epidemiologic studies have not shown a definitive association between environmental exposures and MF [9–11]. However, MF/SS incidence does increase with age with a median age at diagnosis in the mid-50s. Males are affected almost twice as often as females, and there is a higher rate observed in African Americans [7].

Immunopathogenesis

CTCL is characterized by clonal expansion of mature, tissue-resident T-cells. Upon encountering an antigen, naïve T-cells residing in lymph nodes draining from the skin undergo clonal expansion and differentiation into a variety of effector and memory T-cells. During this process, T-cells induce the expression of an E-selectin ligand cutaneous lymphocyte antigen as well as a variety of chemokine receptors (CCR4, CCR8, CXCR6, CCR10) necessary for migration to the skin [12–14]. Effector T-cells migrate to extranodal sites such as the skin, where a small subset of differentiated T-cells will remain as tissue-resident memory cells (T_{RM}). While the majority of T-cells undergoing clonal expansion differentiate into effector T-cells and migrate to the skin, a subset of T-cells differentiate into central memory T-cells (T_{CM}), which retain the ability to access the peripheral blood via CCR7 and L-selectin upregulation [15–17].

Immunophenotyping studies in patients with CTCL have shown that CTCL subtypes arise from separate mature T-cell compartments. Previously, it was believed that SS represented a transformation from MF; however, recent data with respect to molecular expression and genomic alteration provides evidence to the contrary. Biopsy samples from patients with MF have demonstrated clonal T-cell profiles consistent with a T_{RM} phenotype, strongly expressing CCR4 and E-selectin ligand cutaneous lymphocyte antigen [18]. In contrast to a T_{RM} phenotype, patients with SS, which is characterized by leukemic involvement, appear to express CCR7 and L-selectin, resembling the phenotype of T_{CM}. This further supports the theory of separate disease states arising from separate cells of origin. Further evidence supporting subtype-specific cell of origin can be found in gene expression profiling with comparative genomic hybridization. There appears to be a strong discordance with respect to genomic alterations when comparing MF to SS as well as cutaneous anaplastic large-cell lymphoma [19, 20]. Given that disease subtypes within CTCL may develop from specific and differing cells of origin, this may provide rationale for differing clinical presentations, disease behavior, and response to therapy.

Clinical and Histopathologic Features

The diagnosis of MF/SS can be difficult to make and requires consideration of clinical presentation plus histopathologic features. Given the variable clinical presentations, the differential diagnosis for these patients may include psoriasiform dermatitides (e.g., psoriasis, pityriasis rubra pilaris, seborrheic dermatitis), spongiotic dermatitides (e.g., eczema, allergic contact dermatitis), infectious processes (e.g., tinea), or drug eruptions [21]. Initially, limited skin involvement is often presumptively treated as eczema, psoriasis, or other inflammatory dermatitis based on physical appearance. Even once MF is suspected, multiple biopsies are often required to make a definitive diagnosis. The median time from onset of symptoms to diagnosis of MF is approximately 4 years [22].

Mycosis Fungoides

Mycosis fungoides is the most common CTCL and represents approximately 50% of cases. The majority of lesions present in relatively sun-protected locations (e.g., hip girdle, buttocks, skinfolds) [1]. Classic histopathologic findings for MF include epidermotropism (lymphocytes present in the epidermis without spongiosis) as well as formation of epidermal clusters of lymphocytes around Langerhans cells, termed *Pautrier microabscesses* (Fig. 14.1a–c). Proving T-cell clonality is not essential to establishing a diagnosis, however, detection of clonal T-cell receptors (TCRs) from two different biopsy locations is specific for MF. Persistence of a TCR clone over time (when comparing to past biopsy specimens) also strongly supports an MF diagnosis. Immunophenotyping of biopsy samples commonly show an aberrant loss of T-cell antigens such as CD2, CD3, CD5, and CD7 [23, 24].

Although several clinical variants of mycosis fungoides have been described (e.g., bullous, hypopigmented, or poikilodermatous MF), most have a similar clinical behavior to classical MF. However, the WHO-EORTC classification recognizes three variants with distinct clinicohistopathologic features: folliculotropic MF, pagetoid reticulosis, and the extremely rare granulomatous slack skin. Folliculotropic MF is characterized by the presence of malignant T-cell lymphocyte tropism to dermal hair follicles. This variant commonly spares the epidermis, which is typically involved in classical MF (Fig. 14.1d). The clinical presentation is characterized by either grouped follicular papules, acneiform lesions, or indu-

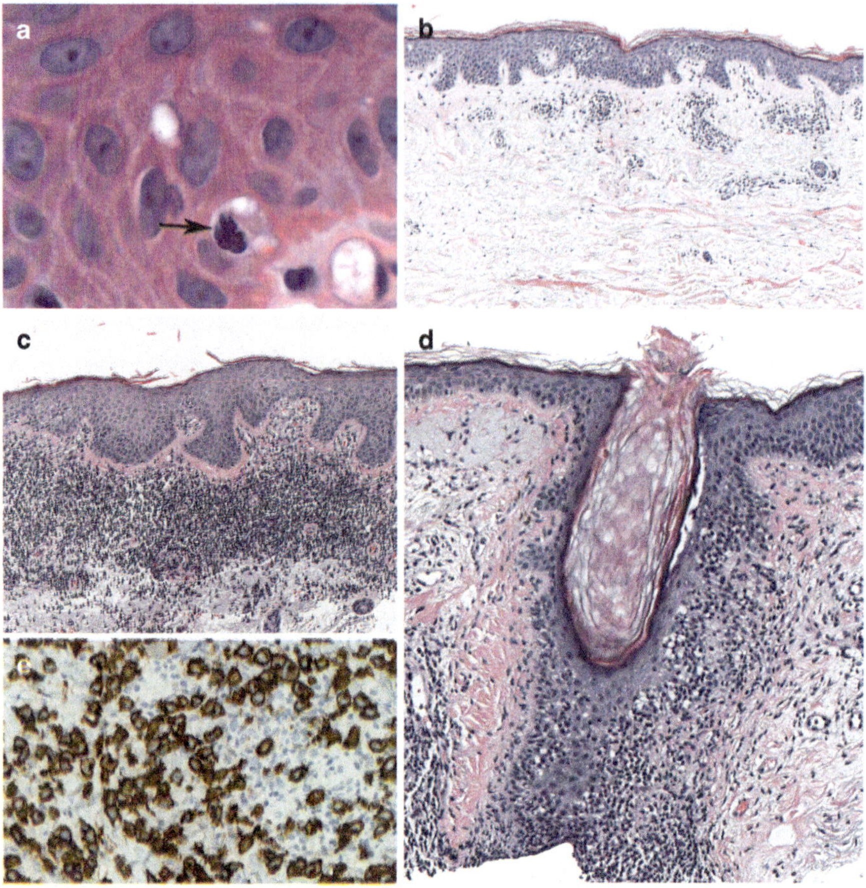

Fig. 14.1 (**a**) Intraepidermal lymphocyte with hyperconvoluted nucleus (arrow). Small- or medium-sized, atypical lymphocytes showing nuclear hyperchromasia and epidermotropism are diagnostic features of cutaneous T-cell lymphoma of the mycosis fungoides pattern. (hematoxylin and eosin, 1000×). (**b**) Patch pattern of mycosis fungoides. Atypical T lymphocytes are present in the papillary dermis and show epidermotropism with Pautrier abscess formation. The deeper dermis and subcutis are minimally uninvolved. (**c**) Plaque pattern of mycosis fungoides. Atypical T lymphocytes fill the papillary dermis and portions of the reticular dermis. Epidermotropism is typically present but may sometimes be minimal. (**d**) Folliculotropic cutaneous T-cell lymphoma. Atypical, hyperchromatic T lymphocytes accumulate within the epithelium of hair follicles. Mucin may also be visible in the follicular epithelium (follicular mucinosis). (**e**) The superposition of accumulations of large atypical T-cells in a patient with mycosis fungoides is termed large-cell transformation. The large cells account for 25% or more of the T-cells in the infiltrate. These large cells sometimes are CD30 positive. (Photos courtesy of Paul Googe, MD)

rated plaques which preferentially involve the head and neck. The presence of plaques involving the eyebrows with associated alopecia is highly specific for folliculotropic MF. The 5-year overall survival (OS) has been found to be approximately 70–80%, which is worse than early-stage MF, and more consistent with tumor-stage MF [25, 26].

Pagetoid reticulosis describes localized patches or plaques with marked intraepidermal proliferation of neoplastic T-cells. Lesions are often solitary and follow an exceptionally indolent course with little to no risk of extracutaneous spread [2] Pagetoid reticulosis should only be used to describe localized disease (Woringer-Kolopp type), as generalized skin involvement should raise suspicion for a more aggressive form of CTCL.

Granulomatous MF is a very rare subtype of MF characterized by diffuse infiltration of malignant T-cell lymphocytes throughout the entire dermis with perivesicular granuloma formation. A minority of patients with granulomatous infiltration develop granulomatous slack skin, characterized by progressive development of pendulous lax skin with predilection for skinfolds, often in the axilla and groin [27–30].

Sézary Syndrome

Sézary syndrome is a rare, although clinically significant, variant accounting for 3–5% of CTCL cases. It has classically been defined by the presence of erythroderma, generalized lymphadenopathy, and neoplastic T-cells (called Sézary cells) in the peripheral blood [31]. Morphologically, Sézary cells are described as large lymphocytes with grooved, lobulated, or cerebriform nuclei [32, 33]. Although previously thought to be a leukemic progression of MF, recent immunophenotyping and genetic studies support that SS exists as a distinct disease process [18–20]. The typical immunophenotype of Sézary cells is CD3+, CD4+, and CD8−. Aberrant loss of CD7 and CD26 has been found in up to 57% and 86% of cases, respectively. In cases where both CD7 and CD26 lack expression, there is a high sensitivity and specificity for SS [34–36]. The presence of Sézary cells is not diagnostic for SS because small numbers of Sézary cells can be found in benign conditions such as actinic reticuloid and drug-induced pseudolymphoma [37–39].

Diagnostic criteria for SS include an absolute Sézary cell count of 1000 cells/mm^3 in peripheral blood, a CD4/CD8 ratio ≥ 10, evidence of a T-cell clone in the peripheral blood, and demonstration of a chromosomally abnormal T-cell clone [40]. Although no minimum criteria must be met to confirm diagnosis, the WHO-EORTC recommends at least establishing TCR clonality as well as one additional criteria above prior to diagnosing SS [2].

Sézary syndrome has a poor overall prognosis. Median survival is 2–4 years with a disease-specific 5-year survival rate of 24% [2]. Due to ineffective T-cell immunity and significant immunosuppression with therapies, infection is a frequent cause of death.

Staging, Risk Stratification, and Prognosis for MF/SS

Staging in CTCL uses a modified tumor, node, metastasis (TNM) classification system [41, 42], which includes a fourth marker, the presence of circulating tumor cells in the blood, termed the B (blood) rating. Stage is determined at diagnosis. However, the patient's updated TNMB classification should be reported throughout treatment to provide information about ongoing tumor burden and response to therapy [43, 44].

Recommended staging studies include physical exam with attention to type and extent of skin disease as well as a thorough lymph node exam. Blood should be sent for a Sézary cell count and/or flow cytometry. Computed tomography (CT) scans and/or a fluorodeoxyglucose (FDG) positron emission tomography (PET) scan should be performed in patients with nodal or blood involvement or ≥ T2 skin disease. Lymph node biopsies should be performed if there is a node ≥1.5 cm in diameter or that is firm, irregular, clustered, or fixed [43].

Skin Stage (T)

Tumor staging of MF is determined by extent of skin involvement, and, therefore, a detailed complete skin exam is a requirement for appropriate staging. T1 is defined as patches, plaques, and papules covering <10% of total body surface area (BSA). T2 is defined as patches, plaques, and papules covering ≥10% of total BSA (Fig. 14.1). These stages can be further stratified into T1a/T2a (patch only disease) and T1b/T2b (plaque disease with or without patches) (Fig. 14.2a). Tumor-stage disease (T3) is defined by the presence of at least one tumor ≥1.5 cm in diameter (Fig. 14.2b). T4 disease is erythrodermic involvement of MF, affecting ≥80% of BSA (Fig. 14.2c) [43].

Patients with T1 disease at diagnosis have an excellent prognosis. The risk of progression at 5 years is only 10% [45], and 10-year OS is similar to matched population controls without MF [46]. In contrast, T4 stage at diagnosis correlates with higher risk of disease progression (48% at 5 years) and lower 10-year OS of only 41% compared to normal controls (Table 14.1) [45, 46].

Node Staging (N)

Nodal staging is based on physical exam and pathologic staging. Peripheral lymph nodes on physical exam that are firm, irregular, clustered, fixed, or >1.5 cm in diameter [43] are considered abnormal. Palpable peripheral lymphadenopathy has been shown in multiple studies to be an independent poor risk factor [47–49]. However, the presence or absence of central lymph node enlargement is not included in N staging. Biopsy of enlarged nodes will frequently demonstrate reactive or dermatopathic nodes without frank involvement by CTCL [50]. Dermatographic nodes without identifiable CTCL involvement are still considered nodal involvement and classified as N1 [51–53].

In the most recent ISCL/EORTC clinical classification guideline, N1–N3 are differentiated by the degree of atypical lymphocyte involvement in the node. There are two separate, validated grading systems for lymph node involvement, the NCI/VA

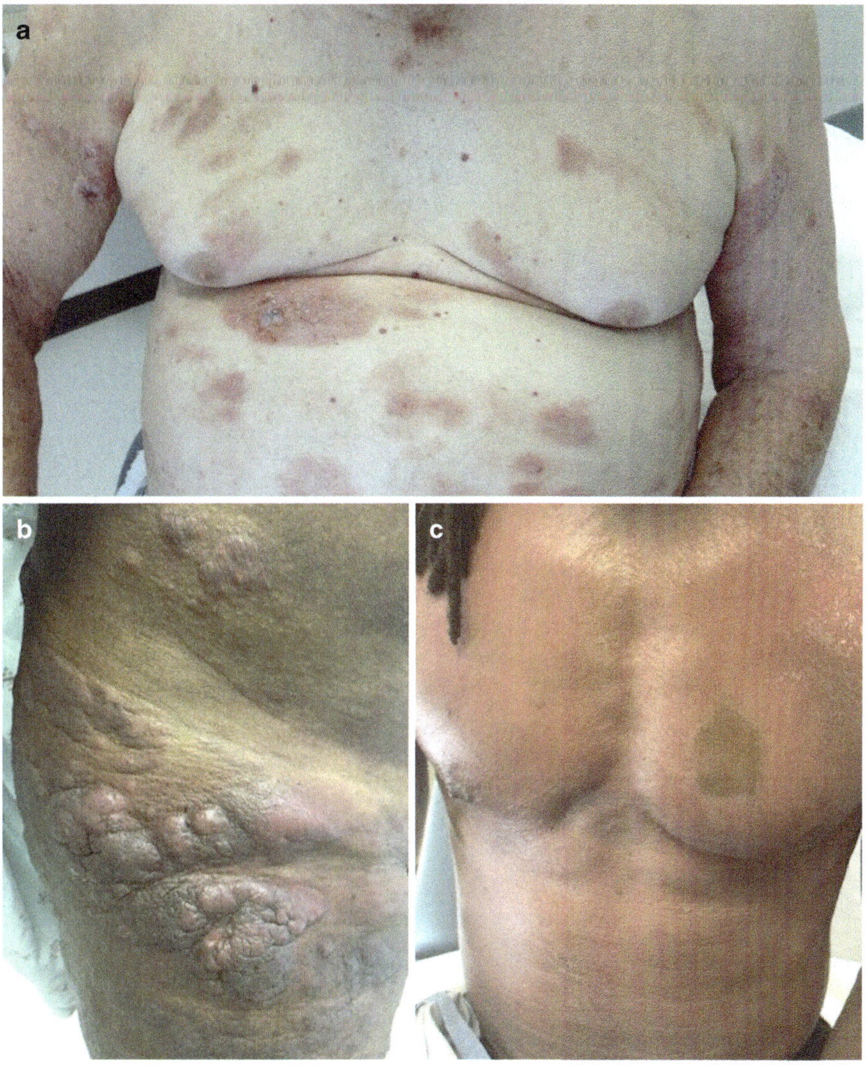

Fig. 14.2 Clinical T stage mycosis fungoides. (**a**) Patches and plaques of mycosis fungoides (Stage T2 disease). (**b**) Tumor-stage (T3) mycosis fungoides. (**c**) Erythroderma associated with mycosis fungoides (Stage T4 disease). (Photos courtesy of Edith Bowers, MD, PhD)

classification system and the Dutch classification system. The NCI/VA system uses a smaller size criteria, defining atypical lymphocytes as ≥6 μm with cerebriform, irregularly folded nuclei. Lymph nodes are then assessed for location of atypical lymphocytes as either occasionally present (LN_1), many atypical lymphocytes or clusters of three to six cells (LN_2), aggregates with preserved nodal architecture (LN_3), or partial to complete effacement of nodal structure by atypical lymphocytes (LN_4) [51, 52]. The Dutch system only considers large atypical cells with an irregular cerebriform nuclei measuring a minimum diameter of 7.5 μm. The Dutch grad-

Table 14.1 ISCL/EORTC clinical staging and overall survival

ISCL/EORTC staging [43, 44]					Overall survival [45, 56, 57]		
Stage	T	N	M	B	Median (years)	5 year (%)	10 year (%)
IA	1	0	0	0–1	35.5	94	88
IB	2	0	0	0–1	21.5	84	70
IIA	1–2	1	0	0–1	15.8	78	47
IIB	3	0–2	0	0–1	4.7–5.6	47–57	34
IIIA	4	0–2	0	0	4.7	47–60	37
IIIB	4	0–2	0	1	3.4–5.2	40–55	25
IVA1	1–4	0–2	0	2	3.8–4.4	37–48	18
IVA2	1–4	3	0	0–2	2.1–2.4	18–32	15
IVB	1–4	0–3	1	0–2	1.4–2.7	18	–

ing is as follows: grade 1 for dermatographic lymphadenopathy, grade 2 with early involvement of atypical lymphocytes, grade 3 with partial effacement of the lymph node, and grade 4 with complete effacement of the lymph node [53].

Prognosis has been clearly linked to either partial or complete effacement of lymph nodes [54]. Therefore, this becomes the major distinction for N1–N3 classification. N1 disease is characterized by the presence of small atypical lymphocytes without effacement (i.e., Dutch grade 1 or NCI/VA LN_1–LN_2). N2 disease is characterized by the presence of large atypical lymphocytes (i.e., Dutch grade 2) or small atypical lymphocyte aggregates without effacement (i.e., NCI/VA LN_3). Finally, N3 disease is classified by any evidence of lymph node effacement (i.e., Dutch grade 3–4 or NCI/VA LN_4). Complicating N staging further, both N1 and N2 can be further subclassified based on the presence of a T-cell clone within the lymph node (e.g., N1 can be either N1a without a clone or N1b with a clone) [43].

Metastatic Staging (M)

Visceral metastases of MF are almost never seen in T1–T3, N0, or B0 disease. Visceral disease is most commonly found as either liver or splenic involvement. The presence of splenomegaly is considered M1 disease and does not require a biopsy. The bone marrow is an infrequent site of metastatic disease in CTCL; therefore, bone marrow biopsies are not routinely performed but can be considered in B2 disease [43, 55].

Blood Staging (B)

In the amended TNMB staging criteria from the ISCL/EORTC in 2007, blood involvement is categorized based on prognostically significant blood involvement by Sézary cells; B0 is the absence of significant blood involvement (≤%5 Sézary cells); B1 represents detectable, but low blood tumor burden (>5% Sézary cells, but does not meet B2 criteria); and B2 is defined as a detection of a clonal TCR rearrangement in the blood and either ≥1000 cells/mm^3 Sézary cells or one of two secondary criteria (CD4/CD8 ratio >10 or increased CD4+ cells with >40% CD4+/CD7− or >30% CD4+/CD26− ratio) [43].

Impact of Staging and Other Factors on Prognosis

Patients with early-stage disease have an excellent survival. Stage IA disease is associated with minimal impact on long-term OS, and patients with less than Stage IIA disease have a median OS greater than 15 years. Stage IIB is an important distinction given the dramatic drop in median OS to only 4.7 years (Table 14.1). The prognosis associated with higher stage CTCL becomes progressively more grim with Stage IVB disease associated with a median OS of only 1.5 years and most deaths attributable to lymphoma [45, 56].

In 2015, the Cutaneous Lymphoma International Consortium (CLIC) published a retrospective study of 1275 patients with advance MF/SS and identified four independent prognostic markers of worse survival: Stage IV disease, age >60 years, large-cell transformation (LCT), and increased lactate dehydrogenase [57]. LCT is defined by an atypical lymphoid infiltrate in either the skin or lymph nodes with >25% of cells characterized as large cells (Fig. 14.1e) [58, 59]. LCT occurs in around 7% of all patients with MF/SS [60] and up to 56–67% of patients with Stage IV MF/SS. Identifying LCT is of clinical importance as it is associated with a median OS of less than 24 months and may require more aggressive treatment with cytotoxic chemotherapy [61–64].

Treatment of MF/SS

The care of patients with MF/SS requires a multidisciplinary team consisting of dermatologists, oncologists, radiation oncologists, pathologists, and wound care specialists.

Skin-directed therapies such as topical steroids, phototherapy, localized radiation therapy, and mechlorethamine are recommended for the first-line management of Stage IA–IIA MF. Second-line therapy for these early disease stages may include systemic retinoids or interferon, total skin electron beam therapy (TSEBT), or low-dose methotrexate (MTX). In Stage IIB–IVB MF, systemic therapies are recommended in the first-line setting [3]. However, even advanced-stage patients on systemic therapy often benefit from concurrent skin-directed therapy such as topical steroids either alone or in combination with phototherapy.

Once systemic treatment is required, most patients will require therapy indefinitely; therefore, it is imperative to balance toxicity of treatment with clinical benefit. Furthermore, because complete remissions are rare, the goals of MF treatment

Table 14.2 Systemic therapy options for CTCL

Systemic treatment	ORR (%)	CR (%)	PFS (months)	FDA approval (as of 1/01/19)
Systemic retinoids [99, 100]	45–66	9–13	3.4–7.3	Approved
Interferon-α + PUVA [79, 103, 104]	80–90	62–74	28–32	Off label
HDACi [108–111]	23–34	5–6	4.9–15	Approved
ECP [112, 113]	36–73	14–26	14–30	Approved
Brentuximab [117]	56	16	16.7	Approved
Alemtuzumab [119–124]	55–84	32–47	6–12	Off label
Mogamulizumab [126, 127]	37–47	3	7.7	Approved
Liposomal doxorubicin [128–130]	41–56	6–20	6–7	Off label
Gemcitabine [131–133]	62–68	8	8–10	Off label
Methotrexate [134, 135]	33–76	12–41	15–22	Approved
Pralatrexate [136]	60	11	12.8	Off label

should focus on improving quality of life and symptoms such as pruritus rather than complete clearance of disease. Minor or partial responses are not considered failures as long as the patient had some clinical benefit from therapy. Even in advanced-stage CTCL, multi-agent chemotherapy has not demonstrated improved survival compared to more conservative therapy [65]; therefore, sequential single-agent therapy is the preferred management approach. Due to the lack of large, randomized clinical trials in CTCL, there is a paucity of data to guide decisions about which therapies should preferentially be used, and in which order. Choices must be made based on provider experience and side effect profile (Table 14.2).

Consensus recommendations of response criteria were created in 2011 by the International Society of Cutaneous Lymphomas. Separate scoring systems are available for skin response, lymph node response, visceral response, and blood response. Skin response is typically assessed by the modified Severity Weighted Assessment Tool (mSWAT) which combines both percent of body surface area involved and a modifier for either plaque-, patch-, or tumor-stage lesions [66]. However, this can be time-consuming and is typically used more in research trials than in clinical practice. Both lymph node and visceral response are typically assessed by serial CT scan. Timing and intervals of CT imaging are determined by each treating physician keeping in mind radiation exposure to recurrent CT imaging. A FDG-PET scan can be useful in selected clinical scenarios but likely results in increased false-positive results from infection and inflammation. Blood response is assessed by either Sézary cell quantification or flow cytometry of T-cell subsets consistent with Sézary cells. Combining these four distinct response scoring systems, a global response score can be determined for overall disease response to therapy [67]. However, decisions about continuation of a particular treatment depend more on clinical response and improvement of symptoms than on the global response score.

Skin-Directed Therapy

Topical Corticosteroids

Topical corticosteroids are an affordable, readily available, and effective choice for many patients. Overall response rates (ORR) >90% and complete response (CR) rates >60% have been reported in Stage T1 patients treated with class I corticosteroids [68, 69].

The choice of topical corticosteroid, both potency and vehicle (e.g., ointment, cream, solution, etc.), depends on the body area being treated and patient preference. Topical corticosteroids are applied once or twice daily to affected areas only. Once clearance is achieved to a given area, they should be stopped and only resumed when patches or plaques recur. Overuse of topical steroids should be avoided to prevent skin atrophy. Response is expected within a few months of use; if control is not achieved within 3 months, alternate therapies should be considered.

Topical Mechlorethamine

Mechlorethamine, commonly known as nitrogen mustard, is an alkylating agent that has been administered topically for the treatment of MF since the 1950s. Approximately 70–80% of patients with Stage T1 disease experience a clinical response, typically achieving skin clearance in 6–10 months [70–73]. Durable remissions lasting at least 10 years occur in 20–25% of patients [72, 73]. Irritant and allergic contact dermatitis are common side effects and are managed by reducing the frequency or strength of application or by using topical corticosteroids. Long-term use of mechlorethamine may lead to the development of secondary cutaneous malignancies, particularly squamous cell carcinoma. However, this is difficult to demonstrate absolutely as many such patients were also treated with other therapies that may alter skin cancer risk, such as phototherapy or radiation [73, 74].

Topical Retinoids

Topical bexarotene is available as a 1% gel and is approved by the US Food and Drug Administration (FDA) for the treatment of patients with Stage IA/IB MF who either have failed or not tolerated other therapies. In patients with Stage IA–IIA MF, ORR of 44–63% has been reported with CR rates of approximately 20% [75, 76]. Initially, it is often administered once daily or every other day, but applications may be titrated up to four times daily if tolerated. Irritant dermatitis at the application site is common and typically limits its use to those patients who have <15% body surface area involvement. Bexarotene is contraindicated in pregnancy.

Phototherapy

Ultraviolet light therapy is widely used and highly efficacious for the treatment of early-stage MF. Phototherapy is particularly advantageous to those patients whose skin involvement is too diffused to practically manage with topical medications. For many patients, phototherapy can also be a safe alternative to systemic treatments. However, treatments are frequent (two to three times per week), and long-term maintenance therapy is often needed, so it may not be a feasible for patients who do not live near a treatment center. Furthermore, phototherapy may not be appropriate for patients with a history of melanoma or extensive non-melanoma skin cancers.

Psoralen Plus Ultraviolet A (PUVA) Photochemotherapy

The combination of psoralen, a plant-derived phototoxic compound, with UVA (320–400 nm) radiation, known as PUVA, has been used for decades to treat MF. The term PUVA typically refers to oral 8-methoxypsoralen (8-MOP) photochemotherapy, although it is sometimes used to describe the topical application of 8-MOP or the use of other psoralen compounds prior to UVA exposure.

Treatment consists of an oral dose of 8-MOP (0.5–0.6 mg/kg) taken 1.5–2 h prior to exposure to UVA light in an office-based phototherapy unit. The entire body is treated, except for a few body areas that are protectively shielded (i.e., eyes and genitalia). Treatments are repeated two to three times per week until clearance is achieved and then gradually tapered.

PUVA is very effective as monotherapy for early-stage MF with reported CR rates of 65–85% [77]. Time to achieve CR is 2–6 months [78, 79], and some patients experience long-term remission of ≥10 years [80]. Complete response rates for advanced-stage disease are much lower: 28% for tumor-stage disease and 43% for erythrodermic MF [77].

Acute complications of PUVA include erythema, photosensitivity, pruritus, blistering, pain, and xerosis. Patients must protect their eyes and skin from sunlight for a minimum of 24 h after 8-MOP intake because of the increased photosensitivity. Patients who are treated long-term with PUVA are at increased risk of developing melanoma [81] and non-melanoma skin cancers [82].

Narrowband Ultraviolet B (UVB)

In patients with patches or thin plaques, narrowband UVB (311 nm) can be used as a safe and effective alternative to PUVA. However, because the depth of penetration of UVB is less than UVA, it is not ideal for patients with thick plaque lesions.

The average CR rate reported in the literature for narrowband UVB as monotherapy is 84% [77]. Similar to PUVA, treatments are administered two to three times weekly until clearance is achieved, after which frequency may be slowly tapered. Acute complications include erythema, but this is shorter-lived and less severe than with PUVA [83]. Although there is a concern for increased photocarcinogenicity, studies have not shown an association between narrowband UVB and skin cancer [84, 85].

Radiation Therapy

Radiation therapy (RT) is one of the most effective treatment modalities for MF and has several different clinical applications. For the rare patient with unilesional disease (or a few clustered lesions), radiation therapy alone is potentially curative. Almost all such patients achieve a complete response (94–100%) with reported 10-year relapse-free survival (RFS) rates of 50–86% [86–88]. A dose of ~30 Gy is recommended in this clinical scenario.

Even patients with more advanced cutaneous disease, with a few symptomatic plaques or tumors, often benefit from local radiation therapy. Several retrospective studies have demonstrated complete response rates >95% for individual MF lesions treated with abbreviated courses of radiation therapy [86–89]. A common fractionation regimen used in low-grade lymphomas (2 Gy × 2, total dose 4 Gy) is not particularly efficacious in mycosis fungoides [90]. However, a slightly more intense regimen (4 Gy × 2, total dose 8 Gy) leads to a complete response in most patients (>90%) [90]. A single 7–8 Gy fraction is similarly efficacious [91]. It has been suggested that more protracted regimens, utilizing total doses of ~30 Gy, are associated with a lower risk of local failure [89]. Thus, the total dose and fractionation scheme should be tailored to the individual circumstances of the patient taking into account the extent and activity of disease, other ongoing treatments, and overall prognosis.

Many patients with MF present with diffuse symptomatic cutaneous disease or will develop such during the course of their illness. Total skin electron beam therapy (TSEBT) can be utilized in such circumstances, particularly in the setting of thick plaques or tumors that may not respond well to other skin-directed therapies. TSEBT is a technically challenging procedure and requires special commissioning (i.e., configuring) of a linear accelerator and significant support from medical physics. Thus, this treatment is generally only available at larger centers that treat many patients a year. As with local radiation therapy, TSEBT is very effective with nearly all patients experiencing significant clinical improvement. For patients with T2 disease, the CR rate has been reported to be 75–85% with 50% RFS at 5 years, but only 10% at 10 years [92–94]. With T3 disease, CR rates of 43–78% have been reported with nearly all patients eventually experiencing recurrent disease [94, 95]. Both conventional courses of TSEBT (30–36 Gy) and low-dose TSEBT (12–15 Gy) are effective, though CR rates are higher with conventional doses.

Systemic Therapies

Systemic Retinoids

Bexarotene, a synthetic retinoid, is FDA approved for use in patients with CTCL refractory to ≥1 systemic therapy. Bexarotene selectively binds and activates RXR nuclear receptors, leading to cell cycle inhibition, decreased proliferation, and increased apoptosis of malignant cells [96–98].

Patients with refractory disease, either early or late stage, treated with bexarotene, have reported ORR of approximately 50% [99, 100]. Recommended dosing is typically 300 mg/m^2 by mouth daily, although some providers start at lower doses and titrate up based on individual patient response and tolerance of side effects.

Similar to other systemic retinoids, bexarotene is teratogenic and is contraindicated in pregnancy. Bexarotene requires frequent lab monitoring of liver function, cell counts, serum lipid levels, and thyroid function throughout therapy. Acquired hypertriglyceridemia and central hypothyroidism, requiring medical management, are common [101]. Other potential side effects include cataracts, xerosis, photosensitivity, myalgias, arthralgias, or headache.

Interferon-α

Interferon-alpha (IFN-α) is commonly prescribed for management of advanced-stage MF and achieves a superior time to next treatment compared to chemotherapy regardless of disease stage [102]. It is administered subcutaneously either daily or three times weekly in doses of 3–9 million units. When used as monotherapy, IFN-α results in an ORR of 64% and CR rate of 27% [79]. Commonly, IFN-α is administered in combination with other skin-directed or systemic therapies. The combination of IFN-α and PUVA has been reported to achieve improved complete response rates of 62–76% with a median duration of response of 28–32 months [79, 103, 104]. Adverse effects of IFN-α include flu-like symptoms, depression, and bone marrow suppression.

Histone Deacetylase Inhibitors (HDACi)

Histone deacetylases (HDACs) are a group of enzymes which function normally to remove acetyl groups form both histone and nonhistone proteins. The epigenetic downregulation of tumor suppressors due to HDACs has been linked to a variety of malignancies [105, 106]. HDAC inhibitors (HDACi) function to maintain histone acetylation and thus transcription of tumor suppressor proteins. HDACi therapy has been found to have clinical activity in advanced-stage MF and SS [107].

Vorinostat is an oral HDACi that is FDA approved, at a dose of 400 mg/day, for recurrent, refractory, or persistent CTCL after ≥2 prior therapies. The ORR in heavily pretreated patients is 24–30% [108, 109]. In clinical trials, the median time to response was 12 weeks, and median time to progression was 30–34 weeks. Romidepsin is an intravenous HDACi that is FDA approved for CTCL after ≥1 prior therapy at a dose of 14 mg/m^2 on days 1, 8, and 15 every 4 weeks. Clinical trials demonstrated an ORR of 34% and CR rate of 6% with a median duration of response (DOR) of 13.7–15 months [110, 111]. Forty-three percent of patients had improvement in pruritus lasting a median of 6 months. Vorinostat and romidepsin have a similar adverse event profile consisting of GI symptoms (nausea, vomiting, and diarrhea) and grade 3 hematologic toxicities (lymphopenia, granulocytopenia, anemia, and thrombocytopenia).

Extracorporeal Photopheresis

Extracorporeal photopheresis (ECP) is FDA approved for use in advanced-stage CTCL patients. ECP involves three distinct steps: separation of a portion of the patient's white blood cells (WBC), which includes the circulating malignant CD4+ cells, through an apheresis procedure, the treatment of the collected white blood cells with 8-methyloxypsoralen and ultraviolet A (UVA) radiation, and reinfusion of treated WBCs to the patient. The mechanism of action is not completely elucidated but is believed to be through induction of antitumor immunity. The 8-MOP intercalates into the WBC DNA which, when exposed to UVA, leads to apoptosis. This causes maturation of monocytes into dendritic cells, which appears to be the cornerstone of the therapy. ECP is also thought to decrease CD4 + FOXP3 + CD25− cells and increase functional CD8+ cells [112].

The reported ORR is 36–73% with CRs in 14–26% of patients. Responses have been associated with shorter duration of disease, fewer circulating malignant cells, and early response of skin lesions to the ECP treatments (>50% regression in 6 months or less) [113].

Typically, one to two treatment cycles of ECP are administered per month with each cycle consisting of two treatments on 2 consecutive days. The median time to maximum response is 5–6 months, but responses have been seen up to 10 months from the start of the therapy. ECP in combination with other modalities has been associated with quicker response time in some cases. Once maximal response is achieved, the interval between treatment cycles can be extended to one cycle every 6–12 weeks. If the patient's disease worsens, the schedule can return to one cycle every 2–4 weeks [113].

ECP is generally very well-tolerated and there are few contraindications. It does not cause systemic immunosuppression. Rarely, during the ECP procedure, hypotension can occur due to volume shifts, and patients can have low-grade fevers a few hours after the procedure. For 24 h after a treatment, the patient is sensitive to light and must wear clothes that cover his/her skin as well as sunscreen and sunglasses [112–114].

Brentuximab Vedotin

Brentuximab vedotin (BV) is an antibody-drug conjugate therapy in which a CD30-directed recombinant IgG1 antibody is conjugated to a microtubule disrupting agent, monomethyl auristatin E [115, 116]. BV is FDA approved for treatment of patients with cutaneous anaplastic large-cell lymphoma (c-ALCL) or CD30+ MF who have received prior systemic therapy.

Approval was largely based on a phase III, randomized trial of BV versus physician choice, of oral methotrexate or bexarotene, in patients with MF or c-ALCL. An ORR lasting at least 4 months occurred in 56% of patients treated with BV versus 12% for physician's choice with CR rates of 16% and 2%, respectively. Median PFS was 15 months in BV and 4 months with physician's choice. Importantly, patient-reported burden of symptoms also showed significantly more improvement in the BV arm. The most frequent toxicity caused by BV is peripheral neuropathy (usually grade 1 or 2) reported in up to 67% of patients [117]. CTCL has significant variation in CD30 expression from strongly expressed to very low expression. Interestingly, the ORR for patients with MF was independent of the level of CD30 expression.

Alemtuzumab

Alemtuzumab is a humanized recombinant IgG1 monoclonal antibody directed against CD52, which is widely expressed by T-cells [118]. Alemtuzumab has been studied in two small phase II studies of patients with Stage IIIA–IVB MF or SS who were administered alemtuzumab 30 mg, three times per week for up to 12 weeks. The ORR was 55–84% with 32–47% CR and a suggestion of more responses in patients with erythroderma and SS [119]. However, there was also a significant rate of infectious complications, approximately 50% either during or shortly after therapy. Infectious complications included reactivation of cytomegalovirus (CMV) in 18% of patients reported in one of the studies [119–122].

With an aim of maintaining efficacy and reducing toxicity, several trials were developed with a reduced dose of alemtuzumab. Bernengo et al. treated 14 patients with SS with a reduced dose of 3 mg subcutaneously on day 1 and then 10 mg on alternating days. ORR was 86% with 21% complete responses. No patients in this reduced dose study developed hematologic toxicity or infections [123]. Furthermore, this dose has subsequently been proven to be safe in elderly patients (80–87 years old) with SS [124]. The clinical responses seen with alemtuzumab are compelling; however, it is imperative that patients are closely monitored for CMV reactivation during therapy.

Mogamulizumab

Mogamulizumab is a humanized monoclonal antibody targeting CC chemokine receptor 4 (CCR4). MF cells strongly express CCR4 (T_{RM} phenotype), which appears to play an important role in T-cell homing to the skin [125]. Mogamulizumab binds with high affinity for CCR4 and is thought to induce cytotoxicity via antibody-dependent cellular toxicity due to NK cell activity.

In August 2018, the international, randomized, phase III study of mogamulizumab versus vorinostat in Stage IB–IV CTCL after at least one prior therapy reported a prolonged median PFS of 7.7 months compared to 3.1 months with vorinostat. This led to FDA approval for all adult patients with relapsed or refractory MF or SS after at least one line of therapy. Mogamulizumab is administered at a dose of 1 mg/kg weekly for 4 weeks and then every 2 weeks as maintenance until disease progression. The best overall global response was 35% for mogamulizumab and only 6% for vorinostat [126]. Responses had previously been reported to be higher in patients with SS (47%). In patients with blood involvement, 94% had a hematologic response [127]. Interestingly, responses were independent of tissue CCR4 expression prior to therapy. Mogamulizumab was very well-tolerated, and the most common adverse events were limited to grade 1–2 nausea, chills, headaches, and infusion reactions.

Cytotoxic Chemotherapy

The role of conventional systemic chemotherapy in the management of CTCL is limited due to short duration of responses and increased toxicities. Therefore, chemotherapy is generally reserved for advanced-stage MF or SS, usually after multiple relapses to other therapeutic agents. Multi-agent chemotherapy has a limited role due to higher rates of significant toxicities with limited improvement in durable responses. However, several drugs such as liposomal doxorubicin, gemcitabine, or folic acid analogs have demonstrated efficacy in MF and SS when administered as single agents.

Pegylated liposomal doxorubicin resulted in ORR of 41–56%, CR rates of 6–20%, and PFS of 6–7 months in patients with relapsed, refractory Stage II–IV MF [128–130]. Gemcitabine has also been studied in advanced MF and SS with an ORR of 62–68% and CR rate of 8% [131–133].

Low-dose oral methotrexate (MTX) has been studied in early-stage MF with an ORR of 33% and a CR rate of 12%. Despite a relatively low response rate in early-stage MF, it can be effective in SS. In patients with SS treated with low-dose oral MTX, high response rates have been reported (ORR 76%; CR rate 41%) [134, 135]. Pralatrexate, which is FDA approved for relapsed/refractory peripheral T-cell lymphoma, has shown some efficacy in MF as well. In a phase I/II study of 34 patients with Stage IV MF, SS, or c-ALCL, the combination of pralatrexate and oral bexarotene showed an ORR of 60% with a 11% CR rate. Furthermore, median progression-free survival was longer than most other systemic therapies, reported at 12.8 months [136].

Hematopoietic Stem Cell Transplant

Hematopoietic stem cell transplantation (SCT) is rarely used in the management of MF/SS. The data available is limited to case reports and retrospective reviews which raises questions about its efficacy, optimal timing in the disease course, and ideal patient population. The evidence for high-dose chemotherapy followed by autologous SCT rescue is limited to a small case series. Results showed a reasonable response rate; however, over half of the patients developed an early relapse [137]. Allogeneic SCT is more frequently used in MF/SS patients but is a high-risk procedure with a reported 1-year non-relapse mortality of 14–40% depending on conditioning regimen and donor type. In one report, patients who underwent allogeneic SCT with a reduced intensity conditioning regimen and a matched-related donor were found to have a 3-year OS of 63% [138]. Responses have been found to be strongly dependent on graft versus lymphoma effect, and many patients required donor lymphocyte infusions after SCT [139]. Given the high treatment-related morbidity and mortality, SCT is typically limited to younger, healthy patients with high-risk disease and a suitable matched donor.

Summary

Cutaneous T-cell lymphomas represent a wide range of clinical entities with differing pathogenesis and responses to treatment. Establishing a clear diagnosis along with staging and risk stratification is critical prior to recommending appropriate therapeutic interventions. Assessments and treatment recommendations are best delivered by a multidisciplinary team involving dermatology, dermatopathology, medical oncology, and radiation oncology. Early-stage CTCL is typically managed with skin-directed therapies, often achieving durable, long-term remissions and disease control. Advanced-stage MF and SS typically require systemic therapy; however, therapy does not typically lead to durable responses. While many new therapies have recently been studied and approved, well-designed clinical trials are needed in the future to optimize disease response and survival.

References

1. Vij A, Duvic M. Prevalence and severity of pruritus in cutaneous T cell lymphoma. Int J Dermatol. 2012;51(8):930–4.
2. Willemze R, Jaffe E, Burg G, Cerroni L, Berti E, Swerdlow SH, et al. WHO-EORTC classification for cutaneous lymphomas. Blood. 2005;105(10):3768–85.
3. Trautinger F, Eder J, Assaf C, Bagot M, Cozzio A, Dummer R, et al. European organisation for research and treatment of cancer consensus recommendations for the treatment of mycosis fungoides/Sézary syndrome – update 2017. Eur J Cancer. 2017;77:57–74.
4. Alibert J-L. Description des maladies de la peau : observées à l'Hôpital Saint-Louis, et exposition des meilleures méthodes suivies pour leur traitement. Barrois l'aîné et fils. Bruxelles: Wahlen; 1825.
5. Sezary A, Bouvrain Y. Erythrodermie avec présence de cellules monstrueses dans le derme et dans lang circulant. Bull Soc Fr Dermatol Syphiligr. 1938;45:254–60.
6. Lutzner M. Cutaneous T-cell lymphomas: the Sézary syndrome, mycosis fungoides, and related disorders. Ann Intern Med. 1975;83(4):534.

7. Criscione V, Weinstock M. Incidence of cutaneous T-cell lymphoma in the United States, 1973–2002. Arch Dermatol. 2007;143(7):854–9.
8. Morales Suárez-Varela MM, Olsen J, Kaerlev L, Guénel P, Arveux P, Wingren G, et al. Are alcohol intake and smoking associated with mycosis fungoides? A European multicentre case–control study. Eur J Cancer. 2001;37(3):392–7.
9. Whittemore AS, Holly EA, Lee I-M, Abel EA, Adams RM, Nickoloff BJ, et al. Mycosis fungoides in relation to environmental exposures and immune response: a case-control study. JNCI J Natl Cancer Inst. 1989;81(20):1560–7.
10. Morales-Suarez-Varela MM, Olsen J, Johansen P, Kaerlev L, Guenel P, Arveux P, et al. Occupational sun exposure and mycosis fungoides: a European multicenter case-control study. J Occup Environ Med. 2006;48(4):390–3.
11. Tuyp E, Burgoyne A, Aitchison T, MacKie R. A case-control study of possible causative factors in mycosis fungoides. Arch Dermatol. 1987;123(2):196–200.
12. Clark RA, Chong B, Mirchandani N, Brinster NK, Yamanaka K –i, Dowgiert RK, et al. The vast majority of CLA+ T cells are resident in normal skin. J Immunol. 2006;176(7):4431–9.
13. Reiss Y, Proudfoot AE, Power CA, Campbell JJ, Butcher EC. CC chemokine receptor (CCR)4 and the CCR10 ligand cutaneous T cell–attracting chemokine (CTACK) in lymphocyte trafficking to inflamed skin. J Exp Med. 2001;194(10):1541–7.
14. Homey B, Alenius H, Müller A, Soto H, Bowman EP, Yuan W, et al. CCL27–CCR10 interactions regulate T cell–mediated skin inflammation. Nat Med. 2002;8(2):157.
15. Marusina AI, Ono Y, Merleev AA, Shimoda M, Ogawa H, Wang EA, et al. CD4+ virtual memory: antigen-inexperienced T cells reside in the naïve, regulatory, and memory T cell compartments at similar frequencies, implications for autoimmunity. J Autoimmun. 2017;77(Supplement C):76–88.
16. Kueberuwa G, Gornall H, Alcantar-Orozco EM, Bouvier D, Kapacee ZA, Hawkins RE, et al. CCR7+ selected gene-modified T cells maintain a central memory phenotype and display enhanced persistence in peripheral blood in vivo. J Immunother Cancer. 2017;5(1):14.
17. Bingaman AW, Patke DS, Mane VR, Ahmadzadeh M, Ndejembi M, Bartlett ST, et al. Novel phenotypes and migratory properties distinguish memory CD4 T cell subsets in lymphoid and lung tissue. Eur J Immunol. 2005;35(11):3173–86.
18. Campbell JJ, Clark RA, Watanabe R, Kupper TS. Sézary syndrome and mycosis fungoides arise from distinct T-cell subsets: a biologic rationale for their distinct clinical behaviors. Blood. 2010;116(5):767–71.
19. Laharanne E, Oumouhou N, Bonnet F, Carlotti M, Gentil C, Chevret E, et al. Genome-wide analysis of cutaneous T-cell lymphomas identifies three clinically relevant classes. J Invest Dermatol. 2010;130(6):1707–18.
20. van Doorn R, van Kester MS, Dijkman R, Vermeer MH, Mulder AA, Szuhai K, et al. Oncogenomic analysis of mycosis fungoides reveals major differences with Sézary syndrome. Blood. 2009;113(1):127–36.
21. Geskin LJ. Cutaneous T-cell lymphoma (mycosis fungoides and Sézary syndrome). In: Kaushansky K, Lichtman MA, Prchal JT, Levi MM, Press OW, Burns LJ, et al., editors. Williams hematology. 9th ed. New York: McGraw-Hill Education; 2015.
22. van Doorn R, Haselen CWV, van Voorst Vader PC, Geerts M-L, Heule F, de Rie M, et al. Mycosis fungoides: disease evolution and prognosis of 309 Dutch patients. Arch Dermatol. 2000;136(4):504–10.
23. Naraghi ZS, Seirafi H, Valikhani M, Farnaghi F, Kavusi S, Dowlati Y. Assessment of histologic criteria in the diagnosis of mycosis fungoides. Int J Dermatol. 2003;42(1):45–52.
24. Pimpinelli N, Olsen EA, Santucci M, Vonderheid E, Haeffner AC, Stevens S, et al. Defining early mycosis fungoides. J Am Acad Dermatol. 2005;53(6):1053–63.
25. Vergier B, Beylot-Barry M, Beylot C, de Mascarel A, Delaunay M, de Muret A, et al. Pilotropic cutaneous T-cell lymphoma without mucinosis. A variant of mycosis fungoides? French Study Group of Cutaneous Lymphomas. Arch Dermatol. 1996;132(6):683–7.

26. van Doorn R, Scheffer E, Willemze R. Follicular mycosis fungoides, a distinct disease entity with or without associated follicular mucinosis: a clinicopathologic and follow-up study of 51 patients. Arch Dermatol. 2002;138(2):191–8.
27. Kempf W, Ostheeren-Michaelis S, Paulli M, Lucioni M, Wechsler J, Audring H, et al. Granulomatous mycosis fungoides and granulomatous slack skin: a multicenter study of the Cutaneous Lymphoma Histopathology Task Force Group of the European Organization for Research and Treatment of Cancer (EORTC). Arch Dermatol. 2008;1:144(12).
28. Li JY, Pulitzer MP, Myskowski PL, Dusza SW, Horwitz S, Moskowitz A, et al. A case-control study of clinicopathologic features, prognosis, and therapeutic responses in patients with granulomatous mycosis fungoides. J Am Acad Dermatol. 2013;69(3):366–374.e4.
29. Clarijs M, Poot F, Laka A, Pirard C, Bourlond A. Granulomatous slack skin: treatment with extensive surgery and review of the literature. Dermatol Basel. 2003;206(4):393–7.
30. van Haselen CW, Toonstra J, van der Putte SJC, van Dongen JJM, van Hees CLM, van Vloten WA. Granulomatous slack skin: report of three patients with an updated review of the literature. Dermatol Basel. 1998;196(4):382–91.
31. Wieselthier JS, Koh HK. Sézary syndrome: diagnosis, prognosis, and critical review of treatment options. J Am Acad Dermatol. 1990;22(3):381–401.
32. Taswell HF, Winkelmann RK. Sézary syndrome – a malignant reticulemic erythroderma. JAMA. 1961;177(7):465–72.
33. Lutzner MA, Jordan HW. The ultrastructure of an abnormal cell in Sézary's syndrome. Blood. 1968;31(6):719–26.
34. Boonk SE, Zoutman WH, Marie-Cardine A, van der Fits L, Out-Luiting JJ, Mitchell TJ, et al. Evaluation of immunophenotypic and molecular biomarkers for Sézary syndrome using standard operating procedures: a multicenter study of 59 patients. J Invest Dermatol. 2016;136(7):1364–72.
35. Klemke CD, Booken N, Weiss C, Nicolay JP, Goerdt S, Felcht M, et al. Histopathological and immunophenotypical criteria for the diagnosis of Sézary syndrome in differentiation from other erythrodermic skin diseases: a European Organisation for Research and Treatment of Cancer (EORTC) Cutaneous Lymphoma Task Force Study of 9. Br J Dermatol. 2015;173(1):93–105.
36. Hristov AC, Vonderheid EC, Borowitz MJ. Simplified flow cytometric assessment in mycosis fungoides and Sézary syndrome. Am J Clin Pathol Chic. 2011;136(6):944–53.
37. Muche JM, Lukowsky A, Asadullah K, Gellrich S, Sterry W. Demonstration of frequent occurrence of clonal T cells in the peripheral blood of patients with primary cutaneous T-cell lymphoma. Blood. 1997;90(4):1636–42.
38. Preesman AH, Schrooyen SJ, Toonstra J, van der Putte SCJ, Rademakers LHPM, Willemze R, et al. The diagnostic value of morphometry on blood lymphocytes in erythrodermic actinic reticuloid. Arch Dermatol. 1995;131(11):1298–303.
39. Rosenthal CJ, Noguera CA, Coppola A, Kapelner SN. Pseudolymphoma with mycosis fungoides manifestations, hyperresponsiveness to diphenylhydantoin, and lymphocyte disregulation. Cancer. 1982;49(11):2305–14.
40. Vonderheid EC, Bernengo MG, Burg G, Duvic M, Heald P, Laroche L, et al. Update on erythrodermic cutaneous T-cell lymphoma: report of the international society for cutaneous lymphomas. J Am Acad Dermatol. 2002;46(1):95–106.
41. Lamberg SI, Bunn PA. Cutaneous T-cell lymphomas: summary of the Mycosis Fungoides Cooperative Group-National Cancer Institute Workshop. Arch Dermatol. 1979;115(9):1103–5.
42. Bunn PA, Lamberg SI. Report of the committee on staging and classification of cutaneous T-cell lymphomas. Cancer Treat Rep. 1979;63(4):725–8.
43. Olsen E, Vonderheid E, Pimpinelli N, Willemze R, Kim Y, Knobler R, et al. Revisions to the staging and classification of mycosis fungoides and Sézary syndrome: a proposal of the International Society for Cutaneous Lymphomas (ISCL) and the cutaneous lymphoma task force of the European Organization of Research and Treatment of Cancer (EORTC). Blood. 2007;110(6):1713–22.

44. Kim YH, Willemze R, Pimpinelli N, Whittaker S, Olsen EA, Ranki A, et al. TNM classification system for primary cutaneous lymphomas other than mycosis fungoides and Sézary syndrome: a proposal of the International Society for Cutaneous Lymphomas (ISCL) and the Cutaneous Lymphoma Task Force of the European Organization of Research and Treatment of Cancer (EORTC). Blood. 2007;110(2):479–84.
45. Kim YH, Liu HL, Mraz-Gernhard S, Varghese A, Hoppe RT. Long-term outcome of 525 patients with mycosis fungoides and Sézary syndrome: clinical prognostic factors and risk for disease progression. Arch Dermatol. 2003;139(7):857–66.
46. Zackheim HS, Amin S, Kashani-Sabet M, McMillan A. Prognosis in cutaneous T-cell lymphoma by skin stage: long-term survival in 489 patients. J Am Acad Dermatol. 1999;40(3):418–25.
47. Sausville EA, Worsham GF, Matthews MJ, Makuch RW, Fischmann AB, Schechter GP, et al. Histologic assessment of lymph nodes in mycosis fungoides/sézary syndrome (cutaneous T-cell lymphoma): clinical correlations and prognostic import of a new classification system. Hum Pathol. 1985;16(11):1098–109.
48. Fuks ZY, Bagshaw MA, Farber EM. Prognostic signs and the management of the mycosis fungoides. Cancer. 1973;32(6):1385–95.
49. Rappaport H, Thomas LB. Mycosis fungoides: the pathology of extracutaneous involvement. Cancer. 1974;34(4):1198–229.
50. Bosse T, Nout RA, McAlpine JN, McConechy MK, Britton H, Hussein YR, et al. Molecular classification of grade 3 endometrioid endometrial cancers identifies distinct prognostic subgroups. Am J Surg Pathol. 2018;42:561–8.
51. Bunn PA. Prospective staging evaluation of patients with cutaneous T-cell lymphomas: demonstration of a high frequency of extracutaneous dissemination. Ann Intern Med. 1980;93(2):223.
52. Clendenning WE, Rappaport HW. Report of the committee on pathology of cutaneous T cell lymphomas. Cancer Treat Rep. 1979;63(4):719–24.
53. Scheffer E, Meijer CJLM, van Vloten WA. Dermatopathic lymphadenopathy and lymph node involvement in mycosis fungoides. Cancer. 1980;45(1):137–48.
54. Vonderheid EC, Diamond LW, Van Vloten WA, Scheffer E, Meijer CJLM, Cashell AW, et al. Lymph node classification systems in cutaneous T-cell lymphoma. Evidence for the utility of the working formulation of non-Hodgkin's lymphomas for clinical usage. Cancer. 1994;73(1):207–18.
55. Sibaud V, Beylot-Barry M, Thiébaut R, Parrens M, Vergier B, Delaunay M, et al. Bone marrow histopathologic and molecular staging in epidermotropic T-cell lymphomas. Am J Clin Pathol. 2003;119(3):414–23.
56. Agar NS, Wedgeworth E, Crichton S, Mitchell TJ, Cox M, Ferreira S, et al. Survival outcomes and prognostic factors in mycosis fungoides/Sézary syndrome: validation of the revised International Society for Cutaneous Lymphomas/European Organisation for Research and Treatment of Cancer Staging Proposal. J Clin Oncol. 2010;28(31):4730–9.
57. Scarisbrick JJ, Prince HM, Vermeer MH, Quaglino P, Horwitz S, Porcu P, et al. Cutaneous lymphoma international consortium study of outcome in advanced stages of mycosis fungoides and Sézary syndrome: effect of specific prognostic markers on survival and development of a prognostic model. J Clin Oncol. 2015;33(32):3766–73.
58. Jawed SI, Myskowski PL, Horwitz S, Moskowitz A, Querfeld C. Primary cutaneous T-cell lymphoma (mycosis fungoides and Sézary syndrome): part I. Diagnosis: clinical and histopathologic features and new molecular and biologic markers. J Am Acad Dermatol. 2014;70(2):205.e1–205.e16.
59. Diamandidou E, Colome-Grimmer M, Fayad L, Duvic M, Kurzrock R. Transformation of mycosis fungoides/Sezary syndrome: clinical characteristics and prognosis. Blood. 1998;92(4):1150–9.
60. Arulogun SO, Prince HM, Ng J, Lade S, Ryan GF, Blewitt O, et al. Long-term outcomes of patients with advanced-stage cutaneous T-cell lymphoma and large cell transformation. Blood. 2008;112(8):3082–7.

61. Benner MF, Jansen PM, Vermeer MH, Willemze R. Prognostic factors in transformed mycosis fungoides: a retrospective analysis of 100 cases. Blood. 2012;119(7):1643–9.
62. Pulitzer M, Myskowski PL, Horwitz SM, Querfeld C, Connolly B, Li J, et al. Mycosis fungoides with large cell transformation: clinicopathological features and prognostic factors. Pathology (Phila). 2014;46(7):610–6.
63. Scarisbrick JJ, Kim YH, Whittaker SJ, Wood GS, Vermeer MH, Prince HM, et al. Prognostic factors, prognostic indices and staging in mycosis fungoides and Sézary syndrome: where are we now? Br J Dermatol. 2014;170(6):1226–36.
64. Talpur R, Sui D, Gangar P, Dabaja BS, Duvic M. Retrospective analysis of prognostic factors in 187 cases of transformed mycosis fungoides. Clin Lymphoma Myeloma Leuk. 2016;16(1):49–56.
65. Kaye FJ, Bunn PA, Steinberg SM, Stocker JL, Ihde DC, Fischmann AB, et al. A randomized trial comparing combination electron-beam radiation and chemotherapy with topical therapy in the initial treatment of mycosis fungoides. N Engl J Med. 1989;321(26):1784–90.
66. Stevens SR, Ke MS, Parry EJ, Mark J, Cooper KD. Quantifying skin disease burden in mycosis fungoides–type cutaneous T-cell lymphomas: the Severity-Weighted Assessment Tool (SWAT). Arch Dermatol [Internet]. 2002 Jan 1 [cited 2019 Jan 16];138(1):42–8. Available from: http://archderm.jamanetwork.com/article.aspx?doi=10.1001/archderm.138.1.42.
67. Olsen EA, Whittaker S, Kim YH, Duvic M, Prince HM, Lessin SR, et al. Clinical end points and response criteria in mycosis fungoides and Sézary syndrome: a consensus statement of the International Society for Cutaneous Lymphomas, the United States Cutaneous Lymphoma Consortium, and the Cutaneous Lymphoma Task Force of the European Organisation for Research and Treatment of Cancer. J Clin Oncol. 2011;29(18):2598–607.
68. Zackheim HS, Kashani-Sabet M, Amin S. Topical corticosteroids for mycosis fungoides: experience in 79 patients. Arch Dermatol. 1998;134(8):949–54.
69. Zackheim HS. Treatment of patch-stage mycosis fungoides with topical corticosteroids. Dermatol Ther. 2003;16(4):283–7.
70. Vonderheid EC, Tan ET, Kantor AF, Shrager L, Micaily B, Van Scott EJ. Long-term efficacy, curative potential, and carcinogenicity of topical mechlorethamine chemotherapy in cutaneous T cell lymphoma. J Am Acad Dermatol. 1989;20(3):416–28.
71. Ramsay DL, Halperin PS, Zeleniuch-Jacquotte A. Topical mechiorethamine therapy for early stage mycosis fungoides. J Am Acad Dermatol. 1988;19(4):684–91.
72. Kim YH, Jensen RA, Watanabe GL, Varghese A, Hoppe RT. Clinical stage IA (limited patch and plaque) mycosis fungoides: a long-term outcome analysis. Arch Dermatol. 1996;132(11):1309–13.
73. Kim YH, Martinez G, Varghese A, Hoppe RT. Topical nitrogen mustard in the management of mycosis fungoides: update of the Stanford experience. Arch Dermatol. 2003;139(2):165–73.
74. Kim YH. Management with topical nitrogen mustard in mycosis fungoides. Dermatol Ther. 2003;16(4):288–98.
75. Heald P, Mehlmauer M, Martin AG, Crowley CA, Yocum RC, Reich SD. Topical bexarotene therapy for patients with refractory or persistent early-stage cutaneous T-cell lymphoma: results of the phase III clinical trial. J Am Acad Dermatol. 2003;49(5):801–15.
76. Breneman D, Duvic M, Kuzel T, Yocum R, Truglia J, Stevens VJ. Phase 1 and 2 trial of bexarotene gel for skin-directed treatment of patients with cutaneous T-cell lymphoma. Arch Dermatol. 2002;138(3):325–32.
77. Olsen EA, Hodak E, Anderson T, Carter JB, Henderson M, Cooper K, et al. Guidelines for phototherapy of mycosis fungoides and Sézary syndrome: a consensus statement of the United States Cutaneous Lymphoma Consortium. J Am Acad Dermatol. 2016;74(1):27–58.
78. Herrmann JJ, Roenigk HH, Hurria A, Kuzel TM, Samuelson E, Rademaker AW, et al. Treatment of mycosis fungoides with photochemotherapy (PUVA): long-term follow-up. J Am Acad Dermatol. 1995;33(2, Part 1):234–42.
79. Roenigk HH, Kuzel TM, Skoutelis AP, Springer E, Yu G, Caro W, et al. Photochemotherapy alone or combined with interferon alpha-2a in the treatment of cutaneous T-cell lymphoma. J Invest Dermatol. 1990;95(6 Suppl):198S–205S.

80. Querfeld C, Rosen ST, Kuzel TM, Kirby KA, Roenigk HH, Prinz BM, et al. Long-term follow-up of patients with early-stage cutaneous T-cell lymphoma who achieved complete remission with psoralen plus UV-A monotherapy. Arch Dermatol. 2005;141(3):305–11.
81. Stern RS, Nichols KT, Väkevä LH. Malignant melanoma in patients treated for psoriasis with methoxsalen (psoralen) and ultraviolet A radiation (PUVA). The PUVA Follow-Up Study. N Engl J Med. 1997;336(15):1041–5.
82. Stern RS. PUVA Follow-Up Study. The risk of squamous cell and basal cell cancer associated with psoralen and ultraviolet A therapy: a 30-year prospective study. J Am Acad Dermatol. 2012;66(4):553–62.
83. Gupta AK, Anderson TF. Psoralen photochemotherapy. J Am Acad Dermatol. 1987;17(5 Pt 1):703–34.
84. Hearn RMR, Kerr AC, Rahim KF, Ferguson J, Dawe RS. Incidence of skin cancers in 3867 patients treated with narrow-band ultraviolet B phototherapy. Br J Dermatol. 2008;159(4):931–5.
85. Lee E, Koo J, Berger T. UVB phototherapy and skin cancer risk: a review of the literature. Int J Dermatol. 2005;44(5):355–60.
86. Wilson LD, Kacinski BM, Jones GW. Local superficial radiotherapy in the management of minimal stage IA cutaneous T-cell lymphoma (mycosis fungoides). Int J Radiat Oncol Biol Phys. 1998;40(1):109–15.
87. Piccinno R, Caccialanza M, Percivalle S. Minimal stage IA mycosis fungoides. Results of radiotherapy in 15 patients. J Dermatol Treat. 2009;20(3):165–8.
88. Micaily B, Miyamoto C, Kantor G, Lessin S, Rook A, Brady L, et al. Radiotherapy for unilesional mycosis fungoides. Int J Radiat Oncol. 1998;42(2):361–4.
89. Cotter GW, Baglan RJ, Wasserman TH, Mill W. Palliative radiation treatment of cutaneous mycosis fungoides – a dose response. Int J Radiat Oncol Biol Phys. 1983;9(10):1477–80.
90. Neelis KJ, Schimmel EC, Vermeer MH, Senff NJ, Willemze R, Noordijk EM. Low-dose palliative radiotherapy for cutaneous B- and T-cell lymphomas. Int J Radiat Oncol Biol Phys. 2009;74(1):154–8.
91. Thomas TO, Agrawal P, Guitart J, Rosen ST, Rademaker AW, Querfeld C, et al. Outcome of patients treated with a single-fraction dose of palliative radiation for cutaneous T-cell lymphoma. Int J Radiat Oncol Biol Phys. 2013;85(3):747–53.
92. Ysebaert L, Truc G, Dalac S, Lambert D, Petrella T, Barillot I, et al. Ultimate results of radiation therapy for T1-T2 mycosis fungoides (including reirradiation). Int J Radiat Oncol Biol Phys. 2004;58(4):1128–34.
93. Jones GW, Kacinski BM, Wilson LD, Willemze R, Spittle M, Hohenberg G, et al. Total skin electron radiation in the management of mycosis fungoides: consensus of the European Organization for Research and Treatment of Cancer (EORTC) Cutaneous Lymphoma Project Group. J Am Acad Dermatol. 2002;47(3):364–70.
94. Navi D, Riaz N, Levin YS, Sullivan NC, Kim YH, Hoppe RT. The Stanford University experience with conventional-dose, total skin electron-beam therapy in the treatment of generalized patch or plaque (T2) and tumor (T3) mycosis fungoides. Arch Dermatol. 2011;147(5):561–7.
95. Quiros PA, Kacinski BM, Wilson LD. Extent of skin involvement as a prognostic indicator of disease free and overall survival of patients with T3 cutaneous T-cell lymphoma treated with total skin electron beam radiation therapy. Cancer. 1996;77(9):1912–7.
96. Budgin JB, Richardson SK, Newton SB, Wysocka M, Zaki MH, Benoit B, et al. Biological effects of bexarotene in cutaneous T-cell lymphoma. Arch Dermatol. 2005;141(3):315–21.
97. Zhang C, Hazarika P, Ni X, Weidner DA, Duvic M. Induction of apoptosis by bexarotene in cutaneous T-cell lymphoma cells: relevance to mechanism of therapeutic action. Clin Cancer Res. 2002;8(5):1234–40.
98. Qu L, Tang X. Bexarotene: a promising anticancer agent. Cancer Chemother Pharmacol. 2010;65(2):201–5.
99. Duvic M, Hymes K, Heald P, Breneman D, Martin AG, Myskowski P, et al. Bexarotene is effective and safe for treatment of refractory advanced-stage cutaneous T-cell lymphoma: multinational phase II-III trial results. J Clin Oncol. 2001;19(9):2456–71.

100. Duvic M, Martin AG, Kim Y, Olsen E, Wood GS, Crowley CA, et al. Phase 2 and 3 clinical trial of oral bexarotene (Targretin capsules) for the treatment of refractory or persistent early-stage cutaneous T-cell lymphoma. Arch Dermatol. 2001;137(5):581–93.
101. Sherman SI, Gopal J, Haugen BR, Chiu AC, Whaley K, Nowlakha P, et al. Central hypothyroidism associated with retinoid X receptor-selective ligands. N Engl J Med. 1999;340(14):1075–9.
102. Hughes CFM, Khot A, McCormack C, Lade S, Westerman DA, Twigger R, et al. Lack of durable disease control with chemotherapy for mycosis fungoides and Sézary syndrome: a comparative study of systemic therapy. Blood. 2015;125(1):71–81.
103. Kuzel TM, Roenigk HH, Samuelson E, Herrmann JJ, Hurria A, Rademaker AW, et al. Effectiveness of interferon alfa-2a combined with phototherapy for mycosis fungoides and the Sézary syndrome. J Clin Oncol. 1995;13(1):257–63.
104. Chiarion-Sileni V, Bononi A, Fornasa CV, Soraru M, Alaibac M, Ferrazzi E, et al. Phase II trial of interferon-alpha-2a plus psolaren with ultraviolet light A in patients with cutaneous T-cell lymphoma. Cancer. 2002;95(3):569–75.
105. Schrump DS. Cytotoxicity mediated by histone deacetylase inhibitors in cancer cells: mechanisms and potential clinical implications. Clin Cancer Res. 2009;15(12):3947–57.
106. Lemoine M, Younes A. Histone deacetylase inhibitors in the treatment of lymphoma. Discov Med. 2010;10(54):462–70.
107. Akilov OE, Grant C, Frye R, Bates S, Piekarz R, Geskin LJ. Low-dose electron beam radiation and romidepsin therapy for symptomatic cutaneous T-cell lymphoma lesions. Br J Dermatol. 2012;167(1):194–7.
108. Duvic M, Talpur R, Ni X, Zhang C, Hazarika P, Kelly C, et al. Phase 2 trial of oral vorinostat (suberoylanilide hydroxamic acid, SAHA) for refractory cutaneous T-cell lymphoma (CTCL). Blood. 2007;109(1):31–9.
109. Olsen EA, Kim YH, Kuzel TM, Pacheco TR, Foss FM, Parker S, et al. Phase IIB multicenter trial of vorinostat in patients with persistent, progressive, or treatment refractory cutaneous T-cell lymphoma. J Clin Oncol. 2007;25(21):3109–15.
110. Piekarz RL, Frye R, Turner M, Wright JJ, Allen SL, Kirschbaum MH, et al. Phase II multi-institutional trial of the histone deacetylase inhibitor romidepsin as monotherapy for patients with cutaneous T-cell lymphoma. J Clin Oncol. 2009;27(32):5410–7.
111. Whittaker SJ, Demierre M-F, Kim EJ, Rook AH, Lerner A, Duvic M, et al. Final results from a multicenter, international, pivotal study of romidepsin in refractory cutaneous T-cell lymphoma. J Clin Oncol. 2010;28(29):4485–91.
112. Schwartz J, Padmanabhan A, Aqui N, Balogun RA, Connelly-Smith L, Delaney M, et al. Guidelines on the use of therapeutic apheresis in clinical practice-evidence-based approach from the Writing Committee of the American Society for apheresis: the seventh special issue: therapeutic apheresis-guidelines 2016. J Clin Apher. 2016;31(3):149–338.
113. Alfred A, Taylor PC, Dignan F, El-Ghariani K, Griffin J, Gennery AR, et al. The role of extracorporeal photopheresis in the management of cutaneous T-cell lymphoma, graft-versus-host disease and organ transplant rejection: a consensus statement update from the UK Photopheresis Society. Br J Haematol. 2017;177(2):287–310.
114. Edelson R, Wu Y, Schneiderman J. American council on ECP (ACE): why now? J Clin Apher. 2018;33:464–8.
115. Katz J, Janik JE, Younes A. Brentuximab vedotin (SGN-35). Clin Cancer Res. 2011;17(20):6428–36.
116. Thomas A, Teicher BA, Hassan R. Antibody–drug conjugates for cancer therapy. Lancet Oncol. 2016;17(6):e254–62.
117. Prince HM, Kim YH, Horwitz SM, Dummer R, Scarisbrick J, Quaglino P, et al. Brentuximab vedotin or physician's choice in CD30-positive cutaneous T-cell lymphoma (ALCANZA): an international, open-label, randomised, phase 3, multicentre trial. Lancet. 2017;390(10094):555–66.

118. Ginaldi L, De Martinis M, Matutes E, Farahat N, Morilla R, Dyer MJ, et al. Levels of expression of CD52 in normal and leukemic B and T cells: correlation with in vivo therapeutic responses to Campath 1H. Leuk Res. 1998;22(2):185–91.
119. Querfeld C, Mehta N, Rosen ST, Guitart J, Rademaker A, Gerami P, et al. Alemtuzumab for relapsed and refractory erythrodermic cutaneous T-cell lymphoma: a single institution experience from the Robert H. Lurie Comprehensive Cancer Center. Leuk Lymphoma. 2009;50(12):1969–76.
120. Lundin J, Hagberg H, Repp R, Cavallin-Ståhl E, Fredén S, Juliusson G, et al. Phase 2 study of alemtuzumab (anti-CD52 monoclonal antibody) in patients with advanced mycosis fungoides/Sézary syndrome. Blood. 2003;101(11):4267–72.
121. Kennedy GA, Seymour JF, Wolf M, Januszewicz H, Davison J, McCormack C, et al. Treatment of patients with advanced mycosis fungoides and Sezary syndrome with alemtuzumab. Eur J Haematol. 2003;71(4):250–6.
122. Thursky KA, Worth LJ, Seymour JF, Prince HM, Slavin MA. Spectrum of infection, risk and recommendations for prophylaxis and screening among patients with lymphoproliferative disorders treated with alemtuzumab. Br J Haematol. 2006;132(1):3–12.
123. Bernengo MG, Quaglino P, Comessatti A, Ortoncelli M, Novelli M, Lisa F, et al. Low-dose intermittent alemtuzumab in the treatment of Sezary syndrome: clinical and immunologic findings in 14 patients. Haematologica. 2007;92(6):784–94.
124. Alinari L, Geskin L, Grady T, Baiocchi RA, Bechtel MA, Porcu P. Subcutaneous alemtuzumab for Sézary syndrome in the very elderly. Leuk Res. 2008;32(8):1299–303.
125. Ni X, Langridge T, Duvic M. Depletion of regulatory T cells by targeting CC chemokine receptor type 4 with mogamulizumab. OncoImmunology. 2015;4(7):e1011524.
126. Kim YH, Bagot M, Pinter-Brown L, Rook AH, Porcu P, Horwitz SM, et al. Mogamulizumab versus vorinostat in previously treated cutaneous T-cell lymphoma (MAVORIC): an international, open-label, randomised, controlled phase 3 trial. Lancet Oncol. 2018;19(9):1192–204.
127. Duvic M, Pinter-Brown LC, Foss FM, Sokol L, Jorgensen JL, Challagundla P, et al. Phase 1/2 study of mogamulizumab, a defucosylated anti-CCR4 antibody, in previously treated patients with cutaneous T-cell lymphoma. Blood. 2015;125(12):1883–9.
128. Quereux G, Marques S, Nguyen J-M, Bedane C, D'incan M, Dereure O, et al. Prospective multicenter study of Pegylated liposomal doxorubicin treatment in patients with advanced or refractory mycosis fungoides or Sézary syndrome. Arch Dermatol. 2008;144(6):727–33.
129. Pulini S, Rupoli S, Goteri G, Pimpinelli N, Alterini R, Tassetti A, et al. Pegylated liposomal doxorubicin in the treatment of primary cutaneous T-cell lymphomas. Haematologica. 2007;92(5):686–9.
130. Dummer R, Quaglino P, Becker JC, Hasan B, Karrasch M, Whittaker S, et al. Prospective international multicenter phase II trial of intravenous pegylated liposomal doxorubicin monochemotherapy in patients with stage IIB, IVA, or IVB advanced mycosis fungoides: final results from EORTC 21012. J Clin Oncol. 2012;30(33):4091–7.
131. Duvic M, Talpur R, Wen S, Kurzrock R, David CL, Apisarnthanarax N. Phase II evaluation of gemcitabine monotherapy for cutaneous T-cell lymphoma. Clin Lymphoma Myeloma. 2006;7(1):51–8.
132. Jidar K, Ingen-Housz-Oro S, Beylot-Barry M, Paul C, Chaoui D, Sigal-Grinberg M, et al. Gemcitabine treatment in cutaneous T-cell lymphoma: a multicentre study of 23 cases. Br J Dermatol. 2009;161(3):660–3.
133. Pellegrini C, Stefoni V, Casadei B, Maglie R, Argnani L, Zinzani PL. Long-term outcome of patients with advanced-stage cutaneous T cell lymphoma treated with gemcitabine. Ann Hematol. 2014;93(11):1853–7.
134. Zackheim HS, Kashani-Sabet M, McMillan A. Low-dose methotrexate to treat mycosis fungoides: a retrospective study in 69 patients. J Am Acad Dermatol. 2003;49(5):873–8.
135. Zackheim HS, Epstein EH. Low-dose methotrexate for the Sézary syndrome. J Am Acad Dermatol. 1989;21(4 Pt 1):757–62.

136. Duvic M, Kim YH, Zinzani PL, Horwitz SM. Results from a phase I/II open-label, dose-finding study of pralatrexate and oral bexarotene in patients with relapsed/refractory cutaneous T-cell lymphoma. Clin Cancer Res. 2017;23(14):3552–6.
137. Bigler RD, Crilley P, Micaily B, Brady LW, Topolsky D, Bulova S, et al. Autologous bone marrow transplantation for advanced stage mycosis fungoides. Bone Marrow Transplant. 1991;7(2):133–7.
138. Duarte RF, Canals C, Onida F, Gabriel IH, Arranz R, Arcese W, et al. Allogeneic hematopoietic cell transplantation for patients with mycosis fungoides and Sézary syndrome: a retrospective analysis of the Lymphoma Working Party of the European Group for blood and marrow transplantation. J Clin Oncol. 2010;28(29):4492–9.
139. Duarte RF, Servitje O, Sureda A. Haematopoietic stem cell transplantation for patients with primary cutaneous T-cell lymphoma. Bone Marrow Transplant. 2008;41(7):597–604.

Index

C. Dittus (ed.), *Novel Therapeutics for Rare Lymphomas*,
https://doi.org/10.1007/978-3-030-25610-4

P

R

The manufacturer's authorised representative in the EU is Springer Nature Customer Service Centre GmbH, Europaplatz 3, 69115 Heidelberg, Germany. If you have any concerns regarding our products, please contact ProductSafety@springernature.com

Printed and bound by CPI Group (UK) Ltd, Croydon, CR0 4YY
30/07/2026
02181675-0001